Hypertension and Nutrition

Hypertension and Nutrition

Editor: Hilary Dawsey

AMERICAN
MEDICAL PUBLISHERS
www.americanmedicalpublishers.com

AMERICAN
MEDICAL PUBLISHERS
www.americanmedicalpublishers.com

Cataloging-in-Publication Data

Hypertension and nutrition / edited by Hilary Dawsey.
p. cm.
Includes bibliographical references and index.
ISBN 978-1-63927-695-0
1. Hypertension. 2. Hypertension--Nutritional aspects. 3. Hypertension--Diet therapy.
4. Dietary supplements. 5. Cardiology. I. Dawsey, Hilary.
RC685.H8 H97 2023
616.132--dc23

American Medical Publishers,
41 Flatbush Avenue,
1st Floor, New York,
NY 11217, USA

ISBN 978-1-63927-695-0 (Hardback)

Contents

Preface

This book was inspired by the evolution of our times; to answer the curiosity of inquisitive minds. Many developments have occurred across the globe in the recent past which has transformed the progress in the field.

Hypertension refers to a type of long-term medical condition where the blood pressure in the arteries is continuously high. Generally, high blood pressure does not show any symptoms. Although, it leads to several diseases such as peripheral arterial disease, dementia, stroke, atrial fibrillation, coronary artery disease, chronic kidney disease, heart failure and vision loss. There are various lifestyle factors which contribute towards risk associated with hypertension, such as smoking, excess salt in the diet, consumption of alcohol and excess body weight. Medications and lifestyle changes may reduce the risk of health complications and help in lowering blood pressure. Healthy diet including fruits, lean meat, cooked hot cereal, vegetables, etc. that are rich in nutrition may improve the condition of hypertension. This book explores all the important aspects of hypertension and its relationship to nutrition. It presents researches and studies performed by experts across the globe. Those in search of information to further their knowledge will be greatly assisted by this book.

This book was developed from a mere concept to drafts to chapters and finally compiled together as a complete text to benefit the readers across all nations. To ensure the quality of the content we instilled two significant steps in our procedure. The first was to appoint an editorial team that would verify the data and statistics provided in the book and also select the most appropriate and valuable contributions from the plentiful contributions we received from authors worldwide. The next step was to appoint an expert of the topic as the Editor-in-Chief, who would head the project and finally make the necessary amendments and modifications to make the text reader-friendly. I was then commissioned to examine all the material to present the topics in the most comprehensible and productive format.

I would like to take this opportunity to thank all the contributing authors who were supportive enough to contribute their time and knowledge to this project. I also wish to convey my regards to my family who have been extremely supportive during the entire project.

Editor

1

Association between the Intake of Fermented Soy Products and Hypertension Risk in Postmenopausal Women and Men Aged 50 Years or Older: The Korea National Health and Nutrition Examination Survey 2013–2018

Dohyun Yoo and Yongsoon Park *

Department of Food and Nutrition, Hanyang University, 222 Wangsimni-ro, Seongdong-gu, Seoul 04763, Korea; dptnsla102@naver.com

* Correspondence: yongsoon@hanyang.ac.kr

Abstract: Sodium intake is positively associated with hypertension risk; however, it is not clear whether there is an association between the intake of fermented soy products, a major source of salt, and blood pressure (BP). This study aimed to investigate the hypothesis that hypertension risk and BP were negatively associated with the intake of fermented soy products but not with the intake of sodium from fermented soy products. This cross-sectional study was performed using data from the Korea National Health and Nutrition Examination Survey (2013–2018). In total, 11,566 men and postmenopausal women aged ≥50 years were divided according to quintiles of sodium or fermented soy product intake. The intake of fermented soy products was negatively associated with hypertension risk (odds ratio: 0.81, 95% confidence interval: 0.66–0.98; *p*-trend = 0.023) and systolic BP (SBP; *p*-trend = 0.043) in postmenopausal women. Mediation analysis showed that the intake of fermented soy products had total and direct effects on SBP; however, there was no indirect effect because soy nutrients, such as protein, fiber, calcium, and potassium, had no significant effects on SBP. Among men, fermented soy product intake was not associated with hypertension risk and BP. Additionally, the intake of sodium from fermented soy products was not significantly associated with hypertension risk and BP in both postmenopausal women and men. This study suggests that hypertension risk and BP were not associated with the intake of sodium from fermented soy products; further, hypertension risk and BP were inversely associated with fermented soy product intake in postmenopausal women. Further clinical studies are needed to confirm the effect of fermented soy product intake on hypertension risk and BP.

Keywords: blood pressure; elderly population; fermented soy products; hypertension; salt intake

1. Introduction

Hypertension is an important risk factor for cardiovascular diseases, which are the major cause of death globally [1]. Blood pressure (BP) increases gradually with age in men and postmenopausal women, and the prevalence of hypertension has been estimated to be approximately 65% among Korean elderly people [2].

Sodium intake is a major modifiable lifestyle risk factor for hypertension [3], and the World Health Organization recommends the consumption of <2000 mg/day of sodium to decrease BP [4]. Most epidemiological studies have reported that salt intake is positively associated with BP and the risk of hypertension [5]. Additionally, a recent meta-analysis of clinical trials showed that a reduction in sodium intake decreased BP in both participants with normotension and hypertension [6]. However, salt from miso, a traditional fermented soy product consumed in Japan, did not increase BP in salt-sensitive rats (compared to a same amount of salt) [7,8]. The use of Doenjang, a Korean fermented soy product, also resulted in lower BP in normotensive rats (compared to the use of the same amount of salt) [9].

The Korea National Health and Nutrition Examination Survey (KNHANES) VI-2 reported that the average daily sodium intake was 5700 mg/day, and the major sources of dietary sodium were table salt, kimchi, and fermented soy products such as soy sauce (Kanjang), soybean paste (Doenjang), and red pepper paste (Gochujang) [2]. Traditional Korean fermented soy products are made using sea salt [10], which not only contains sodium but also contains minerals, such as potassium and calcium [11]. Baek et al. (2015) [12] reported that the use of sea salt decreased BP; however, the use of refined salt did not decrease BP in elderly Korean patients with hypertension.

Furthermore, soybean contains nutrients such as protein, fiber, calcium, and potassium [13]. Previous studies have reported that the supplementation of soy protein [14], calcium [15], potassium [16], and fiber [17] reduced BP in participants with normotension or hypertension. In addition, Nozue et al. (2017) [18] reported that the intake of miso and natto, but not tofu, was negatively associated with the risk of hypertension, defined as systolic blood pressure (SBP) ≥130 mmHg or diastolic blood pressure (DBP) ≥85 mmHg in the Japanese population; this suggests that the intake of fermented soy products had a greater effect on BP than the intake of soy products. Kanda et al. (1999) [19] showed that the consumption of more than two bowls of miso soup per day was negatively associated with the risk of hypertension in elderly Japanese individuals. Although Ito et al. (2017) [20] reported that BP was not significantly different between the groups consuming high and low amounts of miso soup, heart rates were lower in participants of the former group; this suggests that miso intake could attenuate salt-induced BP elevation by lowering heart rate. However, no study has investigated the association between the intake of traditional Korean fermented soy products and hypertension risk and BP. Thus, this study aimed to evaluate the hypothesis that hypertension risk and BP were negatively associated with the intake of fermented soy products but were not associated with the intake of sodium from fermented soy products. In addition, this study determined whether there were direct and indirect relationships between BP and fermented soy product intake.

2. Materials and Methods

2.1. Study Population

This study was based on data from the Korea National Health and Nutrition Examination Survey (KNHANES) VI and VII (2013–2018). The KNHANES is a cross-sectional and nationally representative survey using a stratified and multistage sampling design for the selection of household units. Health interviews and health examinations were conducted by trained medical staff members at mobile examination centers, and the in-person household nutrition survey was conducted by dietitians [21].

Out of a total of 47,217 participants, there were 17,966 men and postmenopausal women aged ≥50 years (Figure 1). The exclusion criteria were as follows: missing data on baseline variables (n = 6032), extreme energy intake (<500 kcal/day or >4000 kcal/day; n = 311), or renal failure (n = 57). Extreme energy intake was defined as age and sex specific total energy intake less than 25% of estimated energy requirements (EER) or more than 200% of EER. After exclusion, 11,566 participants were included in the final analysis.

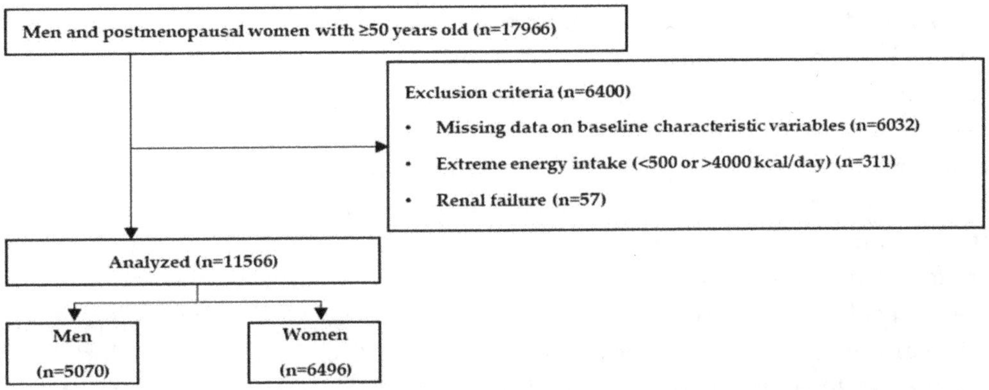

Figure 1. Flowchart of the inclusion and exclusion of participants.

2.2. Data Collection

A health interview was performed to obtain information on age, sex, socioeconomic status, smoking status, drinking status, exercise status and menstruate state. Exercise was defined as walking or strength exercises for >20 min at a time at least 3 times/week or walking or moderate exercise for >30 min at a time at least 5 times/week. Drinking status was categorized into non/light-alcohol drinker or heavy alcohol drinker: men who drank ≥7 alcoholic beverages and women who drank ≥5 alcoholic beverages at a time ≥2 times a week [22]. Postmenopausal status was defined based on a self-reported questionnaire survey containing question for the determination of whether 1 year had passed since the time of last menstruation including hysterectomy.

The intakes of energy, nutrients, and fermented soy products were determined using 1-day 24-h recall and were calculated by multiplying the food code-specific nutrient concentration data by the corresponding weight of each reported food. All the reported items were coded using the Korea Food Composition Table for the KNHANES [23,24], which provided data on nutritional content based on standardized recipes. Fermented soy products include Doenjang (soybean paste fermented for 3–6 month), Chongkukjang (soybean paste fermented for 2–3 days), Kanjang (fermented soy sauce), and Gochujang (fermented red pepper paste) [10].

A health examination survey was performed to obtain information on the levels of fasting plasma glucose (FPG) and lipid profiles (triglyceride, low-density lipoprotein, and high-density lipoprotein) measured directly using a Hitachi Automatic Analyzer 7600 (Hitachi, Tokyo, Japan). The Friedewald equation was used to calculate low-density lipoprotein cholesterol (LDL-C) levels for participants with no data on LDL-C levels [25]. Body mass index (BMI) was calculated using the measured height and weight. BP was measured thrice by trained technicians in the right arm using a standard mercury sphygmomanometer (Baumanometer; W. A. Baum, Copiague, NY, USA). The average of the second and third readings was considered as the final BP. Hypertension was defined as SBP ≥140 mmHg, DBP ≥90 mmHg, or the current use of antihypertensive medications [26].

2.3. Statistical Analysis

All statistical analyses of complex sample survey data were performed using Statistical Package for the Social Sciences (SPSS) version 25.0 (SPSS Inc., Chicago, IL, USA). To ensure that the dataset represented the entire Korean population without biased estimates, sampling weights were applied to each participant's data [27]. The baseline characteristics and risk factors for hypertension in the study population were compared using Student's t-test for continuous variables and the chi-square test for categorical variables. Continuous variables were presented as means and standard errors of the mean, and categorical variables were presented as frequencies and percentages. All groups were subdivided into five groups according to quintiles of sodium and fermented soy product intakes. Analysis of covariance (ANCOVA) with a Bonferroni's post hoc test was used to assess mean differences in BP among the intake quintiles following adjustment for confounders. Multivariate logistic regression models were performed to examine the associations between the intakes of sodium and fermented soy products and the risk for hypertension. The covariates showing p-values <0.20 in the multivariate models were selected as the confounders and included in the fully adjusted model [28]. For men, the covariates were age, LDL-C levels, energy intake, FPG levels, BMI, education levels, drinking status, exercise status, and family history of hypertension; for women, the covariates were age, triglyceride (TG) levels, LDL-C levels, energy intake, FPG levels, BMI, education levels, drinking status, household income, and family history of hypertension.

The p-value for trend was calculated using multivariate logistic regression analyses by handling the median value for each category of sodium intake and fermented soy product intake as a continuous value. A mediation analysis was conducted using the Hayes PROCESS macro (Model 4) to test whether the relationship between fermented soy product intake and BP was mediated by various nutrients [29]. The significance of the mediated effect was evaluated by calculating bias-corrected bootstrap 95% confidence intervals (95% CIs). If the 95% CI did not include zero, the criteria for mediation were met. All statistical tests were two-sided according to a significance level of <0.05.

3. Results

3.1. Characteristics of the Participants

It was observed that men and postmenopausal women with normotension were younger, had lower BMI, lower blood levels of TG, FPG, SBP, and DBP, and a lower prevalence of family history of hypertension and alcohol drinking than those with hypertension but had higher education levels, income, LDL-C levels, and high-density lipoprotein cholesterol (HDL-C) levels (Table 1).

The number of smokers was higher in men with normotension than in men with hypertension, and the number of participants who exercised regularly was higher in women with normotension than in women with hypertension. The energy was higher in men and women with normotension than in those with hypertension, but intake of sodium from fermented soy product was not different between normotension and hypertension in both men and women. Intake of total sodium and fermented soy products was higher in women with normotension than in women with hypertension. However, intake of total sodium and sodium from fermented soy product was not different between normotension and hypertension in men.

3.2. Associations Between the Risk of Hypertension and Intakes of Sodium and Fermented Soy Products

The intakes of total sodium and sodium from fermented soy products were negatively associated with the risk of hypertension in women before, but not after, adjusting for confounders. However, the intake of fermented soy products was negatively associated with the risk of hypertension in women before and after adjusting for confounders (Table 2). In addition, the intakes of total sodium, sodium from fermented soy products, and fermented soy products were negatively associated with the risk of hypertension in men; however, the association disappeared after adjusting for confounders (Table 3).

3.3. Associations Between Blood Pressure and the Intakes of Sodium and Fermented Soy Products

Among women, SBP was negatively associated with the intake of fermented soy products after adjustment for confounders; however, DBP did not show this association (Table 4). In addition, the intakes of total sodium and sodium from fermented soy products were not associated with either SBP or DBP after adjusting for confounders. In men, the intakes of total sodium, sodium from fermented soy products, and fermented soy products were not associated with both SBP and DBP after adjusting for confounders (Table 5). Among postmenopausal women, mediation analysis showed that the intake of fermented soy products had a total and direct effect on SBP but not on DBP; additionally, any nutrients from fermented soy products had no indirect effect (Figure 2, Table 6). Moreover, there were no total, direct, or indirect effects of the intake of fermented soy products on SBP and DBP among men.

Table 1. Baseline characteristics of men and postmenopausal women aged ≥50 years.

Variables	Women		p–Value	Men		p–Value
	Normotensive (n = 3438)	Hypertensive (n = 3058)		Normotensive (n = 2655)	Hypertensive (n = 2415)	
Age (years)	60.07 ± 0.16	65.93 ± 0.19	<0.001	59.72 ± 0.18	63.26 ± 0.23	<0.001
BMI (kg/m^2)			<0.001			<0.001
<18.5	97 (2.9)	34 (1.2)		71 (2.4)	43 (1.6)	
18.5 to <23.0	1504 (45.2)	808 (27.6)		1039 (37.6)	663 (26.1)	
23.0 to <25.0	871 (25.0)	793 (24.7)		775 (29.7)	630 (26.5)	
≥25.0	966 (27.0)	1423 (46.4)		770 (30.3)	1079 (45.8)	
Family history of hypertension, n (%)	964 (29.6)	1166 (40.9)	<0.001	588 (25.8)	815 (37.2)	<0.001
Regular exercise, n (%) [1]	1594 (48.1)	1140 (39.5)	<0.001	1262 (48.4)	1078 (46.0)	0.149
Alcohol drinking, n (%) [2]	50 (1.5)	68 (2.6)	0.007	262 (11.2)	364 (18.0)	<0.001
Smoking, n (%)			0.781			0.020
Never	3263 (94.8)	2897 (94.7)		521 (19.1)	455 (19.2)	
Past	80 (2.3)	81 (2.6)		1343 (48.4)	1343 (52.5)	
Current	95 (3.0)	80 (2.8)		791 (32.5)	617 (28.4)	
Education level, n (%)			<0.001			<0.001
≤ Elementary school	1191 (30.2)	1823 (55.2)		617 (18.7)	686 (25.2)	
Middle school	658 (19.4)	467 (16.3)		425 (14.6)	447 (17.0)	
High school	1040 (33.3)	540 (20.1)		820 (32.7)	752 (32.4)	
≥College	549 (17.2)	228 (8.4)		793 (34.0)	530 (25.4)	
Household income, n (%)			<0.001			<0.001
Low	753 (19.1)	1200 (36.1)		514 (15.0)	663 (22.9)	
Middle-low	917 (25.2)	808 (25.2)		697 (23.6)	644 (24.9)	
Middle-high	806 (25.0)	590 (21.3)		654 (27.1)	542 (24.3)	
High	962 (30.7)	460 (17.5)		790 (34.3)	566 (27.9)	
LDL-C (mmol/L)	3.29 ± 0.02	2.98 ± 0.02	<0.001	3.06 ± 0.02	2.73 ± 0.02	<0.001
HDL-C (mmol/L)	1.39 ± 0.01	1.31 ± 0.01	<0.001	1.21 ± 0.01	1.19 ± 0.01	0.057
TG (mmol/L)	1.38 ± 0.02	1.56 ± 0.02	<0.001	1.75 ± 0.04	1.88 ± 0.04	0.011
FPG (mmol/L)	5.48 ± 0.02	5.95 ± 0.03	<0.001	5.81 ± 0.03	6.13 ± 0.04	<0.001
SBP (mmHg)	114.84 ± 0.24	134.88 ± 0.39	<0.001	116.21 ± 0.26	132.42 ± 0.40	<0.001
DBP (mmHg)	72.78 ± 0.15	78.11 ± 0.26	<0.001	75.38 ± 0.18	80.52 ± 0.31	<0.001
Energy intake (kcal/day)	1681.51 ± 12.61	1569.34 ± 12.33	<0.001	2191.55 ± 16.82	2105.22 ± 17.56	<0.001
Total sodium intake (mg/day)[3]	2928.53 ± 33.92	2820.17 ± 36.30	0.017	4030.34 ± 44.21	4014.40 ± 55.26	0.819
Sodium intake from fermented soy products (mg/day) [3]	690.48 ± 15.33	691.22 ± 15.45	0.971	924.89 ± 20.66	893.00 ± 21.27	0.260
Fermented soy product intake (g/day)	17.47 ± 0.42	16.02 ± 0.38	0.008	23.60 ± 0.59	22.32 ± 0.60	0.117

BMI, body mass index; DBP, diastolic blood pressure; FPG, fasting plasma glucose; HDL-C, high-density lipoprotein cholesterol; LDL-C, low-density lipoprotein cholesterol; SBP, systolic blood pressure; TG, triglyceride. Continuous variables are presented as means ± standard error of the mean, while categorical variables are presented as the subject number (percentage distribution); [1] Regular exercise was defined as vigorous activity for >20 min, >3 times a week or walking or moderate exercise for 30 min, >5 days a week; [2] Alcohol drinking was defined as drinking at least 7 beverages for men and at least 5 beverages for women ≥2 times a week; [3] Adjusted for energy intake.

Table 2. Associations between the risk of hypertension and the intakes of sodium and fermented soy products in postmenopausal women aged ≥50 years.

Variables	Quintiles of Intake					*p*-Trend [1]
	Q1 (*n* = 1299)	Q2 (*n* = 1299)	Q3 (*n* = 1300)	Q4 (*n* = 1299)	Q5 (*n* = 1299)	
Total sodium intake (mg/day)	<1437.25	1437.25 to <2085.23	2085.23 to <2846.36	2846.36 to <3936.08	≥3936.08	
Crude OR (95% CI)	1	0.80 (0.67–0.96)	0.71 (0.59–0.84)	0.63 (0.53–0.76)	0.62 (0.52–0.74)	<0.001
Adjusted OR (95% CI) [2]	1	0.88 (0.71–1.08)	0.83 (0.67–1.02)	0.82 (0.66–1.02)	0.82 (0.64–1.05)	0.183
Sodium intake from fermented soy products (mg/day)	<130.57	130.57 to <354.53	354.53 to <627.84	627.84 to <1076.44	≥1076.44	
Crude OR (95% CI)	1	0.85 (0.72–1.02)	0.82 (0.68–0.98)	0.90 (0.76–1.07)	0.76 (0.64–0.90)	0.011
Adjusted OR (95% CI) [2]	1	0.93 (0.76–1.14)	0.92 (0.76–1.13)	1.02 (0.83–1.25)	0.83 (0.68–1.01)	0.124
Fermented soy product intake (g/day)	<2.85	2.85 to <7.89	7.89 to <14.60	14.60 to <26.39	≥26.39	
Crude OR (95% CI)	1	0.91 (0.76–1.08)	0.85 (0.71–1.02)	0.88 (0.74–1.05)	0.72 (0.61–0.86)	<0.001
Adjusted OR (95% CI) [2]	1	0.97 (0.80–1.19)	1.00 (0.82–1.23)	1.00 (0.82–1.23)	0.81 (0.66–0.98)	0.023

CI, confidence interval; OR, odds ratio, Data are presented as ORs and 95% CIs. The [1] estimated *p*-trend for a linear trend was based on the linear scores derived from the median values from the quintiles of sodium intake and fermented soy product intake among women. [2] Adjusted for age, triglyceride levels, low-density lipoprotein cholesterol levels, energy intake, fasting plasma glucose levels, body mass index, education levels, drinking status, household income, and family history of hypertension.

Table 3. Associations between the risk of hypertension and the intakes of sodium and fermented soy products in men aged ≥50 years.

Variables	Quintiles of Intake					*p*-Trend [1]
	Q1 (*n* = 1014)	Q2 (*n* = 1014)	Q3 (*n* = 1014)	Q4 (*n* = 1014)	Q5 (*n* = 1014)	
Total sodium intake (mg/day)	<2165.32	2165.32 to <3068.22	3068.22 to <4013.82	4013.82 to <5365.74	≥5365.74	
Crude OR (95% CI)	1	0.74 (0.61–0.91)	0.67 (0.55–0.83)	0.78 (0.64–0.94)	0.67 (0.54–0.82)	<0.001
Adjusted OR (95% CI) [2]	1	0.80 (0.64–1.02)	0.78 (0.62–0.98)	0.94 (0.74–1.19)	0.77 (0.60–1.00)	0.209
Sodium intake from fermented soy products (mg/day)	<206.93	206.93 to <493.55	493.55 to <859.18	859.18 to <1469.45	≥1469.45	
Crude OR (95% CI)	1	0.96 (0.79–1.18)	0.84 (0.69–1.03)	0.88 (0.72–1.09)	0.79 (0.65–0.97)	0.020
Adjusted OR (95% CI) [2]	1	1.03 (0.83–1.28)	0.90 (0.73–1.11)	1.01 (0.80–1.27)	0.85 (0.68–1.07)	0.150
Fermented soy product intake (g/day)	<4.66	4.66 to <11.57	11.57 to <20.62	20.62 to <36.34	≥36.34	
Crude OR (95% CI)	1	0.88 (0.72–1.07)	0.88 (0.72–1.08)	0.74 (0.60–0.92)	0.81 (0.66–1.00)	0.043
Adjusted OR (95% CI) [2]	1	0.94 (0.76–1.17)	0.94 (0.75–1.17)	0.84 (0.66–1.05)	0.89 (0.70–1.12)	0.281

CI, confidence interval; OR, odds ratio, data are presented as ORs and 95% CIs. The [1] estimated *p*-trend for a linear trend was based on the linear scores derived from the median values from the quintiles of sodium intake and fermented soy product intake among men; [2] adjusted for age, low-density lipoprotein cholesterol levels, energy intake, fasting plasma glucose levels, body mass index, education levels, drinking status, exercise status, and family history of hypertension.

Table 4. Association between blood pressure and the intakes of sodium and fermented soy products in postmenopausal women aged ≥50 years.

Variables	Quintiles of Intake					p-Trend [1]
	Q1 (n = 1299)	Q2 (n = 1299)	Q3 (n = 1300)	Q4 (n = 1299)	Q5 (n = 1299)	
Total sodium intake (mg/day)	<1437.25	1437.25 to <2085.23	2085.23 to <2846.36	2846.36 to <3936.08	≥3936.08	
SBP (mmHg)	125.44 ± 0.61	124.47 ± 0.57	123.23 ± 0.59	122.74 ± 0.58	122.20 ± 0.57	0.612
DBP (mmHg)	75.16 ± 0.33	74.79 ± 0.31	75.15 ± 0.33	74.96 ± 0.31	75.50 ± 0.31	0.838
Sodium intake from fermented soy products (mg/day)	<130.57	130.57 to <354.53	354.53 to <627.84	627.84 to <1076.44	≥1076.44	
SBP (mmHg)	124.51 ± 0.61	123.48 ± 0.55	123.91 ± 0.64	123.93 ± 0.56	122.25 ± 0.57	0.087
DBP (mmHg)	75.40 ± 0.32	75.16 ± 0.31	75.03 ± 0.33	75.24 ± 0.31	74.74 ± 0.29	0.148
Fermented soy product intake (g/day)	<2.85	2.85 to <7.89	7.89 to <14.60	14.60 to <26.39	≥26.39	
SBP (mmHg)	124.51 ± 0.60	124.05 ± 0.56	123.56 ± 0.61	123.88 ± 0.55	122.05 ± 0.58	0.043
DBP (mmHg)	75.36 ± 0.33	75.21 ± 0.31	75.05 ± 0.32	75.29 ± 0.31	74.65 ± 0.30	0.067

DBP, diastolic blood pressure; SBP, systolic blood pressure, All values are presented as means ± standard error of the mean; [1] p-trend for differences in SBP and DBP according to quintiles of sodium intake and fermented soy product intake after adjustment for confounders, such as age, triglyceride levels, low-density lipoprotein cholesterol levels, energy intake, fasting plasma glucose levels, body mass index, education levels, drinking status, household income, and family history of hypertension.

Table 5. Association between blood pressure and the intakes of sodium and fermented soy products in men aged ≥50 years.

Variables	Quintiles of Intake					p-Trend [1]
	Q1 (n = 1014)	Q2 (n = 1014)	Q3 (n = 1014)	Q4 (n = 1014)	Q5 (n = 1014)	
Total sodium intake (mg/day)	<2165.32	2165.32 to <3068.22	3068.22 to <4013.82	4013.82 to <5365.74	≥5365.74	
SBP (mmHg)	125.51 ± 0.57	123.50 ± 0.60	122.23 ± 0.54	123.41 ± 0.58	122.83 ± 0.58	0.180
DBP (mmHg)	77.70 ± 0.41	77.49 ± 0.39	77.01 ± 0.36	78.59 ± 0.37	78.43 ± 0.39	0.195
Sodium intake from fermented soy products (mg/day)	<206.93	206.93 to <493.55	493.55 to <859.18	859.18 to <1469.45	≥1469.45	
SBP (mmHg)	123.90 ± 0.56	123.93 ± 0.58	122.66 ± 0.60	122.85 ± 0.57	123.96 ± 0.63	0.614
DBP (mmHg)	77.63 ± 0.40	78.16 ± 0.36	77.24 ± 0.39	77.26 ± 0.38	78.10 ± 0.38	0.304
Fermented soy product intake (g/day)	<4.66	4.66 to <11.57	11.57 to <20.62	20.62 to <36.34	≥36.34	
SBP (mmHg)	124.07 ± 0.57	123.43 ± 0.58	123.34 ± 0.57	122.24 ± 0.54	124.22 ± 0.61	0.450
DBP (mmHg)	77.74 ± 0.39	77.70 ± 0.37	77.45 ± 0.36	77.43 ± 0.39	78.07 ± 0.38	0.239

DBP, diastolic blood pressure; SBP, systolic blood pressure, All values are presented as means ± standard error of the mean; [1] p-trend for differences in SBP and DBP according to quintiles of sodium intake and fermented soy product intake after adjustment for confounders, such as age, low-density lipoprotein cholesterol levels, energy intake, fasting plasma glucose levels, body mass index, education levels, drinking status, exercise status, and family history of hypertension.

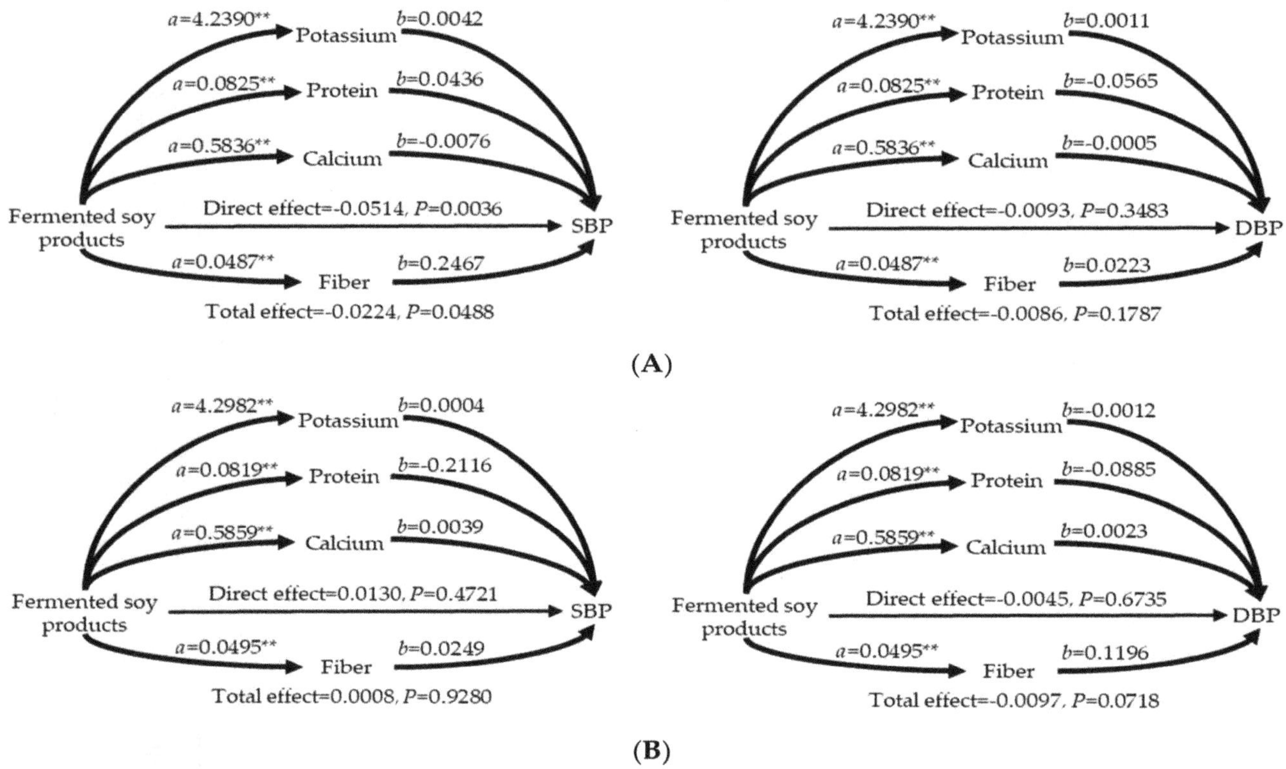

Figure 2. Mediation effects of nutrients on the association between the intake of fermented soy products and blood pressure in postmenopausal women (**A**) and men (**B**) DBP, diastolic blood pressure; SBP, systolic blood pressure. The confounders were age, triglyceride levels, low-density lipoprotein cholesterol levels, energy intake, fasting plasma glucose levels, body mass index, education levels, drinking status, household income, and family history of hypertension in women and age, low-density lipoprotein cholesterol levels, energy intake, fasting plasma glucose levels, body mass index, education levels, drinking status, exercise status, and family history of hypertension in men. Unstandardized coefficients are shown along with their estimated p values using the bootstrapping method. ** $p < 0.001$.

Table 6. Mediating effects of nutrients on the association between the intake of fermented soy products and blood pressure [1]

	SBP		DBP	
	Women	Men	Women	Men
Indirect effect				
Protein	0.0036 (−0.0158, 0.0214)	−0.0173 (−0.0520, 0.0121)	−0.0047 (−0.0238, 0.0017)	−0.0073 (−0.0224, 0.0074)
Fiber	0.0120 (−0.0090, 0.0349)	0.0012 (−0.0216, 0.0236)	0.0011 (−0.0104, 0.0140)	0.0059 (−0.0063, 0.0190)
Calcium	−0.0045 (−0.0209, 0.0123)	0.0023 (−0.0053, 0.0348)	−0.0003 (−0.0080, 0.0093)	0.0014 (−0.0080, 0.0112)
Potassium	0.0179 (−0.0006, 0.0345)	0.0017 (−0.0182, 0.0196)	0.0046 (−0.0056, 0.0143)	−0.0052 (−0.0173, 0.0069)

DBP, diastolic blood pressure; SBP, systolic blood pressure, [1] Data are presented as estimated effect values and bias-corrected bootstrap 95% confidence intervals obtained after mediation analysis, using the Hayes PROCESS macro, adjusted for age, triglyceride levels, low-density lipoprotein cholesterol levels, energy intake, fasting plasma glucose levels, body mass index, education levels, drinking status, household income, and family history of hypertension in women; and adjusted for age, low-density lipoprotein cholesterol levels, energy intake, fasting plasma glucose levels, body mass index, education levels, drinking status, exercise status, and family history of hypertension in men.

4. Discussion

This study shows that the intake of fermented soy products was negatively associated with the risk of hypertension and SBP in postmenopausal women aged ≥50 years but not in men. Consistent with the present study, Kanda et al. (1999) [19] reported that the intake of miso soup (>2 bowls per day) was negatively associated with the risk of hypertension during a 4-year follow-up study in elderly Japanese individuals. Nouze et al. (2017) [18] also reported that the intake of miso or natto was negatively associated with the risk of elevated BP (SBP ≥130 mmHg or DBP ≥85 mmHg) during a 5-year follow-up study in middle-aged Japanese individuals. In addition, dietary patterns characterized by high intakes of natto and tofu were negatively associated with the risk of elevated BP in Japanese individuals [30]. Furthermore, soy intake has been reported to be negatively associated with the risk of hypertension in the China Health and Nutrition Survey [31] and the Korean Multi-Rural Communities Cohort study [32].

The intake of fermented soy products was also negatively associated with SBP in the present study. Ito et al. (2017) [20] reported that there were no significant differences in BP among subjects in the four quartiles of consumption frequency of miso soup (highest quartile: ≥1 bowl per day). Kanda et al. (1999) [19] reported that the consumption of two bowls of miso soup per day was negatively associated with the risk of hypertension; however, the consumption of ≤1 bowl of miso soup per day was not, suggesting that the consumption of at least two bowls of miso soup could have an effect on BP. The present study shows that the intake of fermented soy products in the highest quintile was >26 g, which corresponds to >24 g of miso (present in two bowls of miso soup). Furthermore, previous epidemiologic studies have consistently reported that the intake of soy food was inversely associated with BP in Chinese [33] and American individuals [34,35]. In addition, the supplementation of soy products, such as soy milk [36] and soy nuts [37,38], reduced BP in participants with normotension and hypertension, suggesting that soy nutrients might help decrease BP. Soy contains protein, fiber, and calcium, and potassium [13]. Dietary Approaches to Stop Hypertension diet is an appropriate diet for hypertension, since the diet is rich in protein, fiber, calcium, and potassium [39]. Clinical trials also have shown that BP was reduced in response to supplementation with soy protein [14], fiber [17], calcium [15], and potassium [16] in participants with normotension and hypertension. In the present study, the intakes of protein, fiber, calcium, and potassium from fermented soy products were 1.65 g/day, 0.88 g/day, 11.13 mg/day, and 94 mg/day, respectively. However, those nutrients were only 0.03%, 0.04%, 0.01%, and 0.03% of Korea Dietary Recommended Intake.

In this study, we performed mediation analysis to confirm the indirect effects of soy nutrients on BP; the intake of fermented soy products showed no indirect effects via soy nutrients. During the fermentation of soy, the level of peptides increases [40], and the glycoside form of isoflavone is transformed to aglycone forms, such as daidzein and genistein [41]. Aglycones of isoflavone had a beneficial effect on hepatic lipid metabolism compared with both glycosides of isoflavone and an isoflavone-free diet, indicating that aglycones of isoflavone showed bioavailability [42]. Shin et al. (2001) [43] reported that the injection of isolated peptides from Doenjang inhibited the activity of angiotensin-converting enzyme and thus reduced SBP in spontaneously hypertensive rats. In addition, daidzein and genistein enhanced the activity of endothelial nitric oxide synthase, which improved vascular function and thus reduced SBP in spontaneously hypertensive rats [44]. These studies suggested that the peptide and aglycone forms of isoflavone reduced BP; however, the present study did not include the peptide and aglycone forms of isoflavone in the mediation analysis due to lack of data.

Previous epidemiologic studies have shown that sodium intake is positively associated with the risk of hypertension [45] and with BP [46]. A meta-analysis of clinical trials also showed that BP was decreased after a reduction in sodium intake in both participants with normotension and hypertension [6]. However, the present study shows that the intakes of total sodium and sodium from fermented soy products were not associated with the risk of hypertension and with BP. Fermented soy products are a major source of sodium, and their intake is positively associated with the daily intake of salt among Koreans [2,47]. Previous studies have reported that fermented soy products contain soy nutrients and sea salt, which have beneficial effects on BP [11,12]. Mun et al. (2019) [9] showed that SBP was increased in rats fed 8% salt than in those fed 0.3% salt; however, SBP was observed to be the same in rats fed Doenjang containing 8% salt and 0.3% salt, suggesting that fermented soy products could attenuate salt-induced hypertension by offsetting the side effects of salty fermented soy products.

In this study, the beneficial effects of the intake of fermented soy products on the risk of hypertension and in terms of BP were significant only in women. Yang et al. (2005) [33] showed that soy intake was negatively associated with SBP in postmenopausal women but not in premenopausal women. It is well known that estrogen lowers BP by promoting vasodilation, decreasing vascular inflammation, and improving vascular reactivity [48]; isoflavone acts as an estrogen agonist in a low-estrogen environment [49]. Hooper et al. (2009) [50] showed that supplementation with soy isoflavone increased the blood level of estradiol in postmenopausal women. However, soy intake was negatively correlated with blood estradiol levels in men [51]. Taku et al. (2010) [52] also showed that the supplementation of isoflavones (aglycone equivalents) decreased SBP in postmenopausal women, but not men, with normotension and pre-hypertension.

This study shows that soy intake had beneficial effects on SBP but on DBP. After the age of 50 years, SBP continues to rise but DBP tends to fall, and isolated systolic hypertension is predominant in elderly patients [53]. Additionally, menopause is associated with an accelerated age-related increase in the vascular stiffness of large arteries, which contributes to the rise in SBP [54]. Nestel et al. (2007) [55] also showed that isoflavone supplementation reduced pulse wave velocity, which signified arterial stiffness, and thus reduced SBP in overweight participants, suggesting that isoflavone supplementation had a greater effect on SBP than on DBP.

The major strength of this study lies in the fact that data were gathered from a nationally representative survey; thus, the findings could be generalized to the Korean population. However, the present study has a few limitations. First, due to the cross-sectional design of the study, we were unable to establish a cause-and-effect relationship between the intake of fermented soy products and the risk of hypertension. Second, although adjustments were made for various confounders, certain residual confounders might still remain. Third, although the validated 1-day 24-h recall method was used, 1-day 24-h recall was restricted to reflect the usual intake than the food frequency questionnaire. Finally, sodium intake was estimated by dietary recall but not by 24-h urinary sodium excretion.

5. Conclusions

This study demonstrates that the intake of fermented soy products with a high salt content was inversely associated with the risk of hypertension and with BP in postmenopausal women. However, sodium from fermented soy products was not associated the risk of hypertension and with BP in both men and women, suggesting that salt intake from fermented soy products might not increase hypertension risk and BP. Further clinical studies are needed to confirm the effect of the intake of fermented soy products on the risk of hypertension and on BP.

Author Contributions: D.Y. wrote the paper and performed the statistical analyses. Y.P. designed the study and reviewed the paper. All authors have read and agreed to the published version of the manuscript.

References

1. WHO. *Global Atlas on Cardiovascular Disease Prevention and Control*; Shanthi, M., Pekka, P., Bo, N., Eds.; World Health Organization: Geneva, Switzerland, 2016.
2. Korea Centers for Disease Control and Prevention. *Korea Health Statistics 2016: Korea National Health and Nutrition Examination Survey (KNHANES VII-1)*; Korea Centers for Disease Control and Prevention: Sejong Cheongju, Korea, 2017.
3. Whelton, P.K.; Carey, R.M.; Aronow, W.S.; Casey, D.E., Jr.; Collins, K.J.; Dennison Himmelfarb, C.; DePalma, S.M.; Gidding, S.; Jamerson, K.A.; Jones, D.W.; et al. 2017 ACC/AHA/AAPA/ABC/ACPM/AGS/APA/ASH/ASPC/NMA/PCNA Guideline for the prevention, detection, evaluation, and management of high blood pressure in adults: Executive summary: A report of the American College of Cardiology/American Heart Association task force on clinical practice guidelines. *Circulation* **2018**, *138*, 426–483. [CrossRef]

4. Härtl, G. WHO issues new guidance on dietary salt and potassium. *Cent. Eur. J. Public Health* **2013**, *21*, 16.
5. Mohan, S.; Campbell, N.R. Salt, and high blood pressure. *Clin. Sci.* **2009**, *117*, 1–11. [CrossRef] [PubMed]
6. Graudal, N.; Hubeck-Graudal, T.; Jürgens, G.; Taylor, R.S. Dose-response relation between dietary sodium and blood pressure: A meta-regression analysis of 133 randomized controlled trials. *Am. J. Clin. Nutr.* **2019**, *109*, 1273–1278. [CrossRef] [PubMed]
7. Watanabe, H.; Kashimoto, N.; Kajimura, J.; Kamiya, K. A miso (Japanese soybean paste) diet conferred greater protection against hypertension than a sodium chloride diet in Dahl salt-sensitive rats. *Hypertens. Res.* **2006**, *29*, 731–738. [CrossRef] [PubMed]
8. Yoshinaga, M.; Toda, N.; Tamura, Y.; Terakado, S.; Ueno, M.; Otsuka, K.; Numabe, A.; Kawabata, Y.; Uehara, Y. Japanese traditional miso soup attenuates salt-induced hypertension and its organ damage in Dahl salt-sensitive rats. *Nutrition* **2012**, *28*, 924–931. [CrossRef]
9. Mun, E.G.; Park, J.E.; Cha, Y.S. Effects of doenjang, a traditional Korean soybean paste, with high-salt diet on blood pressure in Sprague-Dawley rats. *Nutrients* **2019**, *11*, 2745. [CrossRef]
10. Shin, D.H.; Jeong, D.Y. Korean traditional fermented soybean products: Jang. *J. Ethn. Foods* **2015**, *2*, 2–7. [CrossRef]
11. Park, J.W.; Kim, S.J.; Kim, S.H.; Kim, B.H.; Kang, S.G.; Nam, S.H.; Jung, S.T. Determination of mineral and heavy metal contents of various salts. *Korean J. Food Sci. Biotechnol.* **2000**, *32*, 1442–1445.
12. Baek, S.H.; Ahn, J.W.; Lee, H.R.; Cho, S.H.; Kim, J.H. Anti-hypertensive effect of a solar salt diet in elderly hypertensive patients: A preliminary randomized, double-blind clinical trial. *Korean J. Health Promot.* **2015**, *15*, 98–107. [CrossRef]
13. Messina, M. Soy and health update: Evaluation of the clinical and epidemiologic literature. *Nutrients* **2016**, *8*, 754. [CrossRef] [PubMed]
14. Dong, J.Y.; Tong, X.; Wu, Z.W.; Xun, P.C.; He, K.; Qin, L.Q. Effect of soya protein on blood pressure: A meta-analysis of randomised controlled trials. *Br. J. Nutr.* **2011**, *106*, 317–326. [CrossRef] [PubMed]
15. van Mierlo, L.A.; Arends, L.R.; Streppel, M.T.; Zeegers, M.P.; Kok, F.J.; Grobbee, D.E.; Geleijnse, J.M. Blood pressure response to calcium supplementation: A meta-analysis of randomized controlled trials. *J. Hum. Hypertens.* **2006**, *20*, 571–580. [CrossRef]
16. Filippini, T.; Naska, A.; Kasdagli, M.I.; Torres, D.; Lopes, C.; Carvalho, C.; Moreira, P.; Malavolti, M.; Orsini, N.; Whelton, P.K.; et al. Potassium intake and blood pressure: A dose-response meta-analysis of randomized controlled trials. *J. Am. Heart Assoc.* **2020**, *9*, e015719. [CrossRef] [PubMed]
17. Hu, X.; Gao, J.; Zhang, Q.; Fu, Y.; Li, K.; Zhu, S.; Li, D. Soy fiber improves weight loss and lipid profile in overweight and obese adults: A randomized controlled trial. *Mol. Nutr. Food Res.* **2013**, *57*, 2147–2154. [CrossRef]
18. Nozue, M.; Shimazu, T.; Sasazuki, S.; Charvat, H.; Mori, N.; Mutoh, M.; Sawada, N.; Iwasaki, M.; Yamaji, T.; Inoue, M.; et al. Fermented soy product intake is inversely associated with the development of high blood pressure: The Japan Public Health Center-Based Prospective Study. *J. Nutr.* **2017**, *147*, 1749–1756. [CrossRef]
19. Kanda, A.; Hoshiyama, Y.; Kawaguchi, T. Association of lifestyle parameters with the prevention of hypertension in elderly Japanese men and women: A four-year follow-up of normotensive subjects. *Asia Pac. J. Public Health* **1999**, *11*, 77–81. [CrossRef]
20. Ito, K.; Miyata, K.; Mohri, M.; Origuchi, H.; Yamamoto, H. The effects of the habitual consumption of miso soup on the blood pressure and heart rate of Japanese adults: A cross-sectional study of a health examination. *Intern. Med.* **2017**, *56*, 23–29. [CrossRef]
21. Kweon, S.; Kim, Y.; Jang, M.J.; Kim, Y.; Kim, K.; Choi, S.; Chun, C.; Khang, Y.H.; Oh, K. Data resource profile: The Korea National Health and Nutrition Examination Survey (KNHANES). *Int. J. Epidemiol.* **2014**, *43*, 69–77. [CrossRef]
22. Williams, B.; Mancia, G.; Spiering, W.; Agabiti Rosei, E.; Azizi, M.; Burnier, M.; Clement, D.; Coca, A.; D Simone, G.; Dominiczak, A.; et al. 2018 Practice guidelines for the management of arterial hypertension of the European Society of Hypertension and the European Society of Cardiology: ESH/ESC task force for the management of arterial hypertension. *J. Hypertens.* **2018**, *36*, 2284–2309. [CrossRef]
23. Rural Development Administration National Institute of Agricultural Sciences. *8th Revision Korean Food Composition Table*; Rural Development Administration National Institute of Agricultural Sciences: Wanju-gun, Jeollabuk-do, Korea, 2011.

24. Rural Development Administration National Institute of Agricultural Sciences. *9th Revision Korean Food Composition Table II*; Rural Development Administration National Institute of Agricultural Sciences: Wanju-gun, Jeollabuk-do, Korea, 2016.
25. Friedewald, W.T.; Levy, R.I.; Fredrickson, D.S. Estimation of the concentration of low-density lipoprotein cholesterol in plasma, without use of the preparative ultracentrifuge. *Clin. Chem.* **1972**, *18*, 499–502. [CrossRef] [PubMed]
26. Lee, H.Y.; Shin, J.; Kim, G.H.; Park, S.; Ihm, S.H.; Kim, H.C.; Kim, K.I.; Kim, J.H.; Lee, J.H.; Park, J.M.; et al. 2018 Korean Society of Hypertension Guidelines for the Management of Hypertension: Part II diagnosis and treatment of hypertension. *Clin. Hypertens.* **2019**, *25*, 20. [CrossRef] [PubMed]
27. Saylor, J.; Friedmann, E.; Lee, H.J. Navigating complex sample analysis using national survey data. *Nurs. Res.* **2012**, *61*, 231–237. [CrossRef] [PubMed]
28. Greenland, S.; Pearce, N. Statistical foundations for model-based adjustments. *Annu. Rev. Public Health* **2015**, *36*, 89–108. [CrossRef]
29. Hayes, A.F. *Introduction to Mediation, Moderation, and Conditional Process Analysis: A Regression-Based Approach*; Guilford Press: New York, NY, USA, 2017.
30. Bahari, T.; Uemura, H.; Katsuura-Kamano, S.; Yamaguchi, M.; Nakamoto, M.; Miki, K.; Ishizu, M.; Arisawa, K. Nutrient-derived dietary patterns and their association with metabolic syndrome in a Japanese population. *J. Epidemiol.* **2018**, *28*, 194–201. [CrossRef] [PubMed]
31. Guo, F.; Zhang, Q.; Yin, Y.; Liu, Y.; Jiang, H.; Yan, N.; Lin, J.; Liu, H.; Ma, L. Legume consumption and risk of hypertension in a prospective cohort of Chinese men and women. *Br. J. Nutr.* **2020**, *123*, 564–573. [CrossRef] [PubMed]
32. Woo, H.W.; Kim, M.K.; Lee, Y.H.; Shin, D.H.; Shin, M.H.; Choi, B.Y. Habitual consumption of soy protein and isoflavones and risk of metabolic syndrome in adults ≥ 40 years old: A prospective analysis of the Korean Multi-Rural Communities Cohort Study (MRCohort). *Eur. J. Nutr.* **2019**, *58*, 2835–2850. [CrossRef]
33. Yang, G.; Shu, X.O.; Jin, F.; Zhang, X.; Li, H.L.; Li, Q.; Gao, Y.T.; Zheng, W. Longitudinal study of soy food intake and blood pressure among middle-aged and elderly Chinese women. *Am. J. Clin. Nutr.* **2005**, *81*, 1012–1017. [CrossRef]
34. Richardson, S.I.; Steffen, L.M.; Swett, K.; Smith, C.; Burke, L.; Zhou, X.; Shikany, J.M.; Rodriguez, C.J. Dietary total isoflavone intake is associated with lower systolic blood pressure: The Coronary Artery Risk Development in Young Adults (CARDIA) study. *J. Clin. Hypertens. (Greenwich)* **2016**, *18*, 778–783. [CrossRef]
35. Papanikolaou, Y.; Fulgoni, V.L., 3rd. Bean consumption is associated with greater nutrient intake, reduced systolic blood pressure, lower body weight, and a smaller waist circumference in adults: Results from the National Health and Nutrition Examination Survey 1999–2002. *J. Am. Coll. Nutr.* **2008**, *27*, 569–576. [CrossRef]
36. Rivas, M.; Garay, R.P.; Escanero, J.F.; Cia, P., Jr.; Cia, P.; Alda, J.O. Soy milk lowers blood pressure in men and women with mild to moderate essential hypertension. *J. Nutr.* **2002**, *132*, 1900–1902. [CrossRef] [PubMed]
37. Welty, F.K.; Lee, K.S.; Lew, N.S.; Zhou, J.R. Effect of soy nuts on blood pressure and lipid levels in hypertensive, prehypertensive, and normotensive postmenopausal women. *Arch. Intern. Med.* **2007**, *167*, 1060–1067. [CrossRef] [PubMed]
38. Acharjee, S.; Zhou, J.R.; Elajami, T.K.; Welty, F.K. Effect of soy nuts and equol status on blood pressure, lipids, and inflammation in postmenopausal women stratified by metabolic syndrome status. *Metabolism* **2015**, *64*, 236–243. [CrossRef] [PubMed]
39. Halla, H.J.; Ameer, M.A.; Uppaluri, K.R. DASH diet to stop hypertension. In *StatPearls*; StatPearls Publishing Copyright © 2020; StatPearls Publishing LLC.: Treasure Island, FL, USA, 2020.
40. Handa, C.L.; Zhang, Y.; Kumari, S.; Xu, J.; Ida, E.I.; Chang, S.K. Comparative study of angiotensin I-converting enzyme (ACE) inhibition of soy foods as affected by processing methods and protein isolation. *Processes* **2020**, *8*, 978. [CrossRef]
41. Da Silva, L.H.; Celeghini, R.M.; Chang, Y.K. Effect of the fermentation of whole soybean flour on the conversion of isoflavones from glycosides to aglycones. *Food Chem.* **2011**, *128*, 640–644. [CrossRef]
42. Kawakami, Y.; Tsurugasaki, W.; Nakamura, S.; Osada, K. Comparison of regulative functions between dietary soy isoflavones aglycone and glucoside on lipid metabolism in rats fed cholesterol. *J. Nutr. Biochem.* **2005**, *16*, 205–212. [CrossRef]

43. Shin, Z.I.; Yu, R.; Park, S.A.; Chung, D.K.; Ahn, C.W.; Nam, H.S.; Kim, K.S.; Lee, H.J. His-His-Leu, an angiotensin I converting enzyme inhibitory peptide derived from Korean soybean paste, exerts antihypertensive activity In Vivo. *J. Agric. Food Chem.* **2001**, *49*, 3004–3009. [CrossRef]
44. Park, E.; Shin, J.I.; Park, O.J.; Kang, M.H. Soy isoflavone supplementation alleviates oxidative stress and improves systolic blood pressure in male spontaneously hypertensive rats. *J. Nutr. Sci. Vitaminol.* **2005**, *51*, 254–259. [CrossRef]
45. Timpka, S.; Stuart, J.J.; Tanz, L.J.; Rimm, E.B.; Franks, P.W.; Rich-Edwards, J.W. Lifestyle in progression from hypertensive disorders of pregnancy to chronic hypertension in Nurses' Health Study II: Observational cohort study. *BMJ* **2017**, *358*, j3024. [CrossRef]
46. Mente, A.; O'Donnell, M.; Rangarajan, S.; McQueen, M.; Dagenais, G.; Wielgosz, A.; Lear, S.; Ah, S.T.L.; Wei, L.; Diaz, R.; et al. Urinary sodium excretion, blood pressure, cardiovascular disease, and mortality: A community-level prospective epidemiological cohort study. *Lancet* **2018**, *392*, 496–506. [CrossRef]
47. Jeong, Y.S.; Lim, H.J.; Kim, S.B.; Kim, H.J.; Son, S.M. Blood pressure and dietary related risk factors associated with high sodium intake assessed with 24-h urine analysis for Korean adults. *Nutr. Res. Pract.* **2014**, *19*, 537–549. [CrossRef]
48. Ashraf, M.S.; Vongpatanasin, W. Estrogen and hypertension. *Curr. Hypertens. Rep.* **2006**, *8*, 368–376. [CrossRef] [PubMed]
49. Hwang, C.S.; Kwak, H.S.; Lim, H.J.; Lee, S.H.; Kang, Y.S.; Choe, T.B.; Hur, H.G.; Han, K.O. Isoflavone metabolites and their in vitro dual functions: They can act as an estrogenic agonist or antagonist depending on the estrogen concentration. *J. Steroid Biochem. Mol. Biol.* **2006**, *101*, 246–253. [CrossRef] [PubMed]
50. Hooper, L.; Ryder, J.J.; Kurzer, M.S.; Lampe, J.W.; Messina, M.J.; Phipps, W.R.; Cassidy, A. Effects of soy protein and isoflavones on circulating hormone concentrations in pre- and post-menopausal women: A systematic review and meta-analysis. *Hum. Reprod. Update* **2009**, *15*, 423–440. [CrossRef] [PubMed]
51. Nagata, C.; Inaba, S.; Kawakami, N.; Kakizoe, T.; Shimizu, H. Inverse association of soy product intake with serum androgen and estrogen concentrations in Japanese men. *Nutr. Cancer* **2000**, *36*, 14–18. [CrossRef] [PubMed]
52. Taku, K.; Lin, N.; Cai, D.; Hu, J.; Zhao, X.; Zhang, Y.; Wang, P.; Melby, M.K.; Hooper, L.; Kurzer, M.S.; et al. Effects of soy isoflavone extract supplements on blood pressure in adult humans: Systematic review and meta-analysis of randomized placebo-controlled trials. *J. Hypertens.* **2010**, *28*, 1971–1982. [CrossRef] [PubMed]
53. Franklin, S.S.; Wong, N.D. Hypertension and cardiovascular disease: Contributions of the Framingham heart study. *Glob. Heart* **2013**, *8*, 49–57. [CrossRef]
54. Staessen, J.A.; van der Heijden-Spek, J.J.; Safar, M.E.; Den Hond, E.; Gasowski, J.; Fagard, R.H.; Wang, J.G.; Boudier, H.A.; Van Bortel, L.M. Menopause and the characteristics of the large arteries in a population study. *J. Hum. Hypertens.* **2001**, *15*, 511–518. [CrossRef]
55. Nestel, P.; Fujii, A.; Zhang, L. An isoflavone metabolite reduces arterial stiffness and blood pressure in overweight men and postmenopausal women. *Atherosclerosis* **2007**, *192*, 184–189. [CrossRef]

Nutrients Intake in Individuals with Hypertension, Dyslipidemia and Diabetes: An Italian Survey

Cecilia Guastadisegni [1,*], Chiara Donfrancesco [1], Luigi Palmieri [1], Sara Grioni [2], Vittorio Krogh [2], Diego Vanuzzo [3], Pasquale Strazzullo [4], Serena Vannucchi [1], Graziano Onder [1] and Simona Giampaoli [1]

1 Department of Cardiovascular, Endocrine-metabolic Diseases and Aging, Istituto Superiore di Sanita, 00161 Rome, Italy; chiara.donfrancesco@iss.it (C.D.); luigi.palmieri@iss.it (L.P.); serena.vannucchi@iss.it (S.V.); graziano.onder@iss.it (G.O.); simona.giampaoli@iss.it (S.G.)
2 Epidemiology and Prevention Unit, Fondazione IRCCS Istituto Nazionale dei Tumori, 20133 Milan, Italy; Sara.Grioni@istitutotumori.mi.it (S.G.); Vittorio.Krogh@istitutotumori.mi.it (V.K.)
3 Associazione Nazionale Medici Cardiologi Ospedalieri (ANMCO), 50121 Florence, Italy; diego50rdc@gmail.com
4 Department of Clinical Medicine and Surgery, ESH Excellence Centre of Hypertension, Federico II University of Naples Medical School, 80131 Naples, Italy; strazzul@unina.it
* Correspondence: cecilia.guastadisegni@iss.it

Abstract: The aim of this study is to evaluate whether nutrients intake in an Italian adult population receiving pharmacological treatment for hypertension, dyslipidemia, and diabetes are within the recommended values proposed by dietary guidelines. Cross-sectional data from the Cardiovascular Epidemiology Observatory/Health Examination Survey in 8462 individuals 35–79 years were used. Food consumption was assessed with a self-administered semi-quantitative food frequency questionnaire. Dietary sodium and potassium intakes were measured in 24-hour urine collection. Recommendations from WHO were used for salt and potassium intakes, those from the Diabetes and Nutrition Study Group for diabetes, and those from the European Society of Cardiology for hypertension and dyslipidemia. Salt intake in urine collection of participants receiving treatment for hypertension was 11.1 ± 4.0 g/day for men and 8.6 ± 3.3 g/day for women, higher than recommended. In participants treated for dyslipidemia, mean saturated fat intake was 11.4% and 11.6% total Kcal in men and women respectively, higher than recommended, while cholesterol intake was higher only in men (365.9 ± 149.6 mg/day). In both men and women receiving treatment for diabetes, mean intake of saturated fats (12.3% and 12.2% of total Kcal), simple carbohydrates (17.5% and 19.8% of total Kcal) and cholesterol (411.0 ± 150.4 and 322.7 ± 111.1 mg/day) were above the recommendations, while fiber intake was below (19.5 ± 6.3 and 17.5 ± 6.2 mg/day). Overall, 70% to 80% of participants treated for these conditions received advice from family doctors on dietary management; however, nutrition is far from being optimal.

Keywords: hypertension; diabetes; dyslipidemia; dietary recommendations

---

1. Introduction

Hypertension, dyslipidemia, and diabetes are known risk factors of cardiovascular diseases (CVD) and a healthy diet is considered as the first approach to treat these conditions [1]. In particular, reduction of salt intake is considered critical for treatment of hypertension, given its positive effect on blood pressure (BP) in hypertensive individuals [2,3]. Also, potassium intake has an effect on lowering BP in both hypertensive and normotensive individuals [2,3].

Similarly, reduction of saturated fatty acids (SFA) intake is fundamental for the treatment of dyslipidemia [4]. It is recognized that SFA increase cardiovascular risk by raising plasma low-density lipoprotein (LDL) cholesterol whereas polyunsaturated fatty acids (PUFA) and monounsaturated fatty acids (MUFA) lower this parameter [5,6]. Finally, nutrition therapy is an integral component of diabetes management and even modest weight loss improves insulin sensitivity in individuals with type 2 diabetes [7,8]. In addition, high fiber intake and low refined carbohydrates are one of the most important interventions for improving glycemic control in individuals with diabetes. The fiber intake recommended for the diabetic population is indeed double that recommended for the general population [9].

The aim of the present study is to evaluate the dietary habits of an Italian population receiving pharmacological treatment for hypertension, dyslipidemia, and diabetes in comparison with the general population not receiving such treatments. In addition, we have assessed whether macronutrients intake and salt and potassium excretion is within the recommended values proposed by current dietary guidelines and we have evaluated how many participants with these conditions receive guidance on dietary recommendations from their family physician.

2. Materials and Methods

2.1. Participants

For the present study we used data from the Cardiovascular Epidemiology Observatory/Health Examination Survey, which was conducted in 2008–2012 in the adult Italian general population [10]. The aim of the survey was to describe lifestyle habits (habitual diet, physical activity, alcohol consumption) and the prevalence of high-risk conditions for CVD. Two hundred and twenty men and women per 1.5 million general population aged 35–79 years and living in 20 Italian regions were randomly selected. An information letter about the project was sent to all the selected participants to explain the research purposes and obtain a signed informed consent to participate. Trained personnel administered questionnaire collecting information on the main characteristics of the participants, including demographics, anthropometric measures and drug treatment, and participants filled out self-administered dietary information. The current study population consisted of people taking drugs for hypertension, dyslipidemia, or diabetes. This variable was assessed by study personnel by specific questions (i.e., 'Are you using any drugs for treatment of . . . ?'). Moreover, study personnel asked the participants, whether their family physician had given advice regarding lifestyle and dietary changes to treat hypertension, dyslipidemia, and diabetes. The Italian National Institute of Health ethical committee approved the survey on 11 November, 2009.

2.2. Assessment of Nutrients Intake

Dietary information was collected by the self-administered Italian version of the food frequency questionnaire (FFQ) of the European Prospective Investigation into Cancer (EPIC), which focused on diet as a major determinant of health. Accuracy and validation of dietary questionnaires was of paramount importance as it was to be applied in several countries and to thousands of study participants [11].The FFQ was designed to capture eating behaviors in the Italian population [12]. Food items were linked using specifically designed software [13] to Italian Food Tables [14] to obtain estimates of daily intake of 37 macro- and micronutrients plus energy (not all nutrients are shown in the tables). Carbohydrates, protein, and fat intakes were classified as percentage of total daily energy intake, dietary cholesterol as mg/day, and dietary fiber, sodium, and potassium as g/day. In addition to using the EPIC questionnaire to assess dietary sodium and potassium intakes, levels were also objectively measured through a 24-hour urine collection in a random sample of 200 people in each region. Participants were provided with a SARSTED plastic container of 3 L with thymol added for urine preservation and assayed centrally.

WHO recommendations were used as the reference for normal salt and potassium intakes [3]. Recommendations from the Diabetes and Nutrition Study Group (DNSG) of the European Association for the Study of Diabetes, endorsed by the Italian Diabetes Society (SID), were used as reference for intake of other nutrients in diabetes [8,15], and European Society of Cardiology (ESC) recommendations were used for hypertension and dyslipidemia [1].

2.3. Study Sample

Of the 8696 men and women aged 35–79 years considered in this analysis, 464 (5.3%) did not complete the dietary questionnaire making it impossible to calculate the total energy intake. We also excluded 176 (2.0%) persons in whom the ratio of total energy intake to basal metabolic rate was at either extreme of the distribution (i.e., energy intake below 400 kcal/day or higher than 5000 kcal/day), leading to a final sample of 8056 participants. For the purpose of the present study, the sample was categorized according to the use of drugs for treatment of hypertension, dyslipidemia, or diabetes. This was done to assess adherence to guidelines and recommendations in persons already receiving pharmacological treatment for these conditions. Urine excretion of sodium and potassium was available for 3513 participants out of 8056; 24-hour urine volume was equal or over 500 ml and its creatinine content referred to body weight was found to be within mean minus/plus 2 standard deviation from the population mean.

2.4. Statistical Analysis

Separate analyses were done for treatment of hypertension (present or not present), hypercholesterolemia (present or not present), and diabetes (present or not present). Each participant may have been included in all three analyses if criteria of inclusion, according to treatment, were met. Hence the number of total persons included in each analysis (hypertension, dyslipidemia, diabetes) was different.

Data are presented, separately for men and women, as mean, standard deviations, and prevalence, with 95% Confidence Intervals (C.I.), standardized by age using the 2013 European standard population age distribution, equal for both men and women. Multivariate regression models were performed for each nutrient; BMI and total energy intake were used to compare treated and not treated groups. Models were adjusted for age, educational level, smoking habit, physical inactivity, and overweight/obesity. Educational level was selected as a proxy for socioeconomic status subdividing participants between low educational level (primary/middle school) and high educational level (high school/university). Smoking was defined as a person smoking one or more cigarettes per day. Physical activity during leisure time was collected through a questionnaire including four levels of exercise (sedentary, mild, moderate, heavy). However, in this analysis, physical activity was considered only as sedentary and non-sedentary. Height and weight were measured following standardized methods; overweight or obesity was defined as BMI above 25 kg/m^2. Further details about procedure and methods used to collect data can be found in the previous publication [10]. Chi-squared test was performed to compare prevalence of treated and not treated groups (supplementary Tables S1–S3). Box plots were used to show the distribution of total energy intake by gender and treatment (supplementary Figure S1–S3). Two sided p-values equal or less than 0.05 were considered statistically significant. Statistical analyses were performed using SAS (9.4 version).

3. Results

Table 1 presents nutritional intake in men and women treated for hypertension as compared with those not receiving treatment. Nutritional recommendations issued by ESC and/or WHO are reported for comparison.

Table 1. Nutrients composition of diet in men and women receiving and not receiving treatment for hypertension. Men and women aged 35–79 years from the Osservatorio Epidemiologico Cardiovascolare/Health Examination Survey of the CUORE Project 2008–2012.

Nutrients	Men					Women					ESC/WHO Recommendations
	Not Treated for Hypertension $n = 2749$		Treated for Hypertension $n = 1280$			Not Treated for Hypertension $n = 2837$		Treated for Hypertension $n = 1174$			
	Mean ± SD	Mean 95% C.I.	Mean ± SD	Mean 95% C.I.	Sign.	Mean ± SD	Mean 95% C.I.	Mean ± SD	Mean 95% C.I.	Sign.	
Proteins (% total Kcal)	16.0 ± 2.5	15.9–16.1	16.3 ± 2.6	16.1–16.4	*	16.5 ± 2.6	16.4–16.6	17.0 ± 2,7	16.8–17.1	ns	10–20%
Total Lipids (% total Kcal)	33.8 ± 5.7	33.7–34.1	34.3 ± 6.4	33.9–34.6	ns	36.5 ± 5.7	36.3–36.7	36.5 ± 6.2	36.1–36.9	ns	20–35%
Saturated fat (% total Kcal)	11.8 ± 2.5	11.7–11.9	11.8 ± 2.6	11.7–11.9	ns	12.7 ± 2.5	12.6–12.8	12.4 ± 2.6	12.2–12.5	*	<10%
Polyunsaturated fat (% total Kcal)	3.9 ± 0.9	3.8–3.9	4.0 ± 1	3.9–4	ns	4.2 ± 0.9	4.1–4.2	4.3 ± 1.1	4.2–4.3	ns	<10%
Carbohydrate (% total Kcal)	46.9 ± 7.9	46.6–47.2	46.0 ± 8.6	45.5–46.5	**	47.6 ± 7.7	47.3–47.9	47.6 ± 8.1	47.1–48	ns	45–60%
Simple carbohydrates (% total Kcal)	19.6 ± 7.0	19.4–19.9	18.6 ± 7.0	18.2–19.0	**	22.6 ± 7.2	22.3–22.8	21.4 ± 7.1	21–21.8	**	<10%
Cholesterol (mg/day)	384.8 ± 164.5	378.7–391	380.5 ± 144.6	372.6–388.4	**	336.7 ± 139.9	331.6–341.9	330.4 ± 135.6	322.6–338.1	ns	<300
Fiber (g/day)	19.4 ± 7.4	19.2–19.7	19.9 ± 6.8	19.5–20.2	*	18.5 ± 7.1	18.2–18.7	18.0 ± 6.8	17.6–18.4	ns	30–45
Sodium (g/day)	2.3 ± 1.1	2.3–2.4	2.5 ± 1.0	2.4–2.5	ns	1.9 ± 0.9	1.9–1.9	1.9 ± 0.9	1.8–1.9	ns	<2
Potassium (g/day)	3.3 ± 1.1	3.2–3.3	3.3 ± 1.0	3.2–3.3	**	3.0 ± 1.0	3–3.1	2.9 ± 1.0	2.9–3	ns	>4
Salt g/day (24hr urine)	10.6 ± 4.1	10.4–10.8	11.1 ± 4.0	10.8–11.4	ns	8.1 ± 3.3	7.9–8.3	8.6 ± 3.3	8.3–8.8	ns	<5
Potassium g/day (24hr urine)	2.5 ± 0.7	2.4–2.5	2.5 ± 0.8	2.4–2.5	ns	2.2 ± 0.7	2.1–2.2	2.2 ± 0.7	2.1–2.2	ns	>3.9
Body Mass Index (kg/m^2)	27.1 ± 4.1	27–27.3	29.4 ± 4.1	29.2–29.7	***	26.3 ± 4.9	26.1–26.5	30.5 ± 5.9	30.1–30.8	***	<25
Energy (Kcal/day)	2297 ± 770	2268–2326	2276 ± 697	2238–2314	**	1899 ± 647	1875–1923	1816 ± 628	1781–1852	ns	

Values are means ± standard deviation. C.I. Confidence Intervals. ESC (European Society of Cardiology). Sign = statistical significance of treatment coefficient in a multivariate regression model adjusted by age, educational level, smoking habit, physical inactivity, and overweight/obesity. *** $p < 0.0001$; ** $p < 0.01$; * $p < 0.05$; ns not statistically significant. Data are standardized by gender and age using the 2013 European population. Number of persons with available salt and potassium g/day (24 hour urine): 1219 untreated and 564 treated men and 1214 untreated and 510 treated women.

There were no significant differences between participants treated and untreated for hypertension in the intake of total lipids, cholesterol, and fiber, while in the treated group a significant lower intake in both total and simple carbohydrates in men and only simple carbohydrates in women was observed. Both men and women of the treated group had a higher BMI as compared with the untreated group and energy intake was slightly reduced in treated as compared with not treated men. Salt excretion in participants receiving treatment for hypertension was higher than untreated participants (11.1 ± 4.0 g/day vs. 10.6 ± 4.1 g/day in men and 8.6 ± 3.3 g/day vs. 8.1 ± 3.3 g/day in women) although not significant. Overall, 70% of the participants treated for hypertension reported to have been advised to reduce salt intake by family doctor as compared to only 6% of the untreated population.

The nutritional intakes of the population under treatment for dyslipidemia together with ESC/WHO recommendations are presented in Table 2.

Intake of SFA was significantly lower in the treated as compared with the untreated sample as well as intake of total cholesterol. Both in men and women, the treated group had a higher BMI and a significant lower energy intake as compared with the untreated group. Saturated fat intake was higher than suggested by ESC recommendations in both men and women. Among treated women, mean cholesterol intake was below the threshold suggested by ESC recommendations, while mean value among men was above the threshold. A high percentage of the population treated for hypercholesterolemia (76.4% men 76.6% women) received recommendations for reducing plasma lipids whereas only 22.1% of men and 21.7% of women untreated received this advice.

Nutrients intake according to diabetes treatment, along with the recent nutritional recommendations issued by DNSG, are presented in Table 3.

In both men and women, treated participants had a higher intake of PUFA and a lower intake of total carbohydrates and simple carbohydrates. Gender differences were observed in the intake of SFA and cholesterol, where treatment was associated with a higher intake of these nutrients in men and with a lower intake in women. Both men and women treated for diabetes had a significantly higher BMI than the untreated population. Total energy intake was significantly lower in the treated than in the untreated sample. In both treated men and women, mean intake of lipids, SFA, simple carbohydrates, and cholesterol was above the threshold suggested by DNSG guidelines, while fiber intake was below the suggested threshold. A high percentage of persons treated for diabetes (80% of men and 86% of women) had received advice from family doctors on lifestyle and nutritional changes.

Table 2. Nutrients composition of the diet in men and women receiving and not receiving treatment for dyslipidemia. Men and women aged 35–79 years from the Osservatorio Epidemiologico Cardiovascolare/Health Examination Survey of the CUORE Project 2008–2012.

Nutrients	Men					Women					ESC/WHO Recommendations
	Not Treated for Dyslipidemia n = 3455		Treated for Dyslipidemia n = 540			Not Treated for Dyslipidemia n = 3456		Treated for Dyslipidemia n = 537			
	Mean ± SD	Mean 95% C.I.	Mean ± SD	Mean 95% C.I.	Sign.	Mean ± SD	Mean 95% C.I.	Mean ± SD	Mean 95% C.I.	Sign.	
Proteins (% total Kcal)	16.0 ± 2.4	15.9–16.1	16.4 ± 2.9	16.2–16.6	**	16.6 ± 2.7	16.5–16.7	16.7 ± 2.8	16.5–16.9	ns	10–20%
Total Lipids (% total Kcal)	33.9 ± 5.9	33.7–34.1	33.2 ± 6.0	32.7–33.7	ns	36.6 ± 5.8	36.4–36.8	36.0 ± 6.0	35.5–36.5	*	20–35%
Saturated fat (% total Kcal)	11.8 ± 2.5	11.8–12	11.4 ± 2.6	11.2–11.7	**	12.7 ± 2.5	12.6–12.8	11.8 ± 2.6	11.5–12	***	<10%
Polyunsaturated fat (% total Kcal)	3.9 ± 0.9	3.9–3.9	3.9 ± 0.9	3.8–3.9	ns	4.2 ± 1.0	4.1–4.2	4.2 ± 1.1	4.1–4.3	ns	<10%
Carbohydrate (% total Kcal)	46.8 ± 8.1	46.5–47	46.6 ± 8.3	45.9–47.3	ns	47.5 ± 7.8	47.3–47.8	47.3 ± 8.2	46.6–48	ns	45–60%
Simple carbohydrates (% total Kcal)	19.5 ± 7.0	19.2–19.7	18.8 ± 6.7	18.2–19.4	*	22.3 ± 7.2	22–22.5	20.9 ± 7.0	20.3–21.5	ns	<10%
Cholesterol (mg/day)	382.9 ± 159.3	377.6–388.3	365.9 ± 149.6	353.3–378.5	**	340.1 ± 139.8	335.4–344.7	294.9 ± 127.9	284–305.7	***	<300
Fiber (g/day)	19.4 ± 7.3	19.1–19.6	19.0 ± 7.0	18.4–19.6	ns	18.5 ± 7.1	18.2–18.7	17.8 ± 6.5	17.3–18.4	ns	30–45
Sodium (g/day)	2.4 ± 1.1	2.4–2.4	2.3 ± 1.0	2.2–2.4	**	1.9 ± 0.9	1.9–2.0	1.7 ± 0.8	1.7–1.8	**	<2
Potassium (g/day)	3.3 ± 1.0	3.2–3.3	3.2 ± 1.1	3.2–3.3	ns	3.0 ± 1.0	3.0–3.0	2.9 ± 1.0	2.8–3	ns	>4
Salt g/day (24hr urine)	10.7 ± 4.1	10.4–10.9	11.3 ± 4.1	10.8–11.8	ns	8.3 ± 3.3	8.1–8.4	7.8 ± 3.0	7.4–8.2	ns	<5
Potassium g/day (24hr urine)	2.5 ± 0.7	2.4–2.5	2.5 ± 0.8	2.4–2.6	ns	2.2 ± 0.7	2.1–2.2	2.0 ± 0.7	2–2.1	ns	>3.9
Body Mass Index (kg/m^2)	27.6 ± 4.1	27.5–27.7	28.5 ± 4.1	28.1—28.8	**	27.1 ± 5.4	27–27.3	28.0 ± 5.2	27.5–28.4	ns	<25
Energy (Kcal/day)	2283 ± 649	2262–2305	2185 ± 726	2124–2246	**	1899 ± 754	1874–1924	1755 ± 585	1706–1805	**	

Values are means ± standard deviations. C.I. = Confidence Intervals. ESC (European Society of Cardiology). Sign = statistical significance of treatment coefficient in a multivariate regression model adjusted by age, educational level, smoking habit, physical inactivity, and overweight/obesity. *** $p < 0.0001$; ** $p < 0.01$; * $p < 0.05$; ns not statistically significant. Data are standardized by gender and age using the 2013 European population. Number of persons with available salt and potassium g/day (24 hour urine): 1530 not treated and 235 treated men, 1474 not treated and 241 treated women.

Table 3. Nutrients composition of the diet in men and women receiving and not receiving treatment for diabetes. Men and women aged 35–79 years from the Osservatorio Epidemiologico Cardiovascolare/Health Examination Survey of the CUORE Project 2008–2012.

Nutrients	Men					Women					DNSG/WHO Recommendations
	Not Treated for Diabetes $n = 3725$		Treated for Diabetes $n = 308$			Not Treated for Diabetes $n = 3820$		Treated for Diabetes $n = 194$			
	Mean ± SD	Mean 95% C.I.	Mean ± SD	Mean 95% C.I.	Sign.	Mean ± SD	Mean 95% C.I.	Mean ± SD	Mean 95% C.I.	Sign.	
Proteins (% total Kcal)	16.0 ± 2,5	15.9–16.0	17.5 ± 2.8	17.2–17.8	***	16.6 ± 2.6	16.5–16.6	17.8 ± 3.0	17.3–18.2	***	10–20%
Total Lipids (% total Kcal)	33.8 ± 5.9	33.6–34.0	35.8 ± 6.2	35.1–36.5	***	36.5 ± 5.8	36.3–36.7	37.5 ± 7.0	36.5–38.5	*	25–35%
Saturated fat (% total Kcal)	11.8 ± 2.6	11.7–11.9	12.3 ± 2.6	12–12.6	*	12.7 ± 2.6	12.6–12.7	12.2 ± 2.5	11.8–12.5	ns	<10%
Polyunsaturated fat (% total Kcal)	3.9 ± 0.9	3.8–3.9	4.2 ± 0.9	4.1–4.3	***	4.2 ± 1.0	4.1–4.2	4.5 ± 1.0	4.3–4.6	*	<10%
Carbohydrate (% total Kcal)	46.8 ± 8.1	46.6–47.1	44.2 ± 8.1	43.3–45.1	**	47.6 ± 7.8	47.4–47.9	45.5 ± 9.5	44.1–46.8	**	45–60%
Simple carbohydrates (% total Kcal)	19.5 ± 7.0	19.3–19.8	17.5 ± 6.2	16.8–18.2	***	22.4 ± 7.1	22.2–22.6	19.8 ± 7.2	18.8–20.8	***	<10
Cholesterol (mg/day)	380.1 ± 159.1	375–385.2	411.0 ± 150.4	394.2–427.7	ns	338.1 ± 140.0	333.6–342.5	322.7 ± 111.1	307–338.3	**	<200
Fiber (g/day)	19.3 ± 7.3	19.1–19.6	19.5 ± 6.3	18.8–20.2	ns	18.5 ± 7.1	18.2–18.7	17.5 ± 6.2	16.7–18.4	ns	>40
Sodium (g/day)	2.4 ± 1.1	2.3–2.4	2.5 ± 1.1	2.4–2.7	ns	1.9 ± 0.9	1.9–1.9	1.8 ± 0.8	1.7–1.9	*	<2
Potassium (g/day)	3.3 ± 1.1	3.2–3.3	3.3 ± 1.0	3.2–3.4	ns	3.0 ± 1.0	3.0–3.0	3.0 ± 1.0	2.8–3.1	ns	>4
Salt g/day (24h urine)	10.6 ± 4.1	10.4–10.8	10.9 ± 3.6	10.3–11.5	ns	8.2 ± 3.3	8.1–8.4	9.2 ± 2.8	8.6–9.8	ns	<5
Potassium g/day (24h urine)	2.5 ± 0.8	2.4–2.5	2.7 ± 0.8	2.6–2.8	ns	2.2 ± 0.7	2.2–2.2	2.3 ± 0.7	2.2–2.5	ns	>3.9
Body Mass Index (kg/m^2)	27.6 ± 4.1	27.4–27.7	29.8 ± 4.3	29.3–30.2	***	27.0 ± 5.2	26.8–27.2	32.1 ± 5.7	31.3–32.9	***	<25
Energy (Kcal/day)	2282 ± 754	2258–2306.4	2205 ± 664	2131–2279.3	***	1896 ± 647	1875.5–1916.5	1735 ± 518	1662.5–1808.3	***	

Values are means ± standard deviations. C.I. = Confidence Intervals. DNSG (Diabetes and Nutrition Study Group). Sign = statistical significance of treatment coefficient in a multivariate regression model adjusted by age, educational level, smoking habit, physical inactivity, and overweight/obesity. *** $p < 0.0001$; ** $p < 0.01$; * $p < 0.05$; ns not statistically significant. Data are standardized by gender and age using the 2013 European population Number of persons with available salt and potassium g/day (24 hour urine): 1657 not treated and 128treated men, 1639 not treated and 85 treated women.

4. Discussion

These data from a national Italian survey show that dietary intake in persons treated for hypertension, dyslipidemia, and diabetes is far from being optimal. Participants treated for hypertension have a higher salt consumption than untreated participants, the mean value of SFA intake in participants treated for dyslipidemia is higher than the <10% recommended level, and only women have the recommended <300 mg/day cholesterol intake. Participants treated for diabetes have mean fiber consumption much lower than recommended.

Data on the dietary salt intake in this Italian population are in line with the results reported in the survey of the MINISAL-GIRCSI study, which showed that salt intake in Italy is high [16]. We showed that excretion of salt by the population under treatment for hypertension was higher than the general population. This finding is in contrast with data from the MINISAL-SIIA study of Italian hypertensive patients that showed a slightly lower sodium intake in comparison with the general population [17]. Indeed, our finding might be explained by the presence of a direct association between BMI and average salt intake, as the hypertensive treated population had a higher BMI than the general population [18]. It was hypothesized that high BMI might be associated with high salt intake due to a greater food and calories consumption. As calories intake is slightly reduced in our hypertensive population, the diuretic treatment for hypertension might have increased sodium excretion [19].

Confirming the results of the previous surveys, potassium intake was, on average, much below the dietary recommended intake of 3.9 g/day. A diet rich in potassium has an antihypertensive effect through various possible mechanisms and, therefore, professional organizations have made recommendations to increase the average intake of potassium as, in many countries, it is relatively low [20]. A concomitant increase in potassium, magnesium, calcium, and dietary fiber and a decrease in salt intake is currently the most recommended essential lifestyle intervention for controlling BP; these recommendations are outlined in the Dietary Approaches to Stop Hypertension [21].

Saturated lipids intake in participants treated for dyslipidemia is higher than recommended in the guidelines. Dietary SFA have a potent plasma LDL cholesterol raising effect, which is a causal risk factor for CVD. The substitution of dietary SFA with PUFA consistently reduces CVD events [4]. Several observational studies and meta-analyses have not demonstrated a significant correlation between SFA consumption and CVD events, but the isoenergetic replacement with PUFA has shown reduced CVD risk [5,6]. Thus, control of LDL cholesterol through reduction of SFA intake remains a cornerstone for management of dyslipidemia and prevention of cardiovascular events [22].

Our data confirm previous findings suggesting that compliance with nutritional recommendations for diabetes is extremely low and that carbohydrates intake in persons receiving treatment for diabetes is lower than the general population [23,24]. In persons with diabetes, complex carbohydrates intake is beneficial and fat-rich and simple sugar-containing foods should be avoided [25].

Despite the fact that between 70% and 80% of the population treated for hypertension, dyslipidemia, and diabetes received suggestions by family doctors on how to change dietary habits, nutrients intake was still not optimum on average. Previous studies have shown that specific intensive interventions based on detailed individualized counseling for lifestyle modification are necessary to achieve dietary modifications [26,27]. This kind of intervention is more effective than metformin in preventing diabetes incidence [28]. It has been shown that individual guidance for physical activity and sessions with nutritionists in persons with impaired glucose tolerance leads to substantial weight loss and a reduction in diabetes incidence [29]. In addition to the individualized interventions, a community-based intervention can also achieve changes in nutrition through the involvement of the local food industry for reducing and modifying the fat and salt content of commonly eaten foods. In Finland, a nation-wide population-based project aimed at improving nutrition through education and social media was shown to impact on dietary habits and to reduce serum cholesterol and BP levels [30].

The major strength of our study is that it is based on a population-based survey, the Cardiovascular Epidemiology Observatory/Health Examination Survey that covers all Italian regions. A major limitation is represented by the limited availability of 24-hour urine samples and the need to rely on the EPIC questionnaire to assess sodium and potassium in the whole study sample. The EPIC questionnaire is considered to be of high standard of accuracy and country specificity. However, the salt commonly added while cooking and the discretionary salt added at table is not calculated in the EPIC questionnaire [12].

5. Conclusions

In conclusion, dietary changes should be considered as the first approach for treatment of hypertension, diabetes, and dyslipidemia, in order to reduce the risk of CVD, but nutritional intakes in persons with these conditions is far from being optimal. Family doctors often advise persons with these conditions on correct dietary approach, but these recommendations are poorly followed.

Supplementary Materials
Figure S1: Distribution of Total energy intake (Kcal/day) in men and women receiving and not receiving hypertension treatment. Men and women aged 35–79 years from Osservatorio Epidemiologico Cardiovascolare/Health Examination Survey of the CUORE Project 2008–2012; Figure S2: Distribution of Total energy intake (Kcal/day) in men and women receiving and not receiving hypercholesterolemia treatment. Men and women aged 35–79 years from Osservatorio Epidemiologico Cardiovascolare/Health Examination Survey of the CUORE Project 2008–2012; Figure S3: Distribution of Total energy intake (Kcal/day) in men and women receiving and not receiving diabetes treatment. Men and women aged 35–79 years from Osservatorio Epidemiologico Cardiovascolare/Health Examination Survey of the CUORE Project 2008–2012; Table S1: Characteristics of men and women receiving and not receiving treatment for hypertension. Men and women aged 35–79 years from Osservatorio Epidemiologico Cardiovascolare/Health Examination Survey of the CUORE Project 2008–2012; Table S2: Characteristics of men and women receiving and not receiving treatment for hypercholesteromia. Men and women aged 35–79 years from Osservatorio Epidemiologico Cardiovascolare/Health Examination Survey of the CUORE Project 2008–2012; Table S3: Characteristics of men and women receiving and not receiving treatment for diabetes. Men and women aged 35–79 years from Osservatorio Epidemiologico Cardiovascolare/Health Examination Survey of the CUORE Project 2008–2012.

Author Contributions: "Conceptualization and design of the survey, S.G., V.K., C.G., C.D.; Formal Analysis, V.K., S.G. Methodology, S.G., D.V., C.D., V.K., P.S.; Investigation D.V., S.G., C.D., L.P., D.V., P.S.; Data Curation and Statistical Analysis, C.D., S.V.; Writing—Original Draft Preparation, CG, SG; Writing—Review and Editing G.O., C.G., C.D.; Project Administration S.V., S.G., D.V.; Funding Acquisition: S.G., D.V.". All authors have read and agreed to the published version of the manuscript.

Acknowledgments: Research group. Associazione Nazionale Medici Cardiologi Ospedalieri/Health Care Foundation (ANMCO/HCF): Diego Vanuzzo (Former Coordinator), Domenico Gabrielli, Michele Massimo Gulizia, Andrea Di Lenarda, Alessandro Boccanelli, Francesco Maria Bovenzi, Francesco Chiarella, Fulvio Colivicchi, Giuseppe Di Pasquale, Pompilio Faggiano, Aldo Pietro Maggioni, Gian Francesco Mureddu, Sergio Pede, Lorenza Pilotto, Salvatore Pirelli, Carmine Riccio, Marino Scherillo, Stefano Urbinati, Massimo Uguccioni, Paolo Verdecchia; Istituto Superiore di Sanità, Roma: Luigi Palmieri (Coordinator), Chiara Donfrancesco (Coordinator), Simona Giampaoli (Former Coordinator), Cinzia Lo Noce, Francesco Dima, Serena Vannucchi, Francesca Romana Meduri, Claudia Meduri; Fondazione IRCCS, Istituto nazionale dei tumori, Milano: Vittorio Krogh, Sara Grioni. Local coordinators of participating centers: Licia Iacoviello (Centro di ricerca e formazione ad alta tecnologia nelle scienze biomediche Giovanni Paolo II, Università Cattolica, Campobasso); Federico Vancheri (Ospedale S. Elia, Caltanissetta); Carlo Alberto Goldoni (Dipartimento di sanità pubblica, Azienda USL, Modena); Carmelo Antonio Caserta (Associazione calabrese di epatologia, Cittanova—Reggio Calabria); Antonio Lopizzo (Ospedale San Carlo, Potenza); Natalino Meloni (USL 4, Loceri—Nuoro); Marinella Gattone (Fondazione S. Maugeri, Veruno—Novara); Giuseppe Salamina (SC Centro controllo malattia, ASL TO1, Torino); Alessandro Boccanelli (Ospedale San Giovanni Addolorata, Roma); Roberto Amici (Ospedale Santa Maria della Pietà, Camerino -Macerata); Gianfranco Alunni (Ospedale SantaMaria dellaMisericordia, Azienda Ospedaliera, Perugia); Giuseppe Favretto (Ospedale rabilitativo di alta specializzazione, Motta di Livenza—Treviso); Mariapiera Vettori (Azienda ULSS 13 del Veneto, Noale—Venezia);Marino Scherillo (Azienda Ospedaliera G. Rummo, Benevento); Pompilio Faggiano (Azienda Ospedaliera Spedali Civili, Brescia); Maria Teresa La Rovere (Fondazione Salvatore Maugeri, Istituto di riabilitazione, Montescano—Pavia); Maria Luisa Biorci (ASL 3 Genovese- PO "La Colletta", Arenzano—Genova); Pasquale Caldarola (Cardiologia, Ospedale di Terlizzi, Centro servizi territoriali della città, Bitonto—Bari); Giovanni Menegoni (Azienda provincial per i servizi sanitari di Trento, Presidio ospedaliero, Borgo Valsugana—Trento); Rosa Maria Teresa Cristaudo (Azienda USL della Valle d'Aosta, Aosta); Andrea Zipoli (Azienda USL 11, Ospedale San Giuseppe, Empoli—Firenze); Paolo Michele Accettura (Laboratorio analisi, Ospedale San Camillo, Atessa—Chieti). Research Group MINISAL-GIRCSI: Pasquale Strazzullo, Ornella Russo, Lanfranco D'Elia, Roberto Iacone, Renato Ippolito, Chiara Donfrancesco, Diego Vanuzzo, Simona Giampaoli.

Research Group CARHES: Luca De Nicola, Chiara Donfrancesco, Roberto Minutolo, Cinzia Lo Noce, Luigi Palmieri, Amalia De Curtis, Licia Iacoviello, Carmine Zoccali, Loreto Gesualdo, Giuseppe Conte, Diego Vanuzzo, Simona Giampaoli. Italian Ministry of health: Giovanna Laurendi, Bianca Maria Polizzi, Daniela Galeone. European Health Examination Survey, Reference Centre: Hanna Tolonen, Kari Kuulasmaa, Paivikki Koponen, Johan Heldan, Susanna Conti, Georg Alfthan.

References

1. Piepoli, M.F.; Hoes, A.W.; Agewall, S.; Albus, C.; Brotons, C.; Catapano, A.L.; Cooney, M.T.; Corrà, U.; Cosyns, B.; Deaton, C.; et al. 2016 European Guidelines on Cardiovascular Disease Prevention in Clinical Practice: The Sixth Joint Task Force of the European Society of Cardiology and Other Societies on Cardiovascular Disease Prevention in Clinical Practice (Constituted by Representatives of 10 Societies and by Invited Experts) Developed with the Special Contribution of the European Association for Cardiovascular Prevention & Rehabilitation (EACPR). *Eur. Heart J.* **2016**, *37*, 2315–2381. [PubMed]
2. Sacks, F.M.; Svetkey, L.P.; Vollmer, W.M.; Appel, L.J.; Bray, G.A.; Harsha, D.; Obarzanek, E.; Conlin, P.R.; Miller, E.R., 3rd; Simons-Morton, D.G.; et al. Effects on Blood Pressure of Reduced Dietary Sodium and the Dietary Approaches to Stop Hypertension (DASH) Diet. DASH-Sodium Collaborative Research Group. *N. Engl. J. Med.* **2001**, *344*, 3–10. [CrossRef] [PubMed]
3. WHO. *Guideline: Sodium Intake for Adults and Children*; World Health Organization (WHO): Geneva, Switzerland, 2012; pp. 1–60.
4. Cha, D.; Park, Y. Association between Dietary Cholesterol and Their Food Sources and Risk for Hypercholesterolemia: The 2012–2016 Korea National Health and Nutrition Examination Survey. *Nutrients* **2019**, *11*, 846. [CrossRef] [PubMed]
5. Ooi, E.M.; Watts, G.F.; Ng, T.W.; Barrett, P.H. Effect of Dietary Fatty acids on Human Lipoprotein Metabolism: A Comprehensive Update. *Nutrients* **2015**, *7*, 4416–4425. [CrossRef]
6. Michas, G.; Micha, R.; Zampelas, A. Dietary Fats and Cardiovascular Disease: Putting together the Pieces of a Complicated Puzzle. *Atherosclerosis* **2014**, *234*, 320–328. [CrossRef]
7. Ojo, O.; Ojo, O.O.; Adebowale, F.; Wang, X.H. The Effect of Dietary Glycaemic Index on Glycaemia in Patients with Type 2 Diabetes: A Systematic Review and Meta-Analysis of Randomized Controlled Trials. *Nutrients* **2018**, *10*, 373. [CrossRef]
8. Mann, J.I.; De Leeuw, I.; Hermansen, K.; Karamanos, B.; Karlström, B.; Katsilambros, N.; Riccardi, G.; Rivellese, A.A.; Rizkalla, S.; Slama, G.; et al. on behalf of the Diabetes and Nutrition Study Group (DNSG) of the European Association for the Study of Diabetes (EASD). Evidence based Nutritional Approaches to the Treatment and Prevention of Diabetes Mellitus. *Nutr. Metab. Cardiovasc. Dis.* **2004**, *14*, 373–394. [CrossRef]
9. Weickert, M.O.; Pfeiffer, A.F.H. Impact of Dietary Fiber Consumption on Insulin Resistance and the Prevention of Type 2 Diabetes. *J. Nutr.* **2018**, *148*, 7–12. [CrossRef]
10. Giampaoli, S.; Palmieri, L.; Donfrancesco, C.; Lo Noce, C.; Pilotto, L.; Vanuzzo, D. Osservatorio Epidemiologico Cardiovascolare/Health Examination Survey Research Group Cardiovascular Health in Italy. Ten-Year Surveillance of Cardiovascular Diseases and Risk Factors: Osservatorio Epidemiologico Cardiovascolare/Health Examination Survey 1998–2012. *Eur. J. Prev. Cardiol.* **2015**, *22*, 9–37.
11. Kaaks, R.; Slimani, N.; Riboli, E. Pilot Phase Studies on the Accuracy of Dietary Intake Measurements in the Epic Project: Overall Evaluation of Results. European Prospective Investigation into Cancer and Nutrition. *Int. J. Epidemiol.* **1997**, *26*, S26–S36. [CrossRef]
12. Pisani, P.; Faggiano, F.; Krogh, V.; Palli, D.; Vineis, P.; Berrino, F. Relative Validity and Reproducibility of a Food Frequency Dietary Questionnaire for Use in the Italian EPIC Centres. *Int. J. Epidemiol.* **1997**, *26*, S152–S160. [CrossRef] [PubMed]
13. Pala, V.; Sieri, S.; Palli, D.; Salvini, S.; Berrino, F.; Bellegotti, M.; Frasca, G.; Tumino, R.; Sacerdote, C.; Fiorini, L.; et al. Diet in the Italian EPIC Cohorts: Presentation of Data and Methodological Issues. *Tumori* **2003**, *89*, 594–607. [CrossRef] [PubMed]
14. Salvini, S.; Parpinel, M.; Gnagnarella, P.; Maissoneuve, P.; Turrini, A. *Banca Dati Composizione Degli Alimenti per Studi Epidemiologici in Italia*; European Institute of Oncology: Milano, Italy, 1998.

15. Gruppo di Studio ADI-AMD-SID "Nutrizione e Diabete". La Terapia Medico-Nutrizionale nel Diabete Mellito. Le Raccomandazioni Nutrizionali 2013 e 2014. Available online: http://www.aemmedi.it/files/LineeguidaRaccomandazioni/2013/RACNUTRIZIONEDEF2013--2014 (accessed on 5 December 2019).
16. Donfrancesco, C.; Ippolito, R.; Lo Noce, C.; Palmieri, L.; Iacone, R.; Russo, O.; Vanuzzo, D.; Galletti, F.; Galeone, D.; Giampaoli, S.; et al. Excess Dietary Sodium and Inadequate Potassium Intake in Italy: Results of the MINISAL Study. *Nutr. Metab. Cardiovasc. Dis.* **2013**, *23*, 850–856. [CrossRef] [PubMed]
17. Galletti, F.; Agabiti-Rosei, E.; Bernini, G.; Boero, R.; Desideri, G.; Fallo, F.; Mallamaci, F.; Morganti, A.; Castellano, M.; Nazzaro, P.; et al. MINISAL-GIRCSI Program Study Group. Excess Dietary Sodium and Inadequate Potassium intake by Hypertensive Patients in Italy: Results of the MINISAL-SIIA Study Program. *J. Hypertens.* **2014**, *32*, 48–56. [CrossRef]
18. Moosavian, S.P.; Haghighatdoost, F.; Surkan, P.J.; Azadbakht, L. Salt and Obesity: A Systematic Review and Meta-Analysis of Observational Studies. *Int. J. Food Sci. Nutr.* **2017**, *68*, 265–277. [CrossRef]
19. Wongboonsin, J.; Thongprayoon, C.; Bathini, T.; Ungprasert, P.; Aeddula, N.R.; Mao, M.A.; Cheungpasitporn, W. Acetazolamide Therapy in Patients with Heart Failure: A Meta-Analysis. *J. Clin. Med.* **2019**, *8*, 349. [CrossRef]
20. Filippini, T.; Violi, F.; D'Amico, R.; Vinceti, M. The Effect of Potassium Supplementation on Blood Pressure in Hypertensive Subjects: A Systematic Review and Meta-Analysis. *Int. J. Cardiol.* **2017**, *230*, 127–135. [CrossRef]
21. Saneei, P.; Salehi-Abargouei, A.; Esmaillzadeh, A.; Azadbakht, L. Influence of Dietary Approaches to Stop Hypertension (DASH) Diet on Blood Pressure: A Systematic Review and Meta-Analysis on Randomized Controlled Trials. *Nutr. Metab. Cardiovasc. Dis.* **2014**, *24*, 1253–1261. [CrossRef]
22. Nettleton, J.A.; Brouwer, I.A.; Geleijnse, J.M.; Hornstra, G. Saturated Fat Consumption and Risk of Coronary Heart Disease and Ischemic Stroke: A Science Update. *Ann. Nutr. Metab.* **2017**, *70*, 26–33. [CrossRef]
23. Castetbon, K.; Bonaldi, C.; Deschamps, V.; Vernay, M.; Malon, A.; Salanave, B.; Druet, C. Diet in 45- to 74-Year-Old Individuals with Diagnosed Diabetes: Comparison to Counterparts without Diabetes in a Nationally Representative Survey (Etude Nationale Nutrition Santé 2006–2007). *J. Acad. Nutr. Diet* **2014**, *114*, 918–925. [CrossRef]
24. Muñoz-Pareja, M.; León-Muñoz, L.M.; Guallar-Castillón, P.; Graciani, A.; López-García, E.; Banegas, J.R.; Rodríguez-Artalejo, F. The Diet of Diabetic Patients in Spain in 2008–2010: Accordance with the Main Dietary Recommendations a Cross-Sectional Study. *PLoS ONE* **2012**, *7*, e39454. [CrossRef] [PubMed]
25. Vitale, M.; Masulli, M.; Rivellese, A.A.; Babini, A.C.; Boemi, M.; Bonora, E.; Buzzetti, R.; Ciano, O.; Cignarelli, M.; Cigolini, M.; et al. Influence of Dietary Fat and Carbohydrates Proportions on Plasma Lipids, Glucose Control and Low-Grade Inflammation in Patients with Type 2 Diabetes-The TOSCA.IT Study. *Eur. J. Nutr.* **2016**, *55*, 1645–1651. [CrossRef] [PubMed]
26. Fountoulakis, N.; Wijesuriya, M.; Gnudi, L.; Gulliford, M.; Karalliedde, J. Reducing the Incidence of Predictors of Cardio-Metabolic Disease and Dysglycaemia with Lifestyle Modification in at-Risk Persons -Results of Further Analyses of DIABRISK-SL in those below 18 Years of Age. *BMC Med.* **2019**, *17*, 162. [CrossRef] [PubMed]
27. Eriksson, M.K.; Franks, P.W.; Eliasson, M. A 3-Year Randomized Trial of Lifestyle Intervention for Cardiovascular Risk Reduction in the Primary Care Setting: The Swedish Björknäs Study. *PLoS ONE* **2009**, *4*, e5195. [CrossRef]
28. Knowler, W.C.; Barrett-Connor, E.; Fowler, S.E.; Hamman, R.F.; Lachin, J.M.; Walker, E.A.; Nathan, D.M. Diabetes Prevention Program Research Group. Reduction in the Incidence of Type 2 Diabetes with Lifestyle Intervention or Metformin. *N. Engl. J. Med.* **2002**, *346*, 393–403.
29. Tuomilehto, J.; Lindström, J.; Eriksson, J.G.; Valle, T.T.; Hämäläinen, H.; Ilanne-Parikka, P.; Keinänen-Kiukaanniemi, S.; Laakso, M.; Louheranta, A.; Rastas, M.; et al. Finnish Diabetes Prevention Study Group. Prevention of Type 2 Diabetes Mellitus by Changes in Lifestyle among Subjects with Impaired Glucose Tolerance. *N. Engl. J. Med.* **2001**, *344*, 1343–1350. [CrossRef]
30. Pekka, P.; Pirjo, P.; Ulla, U. Influencing Public Nutrition for Non-Communicable Disease Prevention: From Community Intervention to National Programme–Experiences from Finland. *Public Health Nutr.* **2002**, *5*, 245–251. [CrossRef] [PubMed]

3

Prospective Association between Whole Grain Consumption and Hypertension: The Furukawa Nutrition and Health Study

Ikuko Kashino [1,*], Masafumi Eguchi [2], Takako Miki [1], Takeshi Kochi [2], Akiko Nanri [1,3], Isamu Kabe [2] and Tetsuya Mizoue [1]

1 Department of Epidemiology and Prevention, Center for Clinical Sciences, National Center for Global Health and Medicine, Tokyo 162-8655, Japan; takakomiki-tky@umin.ac.jp (T.M.); nanri@fwu.ac.jp (A.N.); mizoue@hosp.ncgm.go.jp (T.M.)

2 Department of Health Administration, Furukawa Electric Corporation, Tokyo 100-8322, Japan; masafumi.eguchi@furukawaelectric.com (M.E.); takeshi.kochi@furukawaelectric.com (T.K.); isamu.kabe@kubota.com (I.K.)

3 Department of Food and Health Sciences, International College of Arts and Sciences, Fukuoka Women's University, Fukuoka 813-8529, Japan

* Correspondence: ikukokashino@gmail.com

Abstract: Hypertension has become a major public health issue worldwide. Whole grains contain higher levels and a broader range of nutrients with potential health benefits and may decrease the risk of hypertension. However, no prospective studies have investigated this association in the high-income Asia Pacific region, which has the lowest whole grain intake worldwide. Thus, we examined the prospective association between whole grain consumption and the development of hypertension in Japan. Participants included 944 working Japanese adults aged 19–68 years who had no hypertension at baseline and completed a 3-year follow-up survey. Whole grain consumption was assessed via a self-administered dietary questionnaire. Multivariate logistic regression analysis was carried out to examine the association between whole grain consumption and hypertension, adjusting for potential confounding factors, such as sociodemographic, lifestyle, dietary, and occupational characteristics. After 3 years, 9.4% (86 cases) of the study participants had developed hypertension. More frequent whole grain consumption, classified as an intake frequency of "sometimes or always", was associated with lower odds of hypertension (multivariate-adjusted odds ratio: 0.36; 95% confidence interval: 0.16–0.83; p for trend = 0.04) compared with no consumption. Consuming more whole grains may decrease the risk of developing hypertension.

Keywords: blood pressure; hypertension; whole grain; Asians; Japan; cohort study; epidemiology

1. Introduction

With the increasing number of hypertensive individuals, hypertension has become a major public health issue around the world and results in death and disability via many different causes [1]. In Japan, deaths associated with blood pressure regardless of age or sex increased rapidly between 1990 and 2015 compared with those in western or other high-income Asia-Pacific countries [1]. Although modifiable risk factors associated with hypertension are well known, including unhealthy diets (e.g., excessive salt consumption, high levels of saturated and trans fats, and low intake of fruits and vegetables), physical inactivity, alcohol and tobacco use, and being overweight or obese [2], additional approaches for preventing hypertension should also be explored.

Whole grains, including brown rice, contain more abundant and diverse nutrients with potential health benefits (e.g., fiber, vitamins, and minerals) compared with refined grains, such as white rice. A meta-analysis of four cohort studies conducted in the U.S. showed that whole grain intake was inversely associated with the risk of hypertension [3]. In 2015, the US Dietary Guideline Advisory Committee recommended replacing most refined grains with whole grains in an effort to improve dietary quality among Americans [4]. However, there have been no prospective studies conducted in high-income Asia-Pacific countries including Japan, which has the lowest whole grain intake in the world [5]. Additional evidence from Asia is thus crucial for enhancing the generalizability of the association between hypertension and whole grain intake.

To this end, we prospectively examined the association between dietary habit of whole grain intake and hypertension risk in the Japanese population.

2. Materials and Methods

2.1. Study Procedure

In the Furukawa Nutrition and Health Study, which is part of the Japan Epidemiology Collaboration on Occupational Health Study, factory workers were recruited from two work sites of the same company in Chiba and Kanagawa Prefectures to participate in a survey that was carried out as part of a routine health exam. The survey was conducted both at baseline and 3 years later (April 2012 and 2015 at the work site in Chiba; and May 2013 and 2016 in Kanagawa), as previously described [6]. Prior to these health exams, all employees (n = 2828) were invited to participate and asked to fill out study-specific questionnaires related to diet and general health-related lifestyle. On the day of the health checkup, research staff checked that the questionnaires had been completed and participants were asked to clarify answers if needed. Additional information obtained during the health exams, such as anthropometric and biochemical measurements and dietary history (e.g., alcohol habits), was also evaluated. Informed consent was obtained from the participants, and the study protocol was approved by the Ethics Committee of the National Center for Global Health and Medicine, Japan.

2.2. Participants

Of 2828 workers partaking in the health checkups, 2162 (76%) agreed to participate in the baseline survey, of whom 2151 further completed the baseline questionnaire, including diet and covariate information such as lifestyle characteristics and disease history. Among these participants, we excluded 573 with hypertension and 50 with a history of one or more of the following conditions at baseline: cancer in 11, cardiovascular disease in 8, chronic hepatitis in 2, kidney disease including nephritis in 2 and pancreatitis in 1, and diabetes in 29. We further excluded 32 participants with missing data on covariates and 13 with extreme total energy intake at baseline (i.e., greater than the mean ± 3 standard deviations). Of the remaining 1483 participants, 952 responded to the 3-year follow up survey (response rate: 64.2%). An additional 8 participants with missing blood pressure data at follow-up were excluded from the analysis. In total, 944 participants (834 men and 110 women aged 19–68 years) were analyzed as part of this study (Figure 1).

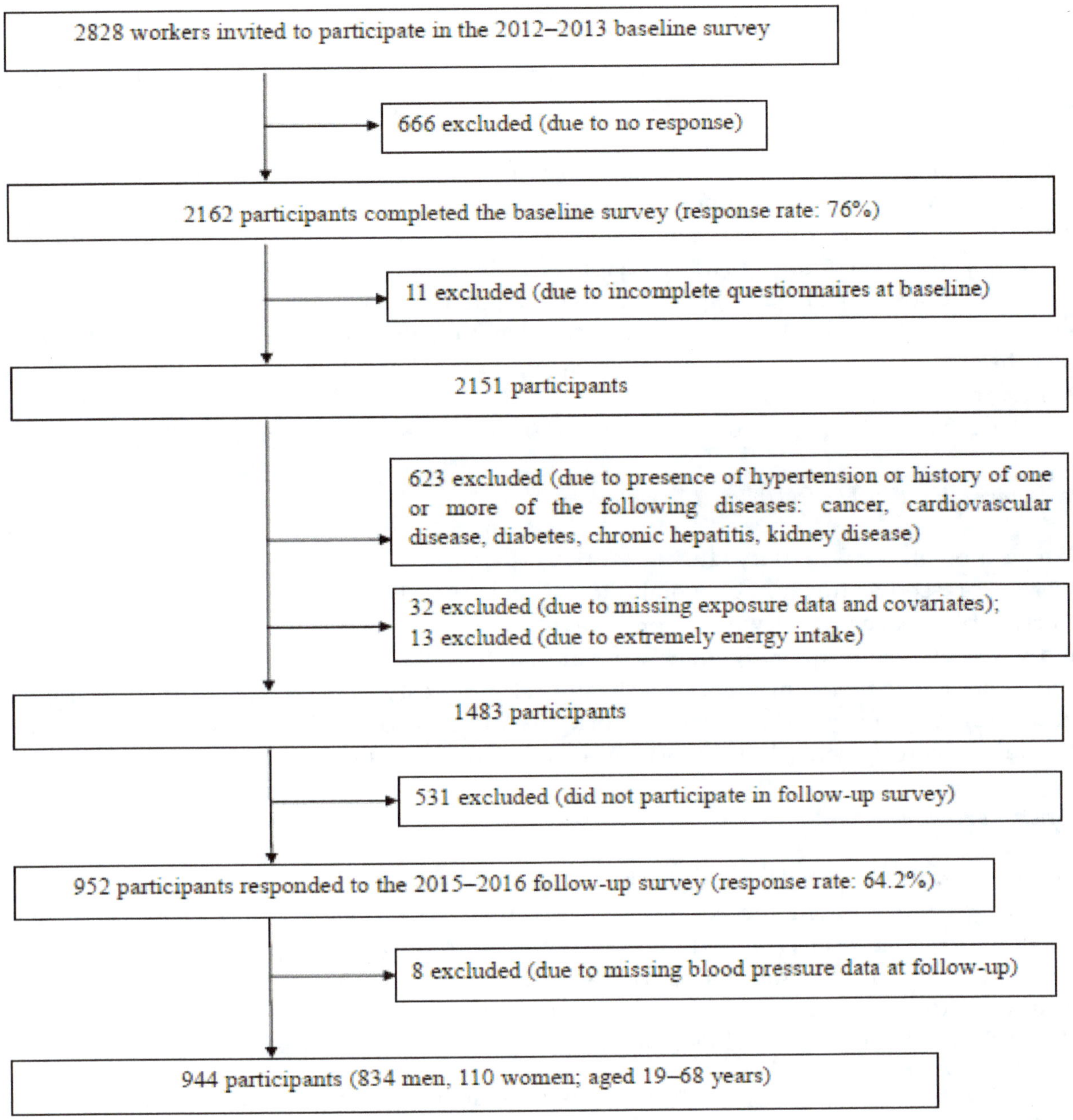

Figure 1. Flowchart of the study population.

2.3. *Definition of Hypertension*

Systolic/diastolic blood pressure was measured using an automated sphygmomanometer (BP 103i II for the 2012 and 2015 survey and HEM-907 for the 2013 and 2016 survey, Omron Health Care Co. Ltd., Kyoto, Japan). Participants underwent a 3-minute rest prior to blood pressure measurement at their work site in Chiba, whereas no such precondition was specified in Kanagawa. Hypertension was defined as systolic blood pressure ≥140 mm Hg and/or diastolic blood pressure ≥ 90 mm Hg or as use of an antihypertensive agent.

2.4. *Assessment of Dietary Intakes*

Dietary intake during the month prior to the health exam was evaluated using the Brief Self-administered Diet History Questionnaire; validation of the questionnaire was previously demonstrated [7,8]. The frequency of whole grain intake was assessed by the question "Do you eat brown rice, germinated rice, or a wheat/millet mix with rice?" Participants selected one of the following four answers: never, rarely, sometimes, or always. Intakes of foods and nutrients, such as rice, bread, noodles, vegetables, fruits, pulses, meats, dairy, soft drinks, sodium, and total energy, were estimated using an *ad hoc* computer algorithm adopted for the Brief Self-administered Diet History Questionnaire and the food composition table for Japan [9]. According to the validation study, Spearman's correlation coefficients for energy-adjusted rice, bread, noodles, vegetables, fruits, pulses, meats, dairy, soft drinks, sodium, and total energy between dietary records and the Brief Self-administered Diet History Questionnaire were 0.66, 0.71, 0.49, 0.62, 0.61, 0.45, 0.67, 0.70, 0.39, 0.61, and 0.45 for women and 0.71, 0.65, 0.47, 0.62, 0.70, 0.55, 0.56, 0.70, 0.49, 0.60, and 0.40 for men, respectively [7,8].

2.5. *Assessment of Other Health-Related Variables*

Exertion of physical activity during work and housework or during commuting and leisure time were expressed as the sum of metabolic equivalent (MET) multiplied by duration of time (in hours) across physical activities with different levels. Body mass index (kg/m^2) was calculated as body weight divided by height squared, which were measured to the nearest 0.1 kg and 0.1 cm, respectively, by trained staff. Participants' answers to the health-related lifestyle questionnaire provided information on night or rotating shift work, overtime work, use of tobacco, alcohol consumption, and physical activity exertion during work, housework, and commuting and leisure time.

2.6. *Statistical Analysis*

To determine the potential bias due to the participants' selection process in this study, we compared baseline characteristics among those who completed the 3-year follow-up survey and those who were lost to follow-up. Participants were divided into three groups according to their whole grain intake frequency: never, rarely, and sometimes, or always. The participants' characteristics were evaluated according to frequency of whole grain intake, using linear regression analysis for the continuous variables and the Mantel–Haenszel test for trend for the categorical variables.

We performed multiple logistic regression analysis to determine the association of intake of whole grains with the likelihood of developing hypertension, estimated as odds ratios (ORs) with 95% confidence intervals (CIs). We used two different models for the analysis and adjusted for potential confounding variables according to the literature [3] and our previous study [10]. Model 1 was adjusted for age, sex, and work site (Chiba vs. Kanagawa). Model 2 was further adjusted for smoking (never smoked, former smoker, current smoker of <20 cigarettes/day, or current smoker of ≥20 cigarettes/day), alcohol consumption (nondrinker, drinker consuming 1–3 days/month, weekly drinker consuming <1, 1 to <2, or ≥2 servings/day; one serving contains 23 g of ethanol), physical activity at work and housework or in commuting to work (<3, 3 to <7, 7 to <20, or ≥20 MET-hours/day), leisure-time physical activity (0, >0 to <3, 3 to <10, or ≥10 MET-hours/week), body mass index (kg/m^2), night or rotating shift work (yes/no), overtime work (<10, 10 to <30, or ≥30 hours/month), total energy intake (kcal/day), and food and nutrient intakes (vegetables, fruits, pulses, meats, dairy, soft drinks, rice, bread, noodles, and sodium) expressed as energy densities. To determine linear trends, the three categories were assigned ordinal values (0–2) and treated as a continuous variable. Furthermore, to examine the association between frequency of repeated whole grain intake over time and development of hypertension, we defined the participants with a consistent whole grain intake frequency of "never" or "sometimes or always" between baseline and the 3-year follow-up as having maintained a low or high intake frequency, respectively. All statistical analyses were performed using the SAS statistical software package, version 9.4 for Windows (SAS Institute Inc., Cary, NC, USA). A two-sided p value < 0.05 was representative of statistical significance in all analyses.

3. Results

Participant characteristics according to frequency of whole grain intake are shown in Table 1. Approximately 20% of participants consumed whole grains either sometimes or always, while 56% of participants did not consume whole grains. Participants with frequent whole grain intake tended to consume more energy, fats, proteins, vegetables, fruits, pulses, and dairy but less carbohydrates, soft drinks, and rice compared with those with less frequent intake (p for trend <0.05 for all). In addition, participants with more frequent whole grain intake were less likely to be current smokers, physically active during work, or night or rotating shift workers but were more likely to be active during leisure time compared with those with less frequent whole grain intake. Compared with those who participated in the follow-up survey, those who did not participate in the follow-up survey were older and more likely to have overtime work and tended to consume lower amounts of pulses, while other characteristics (e.g., whole grain consumption) were similar between both groups (Supplementary Materials Table S1).

At the 3-year follow-up, 89 participants (9.4%) who were not hypertensive at baseline had developed hypertension. Based on the multiple logistic regression model 1, after adjusting for age, sex, and work site, participants that reported consuming whole grains either sometimes or always exhibited lower odds of developing hypertension compared with those who did not consume whole grains (Table 2). In model 2, after additional adjustments for lifestyle, work-related, and dietary factors, the adjusted ORs for developing hypertension were 1.00 (reference), 1.02 (95% CI: 0.57–1.83), and 0.36 (95% CI: 0.16–0.83) for the whole grain intake categories of "never", "rarely", and "sometimes or always", respectively (p for trend = 0.04). A similar but somewhat stronger association was observed in an additional analysis using both baseline and follow-up dietary data (n = 513); the multivariable-adjusted OR of hypertension for those who maintained high consumption was 0.20 (0.05–0.73) compared with participants that maintained low whole grain consumption throughout the entire 3-year study period (Supplementary Materials Table S2).

Table 1. Baseline characteristics of the study population according to frequency of whole grain intake.

	Frequency of Whole Grain Intake			
	Never	Rarely	Sometimes or Always	p_{trend} [1)]
No. of participants	530	221	193	
Age, years (mean ± SD)	39.7 ± 8.7	39.4 ± 8.8	40.9 ± 8.0	0.18
Females, %	10.6	11.3	15.0	0.12
Work site (survey in April 2012), %	56.0	52.9	44.6	0.01
Smoking status (current), %	34.9	28.1	21.8	<0.001
Physical activity during work, housework, or commuting to work (≥20 METs-hours/day), %	28.3	19.5	12.4	<0.001
Leisure-time physical activity (≥10 METs-hours/week), %	24.9	30.3	34.2	0.01
Body mass index (mean ± SD), kg/m^2	22.4 ± 2.8	23.0 ± 3.2	22.4 ± 2.6	0.02
Night or rotating shift work (yes), %	26.8	13.6	8.8	<0.001
Overtime work (≥30 hours/month), %	24.5	26.2	26.9	0.47
Alcohol consumption (current), % [2)]	52.5	47.1	53.9	0.97
Dietary nutrient and food intake (mean ± SD)				
Total energy, kcal/day	1753 ± 484	1854 ± 482	1781 ± 444	0.02
Carbohydrate, % energy	55.3 ± 8.1	55.3 ± 7.4	53.6 ± 7.8	0.03
Fat, % energy	23.7 ± 5.7	24.1 ± 4.8	25.1 ± 5.6	0.01
Protein, % energy	13.4 ± 2.6	13.9 ± 2.3	14.2 ± 2.2	<0.001
Sodium, mg/1000 kcal	2300 ± 473	2322 ± 436	2282 ± 401	0.66
Vegetables, g/1000 kcal	108.5 ± 59.9	129.4 ± 69.4	138.4 ± 71.7	<0.001
Fruits, g/1000 kcal	36.4 ± 44.1	48.4 ± 48.7	51.5 ± 52.2	<0.001
Pulses, g/1000 kcal	24.2 ± 20.1	25.4 ± 17.5	29.7 ± 19.9	0.004
Meats, g/1000 kcal	39.9 ± 18.2	39.4 ± 18.5	38.8 ± 16.2	0.76
Dairy, g/1000 kcal	47.9 ± 51.8	48.1 ± 43.5	62.7 ± 53.0	0.002
Soft drinks, g/1000 kcal	52.1 ± 80.0	41.6 ± 51.0	32.2 ± 51.5	0.003
Rice, g/1000 kcal	186.3 ± 67.0	188.5 ± 60.3	172.8 ± 68.0	0.03
Bread, g/1000 kcal	22.5 ± 18.9	20.1 ± 15.0	22.0 ± 17.9	0.25
Noodles, g/1000 kcal	44.4 ± 31.5	43.6 ± 27.4	41.4 ± 26.8	0.49

Abbreviations: MET, metabolic equivalent. [1)] Based on the Mantel–Haenszel test for categorical variables and linear regression analysis for continuous variables. [2)] Alcohol consumption at least one day per week.

Table 2. Prospective associations between whole grain intake and hypertension.

	Frequency of Whole Grain Intake						
	Never		Rarely		Sometimes or Always		p_{trend} [1)]
Participants (n)	530		221		193		
Cases (n)	57		24		8		
Adjusted odds ratios (95% CI)							
Model 1[2)]	1.00	(Reference)	1.04	(0.62–1.75)	0.35	(0.16–0.77)	0.02
Model 2[3)]	1.00	(Reference)	1.02	(0.57–1.83)	0.36	(0.16–0.83)	0.04

Abbreviations: CI, confidence interval. [1)] Linear trends across the whole grain intake categories were determined using each category as an ordinal variable. [2)] Model 1 adjusted for age (year, continuous), sex, and site (survey in April 2012 or in May 2013). [3)] Model 2 additionally adjusted for smoking (never smoked, former smoke, current smoker consuming <20 cigarettes/day, or current smoker consuming ≥20 cigarettes/day), alcohol consumption (nondrinker, drinker consuming 1–3 days/month, weekly drinker consuming <1, 1 to <2, or ≥2 serving/day; one serving contains 23 g of ethanol), physical activity at work and housework or in commuting to work (<3, 3 to <7, 7 to <20, or ≥20 MET-hour/day), leisure-time physical activity (not engaged, >0 to <3, 3 to <10, or ≥10 MET-hours/week), body mass index (kg/m^2), night or rotating shift work (yes/no), overtime work (<10, 10 to <30, or ≥30 hours/month), total energy intake (kcal/day), and nutrient and food intake expressed as energy density (sodium, vegetables, fruits, pulses, meat, dairy, soft drinks, rice, bread, and noodles).

4. Discussion

This is the first prospective study to address the association between whole grain consumption and hypertension in an Asian population. The results of this study demonstrated about 60% reduced likelihood of developing hypertension among those with a frequent ("sometimes or always") consumption of whole grains compared with no consumption, even after adjusting for numerous potential confounders. These findings are supported by a recent meta-analysis of four cohort studies conducted in the U.S. [3]. In Iran, a cross-sectional study of 827 participants aged 18–74 years showed a 21% lower prevalence of hypertension among adults in the highest quartile compared with the lowest quartile of whole grain intake [11]. In Japan, a randomized controlled study reported that daily supplementation with rice bran, a component of brown rice and by-product of rice polishing, reduced systolic blood pressure in patients with mild hypertension and high-normal blood pressure [12]. The findings from this prospective observational study provide evidence to support the hypothesis that whole grain consumption lowers the risk for hypertension in Asian populations.

The mechanism underlying the beneficial effect of whole grain intake on the risk of hypertension remains unclear; however, data from several mechanistic and experimental studies have been reported. First, in an animal experiment, the potent antihypertensive peptide Leu-Arg-Ala from rice bran protein was shown to exhibit its effects on hypertension via endothelial nitric oxide-mediated vasorelaxation [13]. Second, dietary supplementation with either a Driselase or ethanol fraction of rice bran significantly decreased blood pressure in stroke-prone spontaneously hypertensive rats [14]. Third, a rat experiment suggested that the antihypertensive effect of virgin rice bran oil, which is extracted from the germ and inner husk of rice by the cold-press method, may be mediated by restored hemodynamics, increased nitric oxide bioavailability, and alleviated oxidative stress and inflammation [15]. Finally, injection of gamma-aminobutyric acid, which is commonly produced by germinated brown rice, enhanced the arterial baroreceptor reflex function and adjusted heart rate to reduce blood pressure fluctuations in spontaneously hypertensive rats [16]. Finally, high consumption of fiber rich in whole grain may prevent hypertension through change of gut microbiota [17].

The current study has several strengths including its prospective study design, relatively homogenous study population, and adjustments for a wide range of known and suspected risk factors for hypertension, including work-related factors and nutrients that exhibit a known link to hypertension. There were also some limitations associated with the present study. First, 35.8% of participants did not complete the 3-year follow-up survey; this may have introduced selection bias. However, baseline characteristics were generally similar between participants who completed follow-up and those lost to follow-up. Second, frequency of whole grain intake was ascertained using a single question with simple response options, which did not allow us to estimate the amount of whole grain intake. Third, the dietary measurements taken at baseline might not reflect long-term habitual consumption. Nevertheless, our secondary analysis, which considered both baseline and follow-up dietary data together, also indicated a similar strength of association compared to the primary analysis. Finally, because this study included only workers, the majority of which were men, the generalizability of the findings to the general population in Japan is unclear.

5. Conclusions

Results of this prospective study demonstrate an association between frequent whole grain intake and lower risk of developing hypertension among working individuals in Japan, strengthening the hypothesis that greater consumption of whole grains decreases the risk of hypertension.

Author Contributions: I.K. (Ikuko Kashino) performed the data analyses; I.K. (Ikuko Kashino), M.E., T.K., T.M. (Takako Miki), A.N., I.K. (Isamu Kabe), and T.M. (Tetsuya Mizoue) performed the data acquisition; I.K. (Ikuko

Kashino) drafted the manuscript; and I.K. (Ikuko Kashino) and T.M. (Tetsuya Mizoue) took primary responsibility for the final content. All authors were involved in the interpretation of the results and revision of the manuscript. All authors have read and agreed to the published version of the manuscript.

Acknowledgments: We thank Hiroko Tsuruoka, Rie Ito, and Akiko Makabe (Furukawa Electric Corporation), and Yuriko Yagi (National Center for Global Health and Medicine) for their help in data collection.

References

1. Forouzanfar, M.H.; Liu, P.; Roth, G.A.; Ng, M.; Biryukov, S.; Marczak, L.; Alexander, L.; Estep, K.; Hassen Abate, K.; Akinyemiju, T.F.; et al. Global burden of hypertension and systolic blood pressure of at least 110 to 115 mm Hg, 1990–2015. *JAMA* **2017**, *317*, 165–182. [CrossRef] [PubMed]
2. World Health Organization. Hypertension. Available online: https://www.who.int/news-room/fact-sheets/detail/hypertension (accessed on 1 February 2020).
3. Schwingshackl, L.; Schwedhelm, C.; Hoffmann, G.; Knuppel, S.; Iqbal, K.; Andriolo, V.; Bechthold, A.; Schlesinger, S.; Boeing, H. Food groups and risk of hypertension: A systematic review and dose-response meta-analysis of prospective studies. *Adv. Nutr.* **2017**, *8*, 793–803. [CrossRef] [PubMed]
4. Millen, B.E.; Abrams, S.; Adams-Campbell, L.; Anderson, C.A.; Brenna, J.T.; Campbell, W.W.; Clinton, S.; Hu, F.; Nelson, M.; Neuhouser, M.L. The 2015 Dietary Guidelines Advisory Committee scientific report: Development and major conclusions. *Adv. Nutr.* **2016**, *7*, 438–444. [CrossRef] [PubMed]
5. Micha, R.; Khatibzadeh, S.; Shi, P.; Andrews, K.G.; Engell, R.E.; Mozaffarian, D. Global, regional and national consumption of major food groups in 1990 and 2010: A systematic analysis including 266 country-specific nutrition surveys worldwide. *BMJ Open* **2015**, *5*, e008705. [CrossRef] [PubMed]
6. Miki, T.; Eguchi, M.; Kuwahara, K.; Kochi, T.; Akter, S.; Kashino, I.; Hu, H.; Kurotani, K.; Kabe, I.; Kawakami, N.; et al. Breakfast consumption and the risk of depressive symptoms: The Furukawa Nutrition and Health Study. *Psychiatry Res.* **2019**, *273*, 551–558. [CrossRef] [PubMed]
7. Kobayashi, S.; Murakami, K.; Sasaki, S.; Okubo, H.; Hirota, N.; Notsu, A.; Fukui, M.; Date, C. Comparison of relative validity of food group intakes estimated by comprehensive and brief-type self-administered diet history questionnaires against 16 d dietary records in Japanese adults. *Public Health Nutr.* **2011**, *14*, 1200–1211. [CrossRef] [PubMed]
8. Kobayashi, S.; Honda, S.; Murakami, K.; Sasaki, S.; Okubo, H.; Hirota, N.; Notsu, A.; Fukui, M.; Date, C. Both comprehensive and brief self-administered diet history questionnaires satisfactorily rank nutrient intakes in Japanese adults. *J. Epidemiol.* **2012**, *22*, 151–159. [CrossRef] [PubMed]
9. Science and Technology Agency. *Standard Tables of Food Composition in Japan*, 5th Revised and Enlarged ed.; Printing Bureau of the Ministry of Finance: Tokyo, Japan, 2005. (In Japanese)
10. Akter, S.; Eguchi, M.; Kurotani, K.; Kochi, T.; Pham, N.M.; Ito, R.; Kuwahara, K.; Tsuruoka, H.; Mizoue, T.; Kabe, I.; et al. High dietary acid load is associated with increased prevalence of hypertension: The Furukawa Nutrition and Health Study. *Nutrition* **2015**, *31*, 298–303. [CrossRef] [PubMed]
11. Esmaillzadeh, A.; Mirmiran, P.; Azizi, F. Whole-grain consumption and the metabolic syndrome: A favorable association in Tehranian adults. *Eur. J. Clin. Nutr.* **2005**, *59*, 353–362. [CrossRef] [PubMed]
12. Ogawa, Y.; Shobako, N.; Fukuhara, I.; Satoh, H.; Kobayashi, E.; Kusakari, T.; Suwa, M.; Matsumoto, M.; Ishikado, A. Rice bran supplement containing a functional substance, the novel peptide Leu-Arg-Ala, has anti-hypertensive effects: A double-blind, randomized, placebo-controlled study. *Nutrients* **2019**, *11*, 726. [CrossRef] [PubMed]
13. Shobako, N.; Ishikado, A.; Ogawa, Y.; Sono, Y.; Kusakari, T.; Suwa, M.; Matsumoto, M.; Ohinata, K. Vasorelaxant and antihypertensive effects that are dependent on the endothelial NO system exhibited by rice bran-derived tripeptide. *J. Agric. Food Chem.* **2019**, *67*, 1437–1442. [CrossRef] [PubMed]
14. Ardiansyah; Shirakawa, H.; Koseki, T.; Ohinata, K.; Hashizume, K.; Komai, M. Rice bran fractions improve blood pressure, lipid profile, and glucose metabolism in stroke-prone spontaneously hypertensive rats. *J. Agric. Food Chem.* **2006**, *54*, 1914–1920. [CrossRef] [PubMed]
15. Jan-On, G.; Sangartit, W.; Pakdeechote, P.; Kukongviriyapan, V.; Sattayasai, J.; Senaphan, K.; Kukongviriyapan, U. Virgin rice bran oil alleviates hypertension through the upregulation of eNOS

and reduction of oxidative stress and inflammation in L-NAME-induced hypertensive rats. *Nutrition* **2020**, *69*, 110575. [CrossRef] [PubMed]

16. Ma, P.; Li, T.; Ji, F.; Wang, H.; Pang, J. Effect of GABA on blood pressure and blood dynamics of anesthetic rats. *Int. J. Clin. Exp. Med.* **2015**, *8*, 14296–14302. [PubMed]
17. Marques, F.Z.; Nelson, E.; Chu, P.Y.; Horlock, D.; Fiedler, A.; Ziemann, M.; Tan, J.K.; Kuruppu, S.; Rajapakse, N.W.; El-Osta, A.; et al. High-Fiber Diet and Acetate Supplementation Change the Gut Microbiota and Prevent the Development of Hypertension and Heart Failure in Hypertensive Mice. *Circulation* **2017**, *135*, 964–977. [CrossRef]

4

A Single Dose of Beetroot Juice does not Change Blood Pressure Response Mediated by Acute Aerobic Exercise in Hypertensive Postmenopausal Women

Ana Luiza Amaral [1], Igor M. Mariano [1], Victor Hugo V. Carrijo [1], Tállita Cristina F. de Souza [1], Jaqueline P. Batista [1], Anne M. Mendonça [1,2,3,4], Adriele V. de Souza [5], Douglas C. Caixeta [5], Renata R. Teixeira [5], Foued S. Espindola [5], Erick P. de Oliveira [2] and Guilherme M. Puga [1,*]

1. Laboratory of Cardiorespiratory and Metabolic Physiology, Federal University of Uberlândia, Uberlândia, MG 38400-678, Brazil; anaribeiro.am@gmail.com (A.L.A.); igormmariano@gmail.com (I.M.M.); vilarinhovictorh@gmail.com (V.H.V.C.); tallita_crystina@hotmail.com (T.C.F.d.S.); jaquebpontes@gmail.com (J.P.B.); annemarques.m@hotmail.com (A.M.M.)
2. School of Medicine, Federal University of Uberlândia, Uberlândia, MG 38400-902, Brazil; erick_po@yahoo.com.br
3. Department of Food and Human Nutritional Sciences, University of Manitoba, Winnipeg, MB R3T 2N2, Canada
4. Canadian Centre for Agri-Food Research in Health and Medicine, St. Boniface Hospital Research Centre, Winnipeg, MB R2H 2A6, Canada
5. Laboratory of Biochemistry and Molecular Biology, Institute of Biotechnology, Federal University of Uberlândia, Uberlândia, MG 38400-902, Brazil; adriele_vds@hotmail.com (A.V.d.S.); caixetadoug@gmail.com (D.C.C.); rolandteixeira@yahoo.com (R.R.T.); fsespindola@gmail.com (F.S.E.)

* Correspondence: gmpuga@gmail.com

Abstract: Objective: To verify if acute intake of beetroot juice potentiates post-exercise hypotension (PEH) in hypertensive postmenopausal women. Methods: Thirteen hypertensive postmenopausal women (58.1 ± 4.62 years and 27.4 ± 4.25 kg/m^2) were recruited to participate in three experimental sessions, taking three different beverages: Beetroot juice (BJ), placebo nitrate-depleted BJ (PLA), and orange flavored non-caloric drink (OFD). The participants performed moderate aerobic exercise training on a treadmill, at 65–70% of heart rate reserve (HRR), for 40 min. After an overnight fast, the protocol started at 07h when the first resting blood pressure (BP) was measured. The beverage was ingested at 07h30 and BP was monitored until the exercise training started, at 09h30. After the end of the exercise session, BP was measured every 15 min over a 90-min period. Saliva samples were collected at rest, immediately before and after exercise, and 90 min after exercise for nitrite (NO_2^-) analysis. Results: There was an increase in salivary NO_2^- with BJ intake when compared to OFD and PLA. A slight increase in salivary NO_2^- was observed with PLA when compared to OFD ($p < 0.05$), however, PLA resulted in lower salivary NO_2^- when compared to BJ ($p < 0.001$). There were no changes in salivary NO_2^- with the OFD. Systolic and diastolic BP decreased ($p < 0.001$) on all post exercise time points after all interventions, with no difference between the three beverages. Conclusion: Acute BJ intake does not change PEH responses in hypertensive postmenopausal women, even though there is an increase in salivary NO_2^-.

Keywords: nitrite; nitric oxide; hypertension; menopause; Post Exercise Hypotension

---

1. Introduction

There are several physiological changes in women's body during climacteric period, including reduction of estrogen levels and menstruation cessation (menopause). As estrogen is a cardioprotective hormone [1], subsequent to its reduction, there is an increased risk of developing cardiometabolic diseases, due to reduced vasodilatation, increased blood pressure (BP), oxidative stress, and inflammation [2].

Hypertension is one of the most prevalent cardiometabolic diseases after menopause [3], and pharmacological therapy is the most common treatment approach. However, changes in lifestyle, such as developing healthy dietary habits and performing exercise regularly, are important factors for hypertension prevention and control [3]. The practice of regular physical exercise can reduce resting BP chronically, and induce post-exercise hypotension (PEH), which is a reduction in BP below resting values after exercise training. This phenomenon is clinically relevant in the prevention and treatment of cardiovascular diseases, and in the reduction of cardiovascular events [4]. This cardiovascular regulatory response has been related to endothelium-derived nitric oxide (NO) [4,5]. Exercise-induced shear stress promotes the release of calcium by endothelial cells, from which the calcium binds to calmodulin and stimulates endothelial nitric oxide synthase (eNOS) to reduce L-arginine to NO, where NO is directly involved in vascular tone regulation and homeostasis [5].

During exercise, NO release induces vasodilation, increasing blood flow to skeletal muscles and regulating blood pressure [5]. In addition, consumption of foods containing inorganic nitrate (NO_3^-) can increase NO bioavailability. This increase occurs by the initial conversion of NO_3^- into nitrite (NO_2^-) in the mouth and stomach, through non-enzymatic reactions. The NO_2^- is then released into the systemic circulation for subsequent NO production [6], leading to improvements in hemodynamic regulation. Therefore, consumption of foods rich in NO_3^- may be a good strategy to improve BP regulation in target populations with an increased incidence of cardiometabolic diseases, especially when associated with exercise [7–12], since these two pathways of NO production can complement each other [6].

A common food that has a high NO_3^- concentration is beetroot, and some effects observed with beetroot juice (BJ) consumption are related to improvement in blood flow, vasodilation, and reduction of BP [13–15]. The majority of studies that investigated BJ ingestion are related to sports and exercise performance [16–19], and only a few studies explored BJ consumption in parameters of health, in non-athletic populations, such as evaluating hemodynamic parameters in patients with chronic cardiorespiratory diseases [16,20]. These results are still inconclusive, since one did not find PEH with BJ consumption [20], and the other found PEH only in diastolic BP (DBP) [16]. Moreover, there is a lack of studies evaluating BJ benefits for hypertensive post-menopausal women. This population is of interest because there is a reduction in NO production, both due to hypertension and decreased estrogen levels.

Therefore, the purpose of this study was to verify if BJ ingestion has additional effects on PEH after one aerobic exercise session, and its relationship with salivary NO_2^- in hypertensive postmenopausal women. Our hypothesis was that BJ would improve blood pressure response after exercise in hypertensive postmenopausal women, due to an increase in the NO pathway, measured by salivary NO_2^- levels.

2. Materials and Methods

2.1. Participants

The study intervention was conducted between June and September 2018, at the Laboratory of Cardiorespiratory and Metabolic Physiology of the Federal University of Uberlândia, Uberlândia, MG, Brazil. This study design was approved by the local Ethics Committee (70104717.0.0000.5152) and registered at Clinicaltrials.gov (NCT03620227). All participants agreed and signed an informed consent form prior to admission.

For the inclusion criteria, participants were required to be: in post menopause (amenorrhea for at least 12 months and [FSH] > 40 mIU/mL); diagnosed with hypertension, according to the 7th Brazilian Arterial Hypertension Directive [3], which is defined by baseline blood pressure values greater than or equal to 140 mmHg for systolic BP (SBP) and 90 mmHg for DBP; aged between 50 and 70 years, and able to perform exercises on a treadmill. The exclusion criteria consisted of: use of hormonal therapy; history of food allergies that could compromise the study; sensitivity to NO_3^-; history of stroke or acute myocardial infarction; diagnosis of Diabetes Mellitus; and smoking habits. Although all the volunteers used antihypertensive drugs, they were excluded if they were taking drugs of the β-blocker class. All participants went through a cardiological evaluation with a specialist before the intervention, obtaining a certificate to attest individual suitability for exercise practice. Exclusion criteria also applied to volunteers who failed to perform the protocol test, with some of the reasons, including intolerance to the exercise program, inability to ingest the juice, or inability to go through the fasting time.

The number of volunteers required for this trial was calculated considering BP variation caused by BJ relative to placebo (PLA) as the main variable, with a variation of 5 ± 4 mmHg defined as an acceptable effect [13]. Using online software (OpenEpi), considering a bilateral 95% confidence interval, and power analysis of 80%, a minimum of 11 people were needed for this study. After the calculation, 15 volunteers were recruited to participate in this study. Two out of the 15 volunteers were excluded from the study for inability to adapt to the study protocol, due to an abrupt decrease in blood pressure followed by initial syncope as of 15 min after the beginning of the first exercise session. One of the volunteers had consumed BJ and the other PLA.

The study volunteers answered both an anamnesis and a physical activity questionnaire (IPAQ short version). Anthropometric measures included: body mass (Filizola electronic scale); height (fixed stadiometer Sanny); abdominal circumference (Filizola inelastic tape); and body composition (bioimpedance Inbody 230, Seoul, Coreia do Sul), assessed as previously described [21]. For the body composition measurement, all participants were instructed not to perform vigorous physical exercise 24 h before the test and to avoid alcohol and caffeine consumption 72 h before the test.

2.2. Study Design

The present study was a double blind randomized, placebo-controlled, and crossover trial. The intervention comprised a total of three visits with a minimum wash-out interval of five days in between visits. In each visit, one of the following beverages was taken: Placebo (PLA), non-caloric orange flavor drink (OFD), or Beetroot Juice (BJ). Volunteers arrived in the laboratory at 07:00. and left at 11:40. Figure 1 illustrates the experimental design of the sessions.

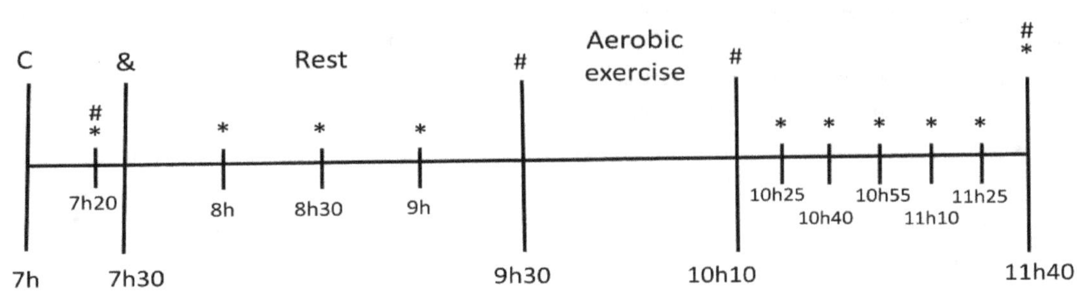

Figure 1. Experimental design of the sessions. (C) Arrival at the laboratory; (*) Blood pressure measurement; (#) Saliva sample collection; (&) Beverage intake.

During all intervention sessions, the volunteers arrived at 07:00, after eight hours of an overnight fast. BP was measured after 20 min of rest in a sitting position (07:20), every 30 min after the beverage intake until the beginning of the exercise (08:00, 08:30, and 09:00), and every 15 min for 90 min after the exercise session. Unstimulated saliva samples were collected after the 20 min of rest (07:20), immediately before (09:30) and after (10:10) exercise, and 90 min after the exercise session was finished (11:40). Heart rate (HR) was measured during the 20 min of rest (between 07:00 and 07:20), during the exercise, and during the 90 min after the exercise session (Polar® RS800CX). The beverage intake took place 10 min after the rest period (07:30), allowing 15 min for the consumption of all the beverage content. The exercise session was 40 min long (from 09:30 to 10:10).

During the sessions, the volunteers were allowed to drink water, but no other drink or food ingestion was permitted. They were instructed to avoid foods and drinks rich in NO_3^- 24 h before the sessions and received a list with the following consumption restrictions: Green vegetables (amaranth, lettuce, cabbage, spinach, broccoli, celery, cauliflower, Chinese radish), beetroot or its juice, sausage, salami, ham, turkey breast, coffee, energy drinks, soft drinks, alcoholic beverages, and to avoid the use of mouthwashes. Before starting each intervention session, volunteers were questioned about these items.

2.3. *Physical Exercise*

The exercise consisted of 40 min of continuous moderate intensity aerobic exercise on a treadmill, allowing the first five minutes to warm-up and the last two minutes to cool down. The treadmill speed could reach 5.5 km/h and the intensity increase was imposed by inclining the treadmill until the volunteer reached the zone between 65% and 70% of HR reserve (HRR) [22]. For the HRR calculation, we used the formula: maximum HR—resting HR. For the participants resting HR, we considered the minimum HR measured during the initial 20 min of rest on the first intervention day, and the maximum HR was estimated by the formula: 220 − age.

HR was monitored during the exercise and the Borg Scale [23] was used to assess the subjective perception of exertion (RPE) for both dyspnea and lower limb fatigue. The measurements for HR and RPE were assessed every two minutes. Whenever the HR was found to be outside of the stipulated zone, the exercise load was readjusted.

2.4. *Intake of Beetroot Juice and Placebo*

The intervention included three different juices: BJ, PLA and OFD, with one beverage assigned to each intervention session. The order of beverage intake was randomly assigned for each of the volunteers using a randomized block design through the website (https://www.random.org/lists/). For the randomization, codes were assigned to each volunteer, each beverage, and each session. Thereafter, the beverage each volunteer would drink on the first session, second and third sessions were randomly allocated in this order. A researcher who did not participate in the data collection process was responsible for assigning a beverage to each code and blinding the drinks, adding each drink to its respective bottle labeled with the volunteer's name.

The BJ had 20.78 mmol/kg of NO_3^- and was prepared using 35 mL of NO_3^- concentrated beetroot juice containing 400 mg of NO_3^- (Beet-It Sport Shot, James White Drinks Ltd., Ipswich, UK), which was diluted in 315 mL of distilled water with 6 g of non-caloric orange juice flavored powder (Clight, Mondelez International, Inc., São Paulo, Brazil), totalizing 350 mL of juice. The PLA had 3.86 mmol/kg of NO_3^- and was prepared by filtering the BJ on an ion exchange resin, capable of depleting the NO_3^- (PA101 OH-, Permution®) [24], similarly to a previous report [25]. Lastly, the OFD was a non-caloric orange flavored drink, prepared using three grams of orange juice powder diluted in 350 mL of distilled water. BJ and PLA were identical in taste, while OFD was slightly different. Each volunteer received the designated drink in a sealed bottle with a lid and a dark straw, making it impossible to visualize or smell the bottle content. The study participants had 15 min to drink the entire beverage.

2.5. *Measurements of Blood Pressure*

BP was measured in a sitting position, without visual or sound stimulation, using OMRON® BP HEM-7113 automatic monitors. Prior to the BP measurement, 20 min of rest was required. BP was measured three times, always in the left arm, and the mean of these measures was calculated for data analysis.

2.6. Salivary Samples Collection and Analysis

Saliva samples were collected using the spit method [26]. All samples were centrifuged at 3000 rpm for 15 min, the supernatant was separated and stored at −80 °C until analysis. The NO_2^- concentration was used to estimate the bioavailability of NO by the Griess method [27].

2.7. Statistical Analysis

Statistical analyses were performed while researchers were blinded regarding the ingested beverage. Results are presented as mean ± standard deviation. The Shapiro-Wilk test was applied to verify data normality, and two-way ANOVA was used to analyze differences between the time points (pre and post exercise) and the treatments (PLA, OFD, BJ), using the Bonferroni post hoc when necessary. The area under the curve (AUC) by the trapezoidal method was used to compare the temporal changes of BP and salivary NO_2^-, separately. One-way ANOVA was used for AUC and exercise analysis, and a Pearson correlation was used to assess BP and NO_2^- effects. Statistical significance was set at $p < 0.05$. All analyses were performed using SPSS version 20 (IBM SPSS, Chicago, IL, USA) and GraphPad Prism 6 (GraphPad Prism Inc., San Diego, CA, USA).

3. Results

This study was completed by 13 postmenopausal women who were overweight, medically treated for hypertension, and physically active. The general characteristics of the volunteers are described in Table 1. There was no difference in exercise intensity between the sessions. For PLA, OFD, and BJ sessions, the HR mean was 125.6 ± 7.2; 126.1 ± 7.8; 126.7 ± 7.4 bpm ($p = 0.658$); the treadmill inclination was 3.4 ± 3.0; 3.5 ± 2.7; 3.3 ± 2.7% ($p = 0.715$); the RPE of dyspnea was 3.7 ± 0.85; 3.4 ± 1.0; 3.4 ± 1.0 ($p = 0.328$); and the RPE of lower limb fatigue was 4.1 ± 1.2; 3.9 ± 1.12; 3.8 ± 1.1 ($p = 0.642$), respectively.

Table 1. General characteristics of the participants. BMI: Body mass index. The general characteristics values are shown as mean ± standard deviation (SD), physical activity level and drugs are shown as: number of subjects (n) and percentage of the total number of subjects (%).

General Characteristics	(Mean ± SD)
Age (years)	58.1 ± 4.6
Body mass (kg)	69.9 ± 9.2
Height (m)	1.57 ± 0.05
BMI (kg/m^2)	27.4 ± 4.2
Waist circumference (cm)	92.9 ± 11.7
Body fat (%)	37.3 ± 6.2
Fat mass (kg)	26.1 ± 6.9
Lean mass (kg)	29.9 ± 9.2
Physical activity level	**(n (%))**
Very Active	2 (15%)
Active	8 (62%)
Irregularly Active	3 (23%)
Drugs	**(n (%))**
Angiotensin 1 Receptor Blockers + Diuretic	6 (46%)
Angiotensin 1 Receptor Blockers	4 (31%)
Diuretic	1 (8%)
Angiotensin Converting Enzyme Inhibitor	1 (8%)
Angiotensin Converting Enzyme Inhibitor + Diuretic	1 (8%)
Statins	3 (23%)
Levothyroxine	4 (31%)

Figure 2 illustrates the results for salivary NO_2^-. Participants had similar values during the sessions for salivary NO_2^- at rest. Before exercise, salivary NO_2^- was slightly increased (1.0 mM) by PLA and greatly increased by BJ (2.6 mM) ($p < 0.05$), while the values remained at a low level with OFD intake (0.1 mM). BJ lead to the highest salivary NO_2^- level (3.3 mM) immediately after exercise when compared to the other beverages (PLA 0.9; OFD 0.1 mM) ($p < 0.01$). Furthermore, salivary NO_2^- remained increased for up to 90 min post exercise with BJ intake when compared to rest (REST = 0.1 ± 0.1; POST 0′ = 3.3 ± 1.3; POST 90′ = 2.5 ± 1.1 mM; $p < 0.001$), but with PLA salivary NO_2^- was only increased until immediately after exercise when compared to rest (REST = 0.2 ± 0.1; POST 0′ = 0.9 ± 0.6; POST 90′ = 0.7 ± 0.4 mM; $p = 0.011$). The AUC for NO_2^- response over time was the highest with BJ when compared to both PLA and OFD ($p < 0.01$), however the response was still higher with PLA when compared to OFD ($p = 0.037$). There was no correlation between salivary NO_2^- and BP (SBP $p = 0.749$, $r = 0.053$; DBP $p = 0.618$, $r = -0.082$).

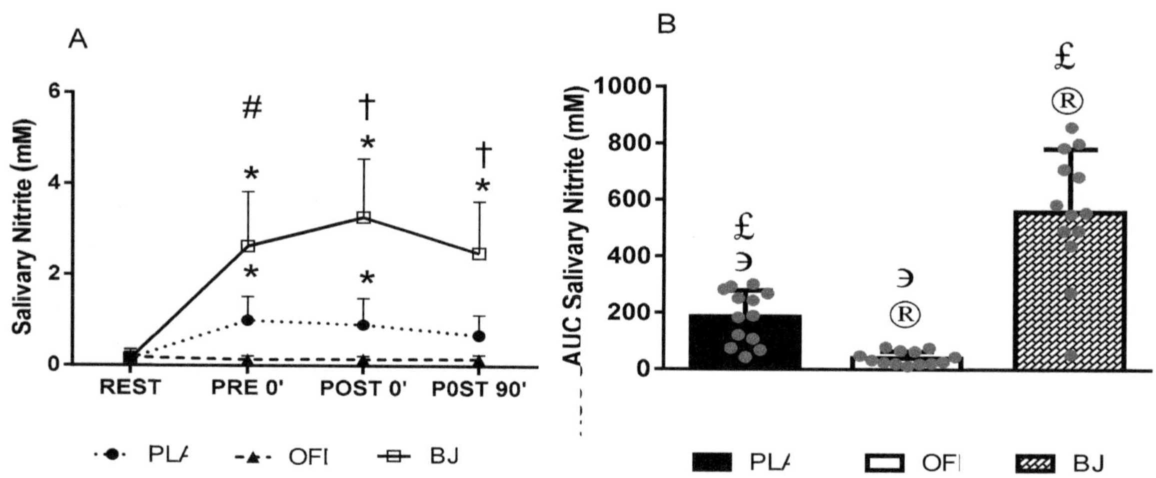

Figure 2. Salivary NO_2^- values from point to point (**A**) and values for the area under the curve (AUC) (**B**). Placebo NO_3^- depleted beetroot juice (PLA); Non-caloric orange flavored drink (OFD); Beetroot juice (BJ). (#) significantly different between all sessions; (†) significantly different when comparing BJ with both PLA and OFD; (*) significantly different when compared to rest (REST); (®) significantly different when compared to PLA; (϶) significantly different when compared to BJ; (£) significantly different when compared to OFD.

Figure 3 shows the SBP, DBP and HR responses throughout the experimental sessions. SBP increased after beverage consumption when compared to rest ($p = 0.001$) and decreased after exercise when compared to both rest and post ingestion time points. DBP also increased after beverage intake ($p = 0.001$) and decreased in the three following time points after exercise when compared to rest ($p = 0.005$). All DBP values decreased after exercise when compared to the pre-exercise value ($p = 0.001$). An increase in HR was observed after exercise when compared to rest ($p = 0.001$). There was no difference in SBP, DBP or HR between the three experimental sessions ($p = 1.000$).

Figure 4 demonstrates the BP variation after exercise in comparison with the BP measured at rest, 30 min before the exercise (at 9:00 am, as shown in Figure 1) and its respective AUC. SBP and DBP decreased in all evaluated time points post-exercise ($p < 0.001$). No difference for the AUC was observed among sessions ($p = 1.000$).

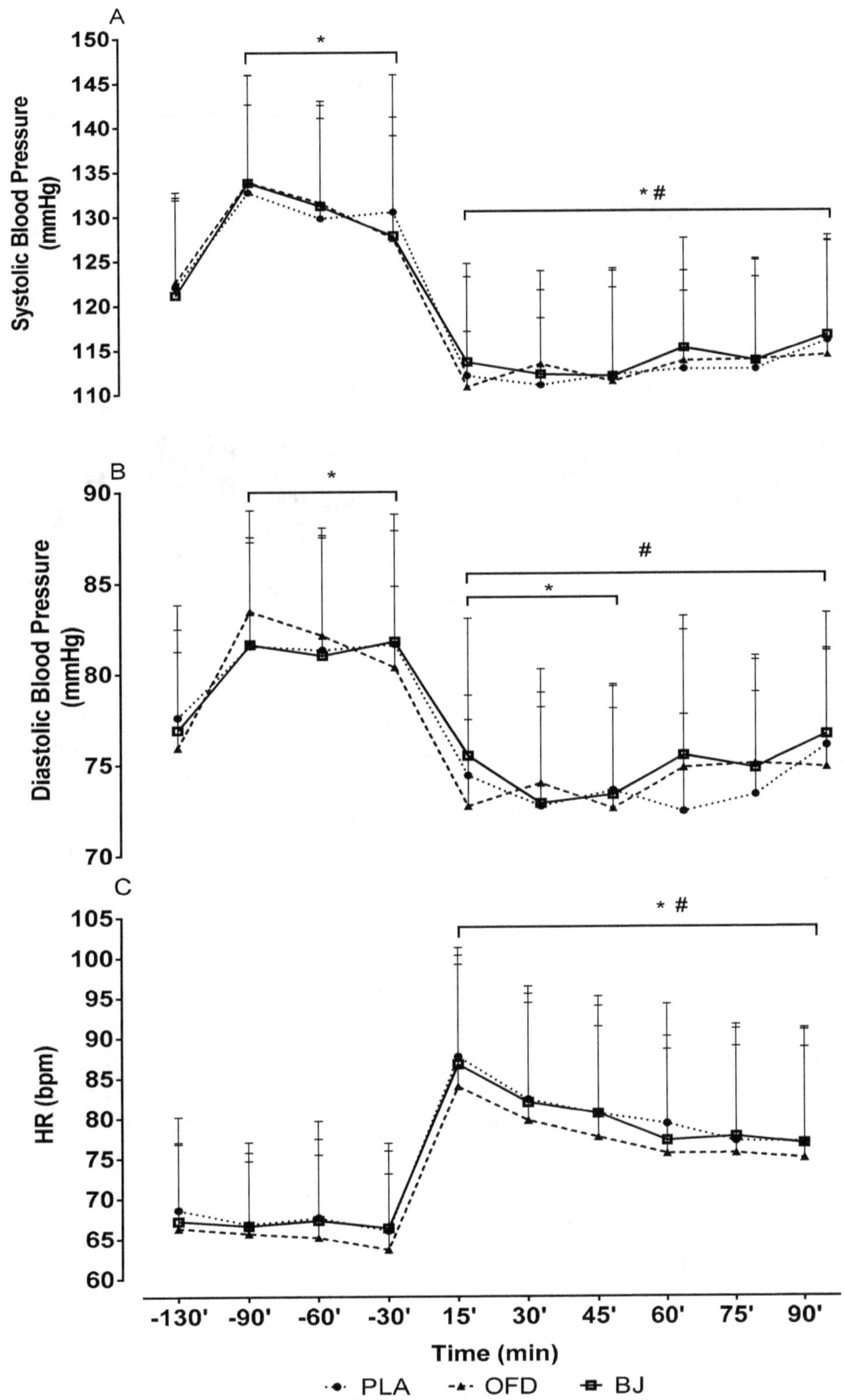

Figure 3. Systolic blood pressure (**A**); diastolic blood pressure (**B**) and point-to-point heart rate (**C**). Placebo NO_3^- depleted beetroot juice (PLA); Non-caloric orange flavor drink (OFD); Beet juice (BJ). The negative time values refer to measurements before exercise. The positive time values refer to measurements after the exercise. (*) significantly different when compared to the −130′ timepoint (resting pre-ingestion); (#) significantly different when compared to the −90′, −60′, −30′ timepoints (post juice intake).

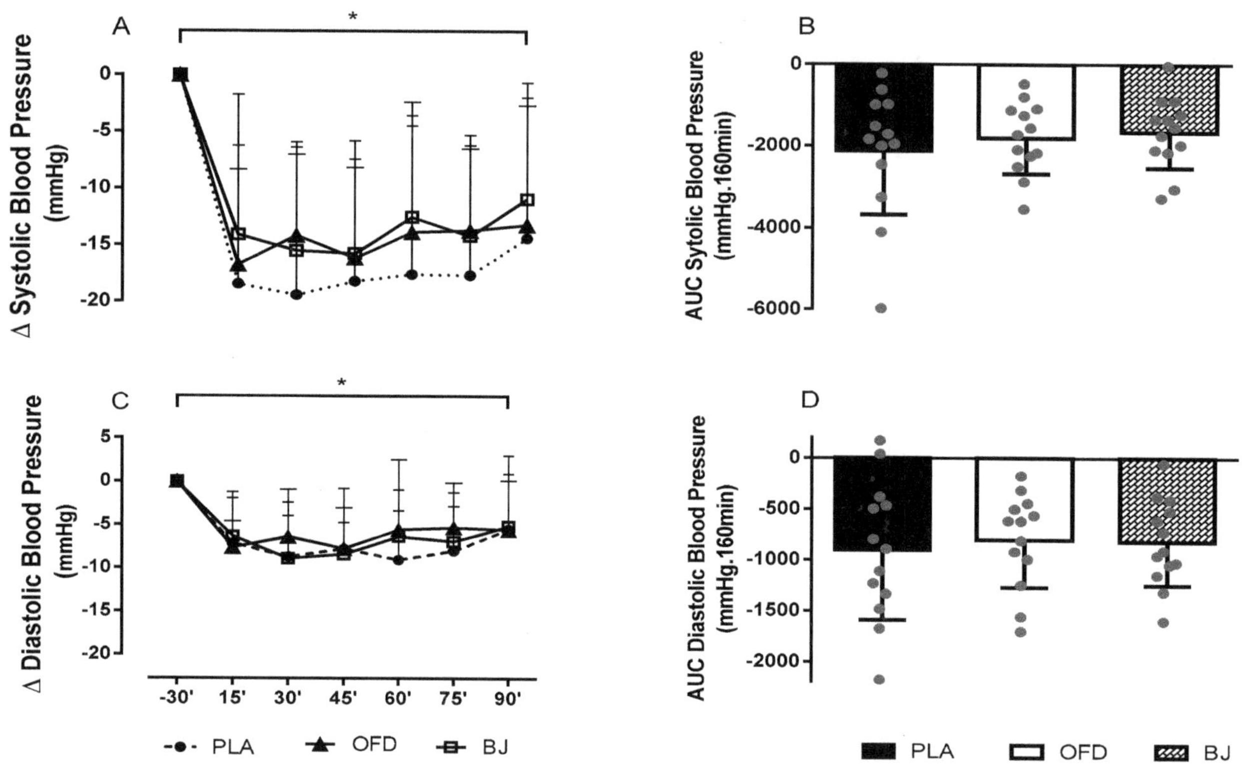

Figure 4. Δ values for systolic blood pressure variation (**A**) and diastolic blood pressure variation (**C**), area under the curve (AUC) for systolic blood pressure (**B**) and for diastolic blood pressure (**D**). Placebo NO_3^- depleted beetroot juice (PLA); Non-caloric orange flavor drink (OFD); Beetroot juice (BJ). The negative time values refer to measurements before exercise. The positive time values refer to measurements after the exercise. (*) significantly different when compared to the −30′ point (pre-exercise).

4. Discussion

The hypothesis underlying this study was that an increase in NO_2^-, due to BJ intake would enhance NO bioavailability, consequently increasing vasodilation and improving BP reduction mediated by exercise in hypertensive postmenopausal women. The main findings of the study were that a moderate-intensity aerobic exercise session was sufficient to cause PEH, and that acute BJ intake did not lead to additional effects on PEH, even though there was an increase in salivary NO_2^-, which could result in enhanced NO bioavailability.

To the best of our knowledge, this is the first study with hypertensive postmenopausal women analyzing acute intake of BJ and its influence on BP. Several other interventions assessing effects of BJ intake have been completed with different populations. Previous studies have investigated chronic [7–12,28] and acute BJ ingestion [16,20,28–30], in athletes [17–19], in healthy non-athletes [31,32], and in patients in disease states [7–12,16,20]. BJ consumption has been analyzed combined with exercise [28,33] and without exercise [34]. Usually, the primary objective of these studies is to evaluate the oxygen consumption and blood flow [28], associated with the analysis of plasma or salivary NO_2^-. Although BJ supplementation may cause a significant reduction in BP and this is usually evaluated as a secondary outcome, we can still cross-compare these studies with ours.

A recent review [6] discussed different study designs for BJ intervention and BP response in non-athlete populations. A meta-analysis showed that elderly people had less accentuated hypotensive responses [35], however, this is not a consensus, since another meta-analysis [13] showed an opposite effect. Other characteristics that may influence these results are both sex (women have less evident responses) and BP level at baseline. In this sense, the present study included middle age to elderly women (58.1 ± 4.6 years), which despite being hypertensive, had medically controlled BP at baseline. Therefore, these characteristics may have masked the hypotensive effects of BJ.

In a previous study with hypertensive patients with chronic obstructive pulmonary disease [16], there was a hypotensive effect in DBP three hours after BJ ingestion containing 12.9 mmol of NO_3^-. Different from the present study, they did not assess BJ consumption in combination with exercise, they used a lower dose of NO_3^- in BJ, and they used a population with compromised cardiorespiratory capacity. In another study [20], patients with insufficient cardiac output using antihypertensive drugs consumed 140 mL of BJ containing 11.2 mmol of NO_3^- and performed a 6 min walk, a maximal strength test, and a fatigue test. Despite evaluating BP post-exercise, they did not find a hypotensive effect associated with exercise or BJ supplementation. It should be noted that this evaluation occurred only 10 min after exercise, and the exercise protocol had more similarities to resistance exercise of high relative intensity. These characteristics differ greatly from the present study and may explain the absence of PEH, since this effect is better reported in post-aerobic exercise [36]. The amount of NO_3^- used in our study was based on previous studies investigating different doses of beetroot/NO_3^- and blood pressure responses [37]. Wylie and colleagues [37] found that consumption of NO_3^- of up to 8.4 mmol had dose dependent lowering effects on BP, but higher doses had no additional effects on BP. Therefore, the dose used in our study should be enough to increase NO availability and increase blood flow.

After exercise, local vasodilator mechanisms contribute to BP reduction, leading to a sustained vasodilatation response [4]. There are studies suggesting that NO released by endothelium could lead to this effect, even though this is not the main cause of PEH [16]. Thus, nitric oxide could be considered a potential contributor to sustained post-exercise vasodilatation and could be involved in PEH. It is known that shear stress and activation of endothelial receptors cause NO release by eNOS and the capacity of this pathway depends on the interaction of neuropeptide and mechanical stimuli [38]. PEH is more evident after moderate intensity aerobic exercise in people with hypertension [39]. Considering the initial level of BP as one of the factors that determines the magnitude of PEH [39,40], the use of antihypertensive drugs before exercise could mitigate this response. However, we found a PEH response even with antihypertensive drug use, which highlights the importance of exercise even in hypertensive patients under pharmacological therapy.

Additionally, the local vasodilatory response is not the only mechanism leading to PEH. Halliwill et al. [4] highlighted the possible explanations to PEH as: an adjustment of the baroreflex control to maintain a lower BP after exercise; a reduction in sympathetic nerve activity; a thermoregulatory readjustment; a vasodilation caused by release of NO and prostaglandins, which also cause reduction in α-adrenergic sensitivity; and a vasodilation caused by the action of histamines. It is possible that one or more of these pathways could be the main cause of PEH rather than NO bioavailability. Interestingly, BJ has a notable influence on the bioavailability of NO, and although this pathway does not seem to be the most important cause of PEH [4], some studies have shown that BJ intake can decrease BP [16,28,33,37]. Therefore, there is a possibility that increasing NO bioavailability by BJ consumption could change BP response. However, when considered along with other mechanisms causing PEH, there might be an attenuation or inhibition of other pathways involved that do not allow a significant additional effect in BP reduction.

In postmenopausal women, there is an increase in oxidative stress, due to the reduction in estrogen synthesis, impairing both vascular cell integrity and activity of antioxidant enzymes [41]. Furthermore, the impairment of oxidative balance has an important role in the pathogenesis of hypertension and may lead to impaired endothelium-dependent relaxation [42]. This decrease in relaxation capacity is associated with decreased NO production, increased cyclooxygenase-2 (COX-2) expression, and increased nicotinamide adenine dinucleotide phosphate oxidase (NADPH oxidase), of which COX-2 and NADPH oxidase are involved in stimulating the production of reactive oxygen species [42]. Thus, hypertensive women after menopause, have compromised blood vessel integrity, leading to endothelial dysfunction [42]. Ingestion of BJ [43] could be a clinically valid strategy to reduce the oxidative imbalance in this population, to increase the activity of antioxidant enzymes and blood flow, and to improve vascular relaxation dependent on shear stress derived from exercise.

A study [25] compared the responses to BJ intake in plasma, saliva, and urine and found that saliva is more sensitive to NO_3^-, with the NO_2^- concentration increasing seven times in saliva, three times in plasma, and four times in urine when compared to placebo. In agreement with these findings, in the current study there was a slight increase in salivary NO_2^- with PLA intake, showing that even with the low concentration of NO_3^- present in PLA, saliva is sensitive enough to respond to this stimulus [25]. This is likely due to the initial conversion of NO_3^- to NO_2^- that occurs in the mouth by salivary components [25,44], especially by oral microbiome [45]. The bacteria genus *Veillonella* spp. is of importance, increasing the conversion of NO_3^- to NO_2^- in the oral cavity, thus, assisting with the reintroduction of NO_2^-/NO_3^- in the pathway of NO production [45]. Recently, the clinical importance of the oral microbiome has been demonstrated in a hypertensive population by the use of antibacterial mouthwashes, which decreased the oral reduction of NO_3^- and increased blood pressure in this population [46]

Based on our results, there are other possibilities to explain the lack of an additional effect on PEH with BJ ingestion. The literature shows that the amount of NO_3^- consumed is sufficient to cause a hypotensive response in healthy individuals [37], however, the NO_3^- dose response could vary among different populations. Therefore, this dose may not have been enough for hypertensive postmenopausal women. Although there are indications that increased bioavailability of NO_2^- is associated with the increased bioavailability of NO [47,48], this conversion may not have been satisfactory to generate enough NO to potentiate vasodilation. In addition, the endothelium status of the participants is not known. As all participants have been diagnosed with hypertension for more than one year, there may be a deficiency in the production of eNOS, which could reduce NO production [49]. Thus, it is important to evaluate the NO response, to determine NO_3^- dose responses in different populations, and evaluate chronic consumption of BJ. Although there are no studies evaluating the interaction of antihypertensives and blood pressure response with exercise [50], it is important to consider that the study volunteers had pharmacologically controlled hypertension, and these drugs could influence blood pressure response after exercise. Furthermore, the bioavailability of NO may not be the main cause of PEH, and other mechanisms causing PEH were not evaluated in the present study, of which we highlight the activity of baroreflex and vasodilation caused by other substances, such as histamine and prostaglandins [4].

This study had limitations, since blood flow was not measured, and BJ intake and BP measurements were assessed in a short term, thus, our results cannot be extrapolated to chronic settings. The study participants were taking different anti-hypertensive medication, which could mask the effect of NO_3^- on blood pressure. Our results suggest that moderate aerobic exercise is a good strategy to induce PEH and may be helpful for hypertension treatment. However, only one dose of BJ is not sufficient to cause an additional effect on PEH.

5. Conclusions

In conclusion, acute intake of beetroot juice does not change BP response mediated by moderate intensity aerobic exercise in hypertensive postmenopausal women, even though there is an increase in the bioavailability of salivary NO_2^-/NO.

Author Contributions: A.L.A. participated in the data collection and analysis, performed statistical analysis, and wrote the manuscript; I.M.M. participated in the data collection and analysis, performed statistical analysis and contributed with the revision of the manuscript; V.H.V.C., T.C.F.d.S. and J.P.B. participated in the data collection, and contributed with the revision of the manuscript; A.M.M. contributed with the manuscript and English review; A.V.d.S., D.C.C., R.R.T. and F.S.E. participated in the data analysis, performed statistical analysis and contributed with the revision of the manuscript, E.P.d.O. participated in the study design, elaboration of the discussion and with the revision of the manuscript; G.M.P. contributed with the study design, data collection and analysis, statistical analysis, and with the manuscript elaboration and review. All authors read and approved the final manuscript.

References

1. Lagranha, C.J.; Silva, T.L.A.; Silva, S.C.A.; Braz, G.R.F.; da Silva, A.I.; Fernandes, M.P.; Sellitti, D.F. Protective effects of estrogen against cardiovascular disease mediated via oxidative stress in the brain. *Life Sci.* **2018**, *192*, 190–198. [CrossRef]
2. Coylewright, M.; Reckelhoff, J.F.; Ouyang, P. Menopause and Hypertension An Age-Old Debate. *Hypertension* **2008**, *51*, 952–959. [CrossRef]
3. Malachias, M.; Souza, W.; Plavnik, F.; Rodrigues, C.; Brandão, A.; Neves, M.; Bortolotto, L.; Franco, R.; Poli-de-Figueiredo, C.; Jardim, P.; et al. 7ª Diretriz Brasileira De Hipertensão Arterial. In *Arquivos Brasileiros de Cardiologia*; 2016; Volume 107, ISBN 1435-232X (Electronic)r1434-5161 (Linking). Available online: http://publicacoes.cardiol.br/2014/diretrizes/2016/05_HIPERTENSAO_ARTERIAL.pdf (accessed on 3 November 2018).
4. Halliwill, J.R.; Buck, T.M.; Lacewell, A.N.; Romero, S.A. Postexercise hypotension and sustained postexercise vasodilatation: What happens after we exercise? *Exp. Physiol.* **2013**, *98*, 7–18. [CrossRef]
5. Farah, C.; Nascimento, A.; Bolea, G.; Meyer, G.; Gayrard, S.; Lacampagne, A.; Cazorla, O.; Reboul, C. Key role of endothelium in the eNOS-dependent cardioprotection with exercise training. *J. Mol. Cell. Cardiol.* **2017**, *102*, 26–30. [CrossRef]
6. Ocampo, D.A.B.; Paipilla, A.F.; Marín, E.; Vargas-Molina, S.; Petro, J.L.; Pérez-Idárraga, A. Dietary Nitrate from Beetroot Juice for Hypertension: A Systematic Review. *Biomolecules* **2018**, *8*, 134. [CrossRef]
7. Eggebeen, J.; Kim-Shapiro, D.B.; Haykowsky, M.; Morgan, T.M.; Basu, S.; Brubaker, P.; Rejeski, J.; Kitzman, D.W. One Week of Daily Dosing With Beetroot Juice Improves Submaximal Endurance and Blood Pressure in Older Patients With Heart Failure and Preserved Ejection Fraction. *JACC Heart Fail.* **2016**, *4*, 428–437. [CrossRef]
8. Kenjale, A.A.; Ham, K.L.; Stabler, T.; Robbins, J.L.; Johnson, J.L.; VanBruggen, M.; Privette, G.; Yim, E.; Kraus, W.E.; Allen, J.D. Dietary nitrate supplementation enhances exercise performance in peripheral arterial disease. *J. Appl. Physiol.* **2011**, *110*, 1582–1591. [CrossRef]
9. Kelly, J.; Fulford, J.; Vanhatalo, A.; Blackwell, J.R.; French, O.; Bailey, S.J.; Gilchrist, M.; Winyard, P.G.; Jones, A.M. Effects of short-term dietary nitrate supplementation on blood pressure, O2 uptake kinetics, and muscle and cognitive function in older adults. *AJP Regul. Integr. Comp. Physiol.* **2013**, *304*, R73–R83. [CrossRef]
10. Bock, J.M.; Treichler, D.P.; Norton, S.L.; Ueda, K.; William, E.; Casey, D.P. Inorganic nitrate supplementation enhances functional capacity and lower-limb microvascular reactivity in patients with peripheral artery disease. *Nitric Oxide* **2018**, *80*, 45–51. [CrossRef]
11. Siervo, M.; Oggioni, C.; Mathers, J.C.; Celis-Morales, C.; Ashor, A.W.; Jakovljevic, D.G.; Trenell, M.; Houghton, D.; Trenell, M.; Mathers, J.C.; et al. Dietary nitrate does not affect physical activity or outcomes in healthy older adults in a randomized, cross-over trial. *Nutr. Res.* **2016**, *36*, 1361–1369. [CrossRef]
12. Woessner, M.; VanBruggen, M.D.; Pieper, C.F.; Sloane, R.; Kraus, W.E.; Gow, A.J.; Allen, J.D. Beet the Best? *Circ. Res.* **2018**, *123*, 654–659. [CrossRef]
13. Bahadoran, Z.; Mirmiran, P.; Kabir, A.; Azizi, F.; Ghasemi, A. The Nitrate-Independent Blood Pressure-Lowering Effect of Beetroot Juice: A Systematic Review and Meta-Analysis. *Adv. Nutr.* **2017**, *8*, 830–838. [CrossRef]
14. Jackson, J.K.; Patterson, A.J.; Macdonald-wicks, L.K.; Oldmeadow, C.; Mcevoy, M.A. The role of inorganic nitrate and nitrite in cardiovascular disease risk factors: A systematic review and meta-analysis of human evidence. *Nutr. Rev.* **2018**, *76*, 348–371. [CrossRef]
15. Stanaway, L.; Rutherfurd-Markwick, K.; Page, R.; Ali, A. Performance and health benefits of dietary nitrate supplementation in older adults: A systematic review. *Nutrients* **2017**, *9*, 1171. [CrossRef]
16. Curtis, K.J.; O'Brien, A.K.; Tanner, R.J.; Polkey, J.I.; Minnion, M.; Feelisch, M.; Polkey, M.I.; Edwards, M.; Hopkinson, N.S. Acute dietary nitrate supplementation and exercise performance in COPD: A double-blind, placebo-controlled, randomised controlled pilot study. *PLoS ONE* **2015**, *10*, e0144504. [CrossRef]
17. Lansley, K.E.; Winyard, P.G.; Bailey, S.J.; Vanhatalo, A.; Wilkerson, D.P.; Blackwell, J.R.; Gilchrist, M.; Benjamin, N.; Jones, A.M. Acute dietary nitrate supplementation improves cycling time trial performance. *Med. Sci. Sports Exerc.* **2011**, *43*, 1125–1131. [CrossRef]
18. Thompson, C.; Vanhatalo, A.; Jell, H.; Fulford, J.; Carter, J.; Nyman, L.; Bailey, S.J.; Jones, A.M. Dietary nitrate supplementation improves sprint and high-intensity intermittent running performance. *Nitric Oxide* **2016**, *61*, 55–61. [CrossRef]

19. Clifford, T.; Berntzen, B.; Davison, G.W.; West, D.J.; Howatson, G.; Stevenson, E.J. Effects of beetroot juice on recovery of muscle function and performance between bouts of repeated sprint exercise. *Nutrients* **2016**, *8*, 506. [CrossRef]
20. Coggan, A.R.; Leibowitz, J.L.; Spearie, C.A.; Kadkhodayan, A.; Thomas, D.P.; Ramamurthy, S.; Mahmood, K.; Park, S.; Waller, S.; Farmer, M.; et al. Acute Dietary Nitrate Intake Improves Muscle Contractile Function in Patients with Heart Failure: A Double-Blind, Placebo-Controlled, Randomized Trial. *Circ. Heart Fail.* **2015**, *8*, 914–920. [CrossRef]
21. Barbosa, C.D.; Costa, J.G.; Giolo, J.S.; Rossato, L.T.; Nahas, P.C.; Mariano, I.M.; Batista, J.P.; Puga, G.M.; de Oliveira, E.P. Isoflavone supplementation plus combined aerobic and resistance exercise do not change phase angle values in postmenopausal women: A randomized placebo-controlled clinical trial. *Exp. Gerontol.* **2019**, *117*, 31–37. [CrossRef]
22. Karvonen, M.J.; Kentala, E.; Mustala, O. The effects of training on heart rate; a longitudinal study. *Ann. Med. Exp. Biol. Fenn.* **1957**, *35*, 307–315.
23. Borg, G.A. Psychophysical bases of perceived exertion. *Med. Sci. Sports Exerc.* **1982**, *14*, 377–381. [CrossRef]
24. De Castro, T.F.; Manoel, F.D.A.; Figueiredo, D.H.; Figueiredo, D.H.; Machado, F.A. Effect of beetroot juice supplementation on 10-km performance in recreational runners. *Appl. Physiol. Nutr. Metab.* **2018**, *44*, 90–94. [CrossRef]
25. Bondonno, C.P.; Liu, A.H.; Croft, K.D.; Ward, N.C.; Shinde, S.; Moodley, Y.; Lundberg, J.O.; Puddey, I.B.; Woodman, R.J.; Hodgson, J.M. Absence of an effect of high nitrate intake from beetroot juice on blood pressure in treated hypertensive individuals: A randomized controlled trial. *Am. J. Clin. Nutr.* **2015**, *102*, 368–375. [CrossRef]
26. Navazesh, M. Methods for Collecting Saliva. *Ann. N. Y. Acad. Sci.* **1993**, *694*, 72–77. [CrossRef]
27. Kurose, I.; Wolf, R.; Grisham, M.B.; Granger, D.N. Effects of an endogenous inhibitor of nitric oxide synthesis on postcapillary venules. *Am. J. Physiol.* **1995**, *268*, H2224–H2231. [CrossRef]
28. Vanhatalo, A.; Bailey, S.J.S.; Blackwell, J.R.J.; DiMenna, F.J.F.; Pavey, T.G.; Wilkerson, D.P.; Benjamin, N.; Winyard, P.G.P.; Jones, A.M. Acute and chronic effects of dietary nitrate supplementation on blood pressure and the physiological responses to moderate-intensity and incremental exercise. *Am. J. Physiol. Regul. Integr. Comp. Physiol.* **2010**, *299*, R1121–R1131. [CrossRef]
29. Betteridge, S.; Bescós, R.; Martorell, M.; Pons, A.; Garnham, A.P.; Stathis, C.C.; McConell, G.K. No effect of acute beetroot juice ingestion on oxygen consumption, glucose kinetics, or skeletal muscle metabolism during submaximal exercise in males. *J. Appl. Physiol.* **2016**, *120*, 391–398. [CrossRef]
30. Kim, J.-K.; Moore, D.J.; Maurer, D.G.; Kim-Shapiro, D.B.; Basu, S.; Flanagan, M.P.; Skulas-Ray, A.C.; Kris-Etherton, P.; Proctor, D.N. Acute dietary nitrate supplementation does not augment submaximal forearm exercise hyperemia in healthy young men. *Appl. Physiol. Nutr. Metab.* **2015**, *40*, 122–128. [CrossRef]
31. Bond, V., Jr.; Curry, B.H.; Adams, R.G.; Haddad, G.E. Cardiorespiratory function associated with dietary nitrate supplementation. *Appl. Physiol. Nutr. Metab.* **2014**, *39*, 168–172. [CrossRef]
32. Dos Santos Baião, D.; Conte-Junior, C.A.; Paschoalin, V.M.F.; Alvares, T.S. Beetroot juice increase nitric oxide metabolites in both men and women regardless of body mass. *Int. J. Food Sci. Nutr.* **2016**, *67*, 40–46. [CrossRef]
33. Berry, M.J.; Justus, N.W.; Hauser, J.I.; Case, A.H.; Helms, C.C.; Basu, S.; Rogers, Z.; Lewis, M.T.; Miller, G.D. Dietary nitrate supplementation improves exercise performance and decreases blood pressure in COPD patients. *Nitric Oxide-Biol. Chem.* **2015**, *48*, 22–30. [CrossRef]
34. Hohensinn, B.; Haselgrübler, R.; Müller, U.; Stadlbauer, V.; Lanzerstorfer, P.; Lirk, G.; Höglinger, O.; Weghuber, J. Sustaining elevated levels of nitrite in the oral cavity through consumption of nitrate-rich beetroot juice in young healthy adults reduces salivary pH. *Nitric Oxide-Biol. Chem.* **2016**, *60*, 10–15. [CrossRef]
35. Siervo, M.; Lara, J.; Jajja, A.; Sutyarjoko, A.; Ashor, A.W.; Brandt, K.; Qadir, O.; Mathers, J.C.; Benjamin, N.; Winyard, P.G.; et al. Ageing modifies the effects of beetroot juice supplementation on 24-h blood pressure variability: An individual participant meta-analysis. *Nitric Oxide-Biol. Chem.* **2015**, *47*, 97–105. [CrossRef]
36. Cornelissen, V.A.; Smart, N.A. Exercise Training for Blood Pressure: A Systematic Review and Meta-analysis. *J. Am. Heart Assoc.* **2013**, 2, e004473. [CrossRef]

37. Wylie, L.J.; Kelly, J.; Bailey, S.J.; Blackwell, J.R.; Skiba, P.F.; Winyard, P.G.; Jeukendrup, A.E.; Vanhatalo, A.; Jones, A.M. Beetroot juice and exercise: Pharmacodynamic and dose-response relationships. *J. Appl. Physiol.* **2013**, *115*, 325–336. [CrossRef]
38. Quillon, A.; Fromy, B.; Debret, R. Endothelium microenvironment sensing leading to nitric oxide mediated vasodilation: A review of nervous and biomechanical signals. *Nitric Oxide-Biol. Chem.* **2015**, *45*, 20–26. [CrossRef]
39. Gomes Anunciação, P.; Doederlein Polito, M. A review on post-exercise hypotension in hypertensive individuals. *Arq. Bras. Cardiol.* **2011**, *96*, 100–109.
40. Reboussin, D.M.; Allen, N.B.; Griswold, M.E.; Guallar, E.; Hong, Y.; Lackland, D.T.; Miller, E.P.R.; Polonsky, T.; Thompson-Paul, A.M.; Vupputuri, S. Systematic Review for the 2017 ACC/AHA/AAPA/ABC/ACPM/AGS/APhA/ASH/ASPC/NMA/PCNA Guideline for the Prevention, Detection, Evaluation, and Management of High Blood Pressure in Adults: A Report of the American College of Cardiology/American Heart Association. *J. Am. Coll. Cardiol.* **2018**, *71*, 2176–2198. [CrossRef]
41. Jarrete, A.P.; Novais, I.P.; Nunes, H.A.; Puga, G.M.; Delbin, M.A.; Zanesco, A. Influence of aerobic exercise training on cardiovascular and endocrine-inflammatory biomarkers in hypertensive postmenopausal women. *J. Clin. Transl. Endocrinol.* **2014**, *1*, 108–114. [CrossRef]
42. Korsager Larsen, M.; Matchkov, V.V. Hypertension and physical exercise: The role of oxidative stress. *Medicina* **2016**, *52*, 19–27. [CrossRef] [PubMed]
43. Clifford, T.; Howatson, G.; West, D.J.; Stevenson, E.J. The potential benefits of red beetroot supplementation in health and disease. *Nutrients* **2015**, *7*, 2801–2822. [CrossRef] [PubMed]
44. Bedale, W.; Sindelar, J.J.; Milkowski, A.L. Dietary nitrate and nitrite: Benefits, risks, and evolving perceptions. *Meat Sci.* **2016**, *120*, 85–92. [CrossRef] [PubMed]
45. Blekkenhorst, L.C.; Bondonno, N.P.; Liu, A.H.; Ward, N.C.; Prince, R.L.; Lewis, J.R. Nitrate, the oral microbiome, and cardiovascular health: A systematic literature review of human and animal studies. *Am. J. Clin. Nutr.* **2018**, *107*, 504–522. [CrossRef] [PubMed]
46. Bondonno, C.P.; Liu, A.H.; Croft, K.D.; Considine, M.J.; Puddey, I.B.; Woodman, R.J.; Hodgson, J.M. Antibacterial Mouthwash Blunts Oral Nitrate Reduction and Increases Blood Pressure in Treated Hypertensive Men and Women. *Am. J. Hypertens.* **2015**, *28*, 572–575. [CrossRef] [PubMed]
47. Duncan, C.; Dougall, H.; Ohnston, P.; Green, S.; Brogan, R.; Leifer, C.; Smith, L.; Gowen, M.; Benjamin, N. Chemical generation of nitric oxide in the mouth from the enterosalivary circulation of dietary nitrate. *Nat. Med.* **1995**, *1*, 546. [CrossRef] [PubMed]
48. Kim-Shapiro, D.B.; Gladwin, M.T. Mechanisms of Nitrite Bioactivation. *Nitric Oxide* **2014**, *38*, 58–68. [CrossRef]
49. Förstermann, U. Nitric oxide and oxidative stress in vascular disease. *Eur. J. Physiol.* **2010**, *459*, 923–939. [CrossRef]
50. Naci, H.; Salcher-konrad, M.; Dias, S.; Blum, M.R.; Sahoo, S.A.; Nunan, D.; Ioannidis, J.P.A. How does exercise treatment compare with antihypertensive medications ? A network meta-analysis of 391 randomised controlled trials assessing exercise and medication effects on systolic blood pressure. *Brith J. Sprots Med.* **2018**, 1–12. [CrossRef]

5

The Inhibitory Effect of Ojeoksan on Early and Advanced Atherosclerosis

Byung Hyuk Han [1,2], Chang Seob Seo [3], Jung Joo Yoon [1,2], Hye Yoom Kim [1,2], You Mee Ahn [1,2], So Young Eun [1,5], Mi Hyeon Hong [1,2], Jae Geon Lee [1,4], Hyeun Kyoo Shin [3], Ho Sub Lee [1,2], Yun Jung Lee [1,2,*] and Dae Gill Kang [1,2,*]

1 Hanbang Cardio-Renal Syndrome Research Center, Wonkwang University, 460, Iksan-daero, Iksan, Jeonbuk 54538, Korea; arum0924@nate.com (B.H.H.); mora16@naver.com (J.J.Y.); hyeyoomc@naver.com (H.Y.K.); aum2668@naver.com (Y.M.A.); eunsoyg@wku.ac.kr (S.Y.E.); mihyeon123@naver.com (M.H.H.); john1027@snu.ac.kr (J.G.L.); host@wku.ac.kr (H.S.L.)

2 College of Oriental Medicine and Professional Graduate School of Oriental Medicine, Wonkwang University, 460, Iksan-daero, Iksan, Jeonbuk 54538, Korea

3 K-herb Research Center, Korea Institute of Oriental Medicine, 1672 Yuseong-daero, Yuseong-gu, Daejeon 34054, Korea; csseo0914@kiom.re.kr (C.S.S.); hkshin@kiom.re.kr (H.K.S.)

4 Department of Physiology, Seoul National University College of Medicine, 103, Daehak-ro, Jongno-gu, Seoul 03080, Korea

5 Department of Dental Pharmacology, School of Dentistry and Institute of Oral Bioscience, BK21 Plus, Chonbuk National University, 567 Baekje-daero, Jeonju, Jeonbuk 54896, Korea

* Correspondence: shrons@wku.ac.kr (Y.J.L.); dgkang@wku.ac.kr (D.G.K.)

Abstract: Atherosclerosis is closely related to vascular dysfunction and hypertension. Ojeoksan (OJS), originally recorded in an ancient Korean medicinal book named "Donguibogam", is a well-known, blended herbal formula. This study was carried out to investigate the beneficial effects of OJS on atherosclerosis in vitro and in vivo. Western-diet-fed apolipoprotein-E gene-deficient mice (ApoE −/−) were used for this study for 16 weeks, and their vascular dysfunction and inflammation were analyzed. OJS-treated ApoE −/− mice showed lowered blood pressure and glucose levels. The levels of metabolic parameters with hyperlipidemia attenuated following OJS administration. Hematoxylin and eosin (H&E) staining revealed that treatment with OJS reduced atherosclerotic lesions. OJS also suppressed the expression of adhesion molecules and matrix metalloproteinases (MMPs) compared to Western-diet-fed ApoE −/− mice and tumor necrosis factor-alpha (TNF-α)-stimulated human umbilical vein endothelial cells (HUVECs). Expression levels of MicroRNAs (miRNA)-10a, -126 3p were increased in OJS-fed ApoE −/− mice. OJS significantly increased the phosphorylation of endothelial nitric oxide synthase (eNOS) and protein kinase B (Akt), which are involved in nitric oxide (NO) production. OJS also regulated eNOS coupling by increasing the expression of endothelial GTP Cyclohydrolase-1 (GTPCH). Taken together, OJS has a protective effect on vascular inflammation via eNOS coupling-mediated NO production and might be a potential therapeutic agent for both early and advanced atherosclerosis.

Keywords: Ojeoksan; atherosclerosis; vascular inflammation; vasodilation; hypertension; adhesion molecule

---

1. Introduction

Inflammatory disorder is commonly known to be a major cause of Atherosclerosis [1] and characterized as a chronic inflammatory disease of the arterial wall [2]. The main reasons of early stage of atherosclerosis are hyperglycemia, high blood serum triglyceride levels, low concentration of high-density lipoprotein (HDL) cholesterol, high blood pressure, and central obesity [3]. Acetylcholine (ACh)-induced endothelium-dependent vasorelaxation is mediated by nitric oxide (NO), which acts via soluble guanylyl cyclase and cyclic Guanosine monophosphate (GMP). Endothelial dysfunction is a key marker of early stage of atherosclerosis. This process is mainly regulated by the expressions of cellular adhesion molecules on the endothelium.

The expression of adhesion molecules increases in atherosclerotic lesion sites and can be the cause for vascular dysfunction and advanced atherosclerosis [4]. Mediated signaling by cytokines, such as tumor necrosis factor alpha (TNF-α), induce the expression levels of cell adhesion molecules, which is an important mediator in the pre-inflammatory process [5]. MicroRNAs (miRNAs) are single-stranded, non-coding, small RNAs that regulate gene expression by destabilizing target mRNAs and/or inhibiting translation. For example, miR-126 was well known to reduce the expression of adhesion molecules, such as intracellular adhesion molecule-1 (ICAM-1), vascular cell adhesion molecule-1 (VCAM-1), and endothelial cell selectin (E-selectin), by directly targeting the 3′ untranslated region (3′UTR) of these genes [6,7]. In addition, micro RNA-10a (MiR-10a) regulated the expression of Mitogen-Activated Protein Kinase Kinase Kkinase 7 (MAP3K7) and Transforming growth factor beta-activated kinase 1 (TAK1), and both of which regulate Inhibitor of NF-kappa B (IκB) degradation [8]. Adhesion molecules such as ICAM-1 and VCAM-1 play key roles in the process of atherosclerosis. Endothelial dysfunction is thought to be the cause of the development of atherosclerosis [9]. All vascular cells including endothelial cells and macrophages secrete matrix metalloproteinases (MMPs), especially MMP-2 and MMP-9, which are synthesized in atheroma plaques, and are particularly prevalent in rupture-prone shoulder regions [10]. MMPs degrade collagen and allow for smooth-muscle cell migration within a vessel. Moreover, this begets an accumulation of other cellular material, resulting in atherosclerosis and ischemic events to tissues [11].

Endothelial NO synthase (eNOS) produces NO, which is a key regulator in the vasodilation process. NO regulates early stages of inflammatory processes by downregulating nuclear factor Nuclear factor-kappa B (NF-κB) [12,13]. Cardiovascular disease has a variety of causes, involving uncoupled eNOS signaling [14]. Studies with endothelial cells and isolated vessels supported the important role of eNOS coupling, showing that the inhibition of GTP cyclohydrolase-1 (GTPCH) results in reduced NO synthesis. In vascular disorders such as atherosclerosis, NO activity is decreased, whereas oxidative stress is upregulated and results in endothelial dysfunction. Enzymatic eNOS coupling by the cofactor tetrahydrobiopterin (BH4) plays a key role in maintaining endothelial function [15]. In the case of cardiovascular risk, the availability of BH4 decreased in the vessel wall with subsequent eNOS dysfunction may be a crucial determinant of impaired NO-mediated endothelial function. Protein kinase B (Akt) can activate eNOS, which leads to NO production. Additionally, the Phosphoinositide 3-kinase (PI3K)/Akt/eNOS pathway plays a key role in NO production [16,17].

Ojeoksan (OJS; Wuji-san in Chinese, Goshaku-san in Japanese) is composed of 17 herbal medicines (Table 1). OJS has been documented in a traditional Korean medical book named "Donguibogam" and in a traditional Chinese medical book named "Tae-Pyung-Hye-Min-Hwa-Je-Guk-Bang". According to records, OJS has been used as a pain-relieving agent and used to manage rash caused by circulation disadvantage of qi (氣) and blood (血), food (食), cold (寒), and congestion (痰). This study focused on the effects of OJS on blood (血) circulation disorders. In Korea, OJS is ranked first in terms of oriental health treatment medicated days and medical expenses, as it is included in 56 prescription drugs [18]. A previous study has determined whether OJS can alleviate liver inflammation induced by liver toxicity [19]. However, there are no reports regarding the protective effects of OJS against cardiovascular disease. Apolipoprotein-E gene-deficient mice (ApoE −/− mice) have been shown to develop hyperlipidemia and atherosclerosis as well as hypertension and endothelial dysfunctions [20]. Therefore, the present study was carried out to investigate whether OJS has a protective role in vascular inflammation and suppresses atherosclerotic lesions in ApoE $^{-/-}$ mice.

Table 1. Decoction of Ojeoksan (OJS).

Latin Name	Scientific Name	Amount (g)	Origin
Atractylodis Rhizoma	*Atractylodes lancea* DC	7.5	China
Ephedrae Herba	*Ephedra sinica* Stapf	3.7	China
Citri unshii Percarpium	*Citrus reticulata* Blanco	3.7	Jeju, Korea
Magnoliae Cortex	*Magnolia officinalis* Rehder & E.H. Wilson	3.0	China
Platycodi Radix	*Platycodon grandiflorus* (Jacq.) A. DC	3.0	Yeongcheon, Korea
Aurantii Fructus Immaturus	*Citrus aurantium* L	3.0	China
Angelicae Gigantis Radix	*Angelica gigas* Nakai	3.0	Pyeongchang, Korea
Zingiberis Rhizoma	*Zingiber officinale* Roscoe	3.0	Yeongcheon, Korea
Paeoniae Radix	*Paeonia lactiflora* Pall	3.0	Hwasun, Korea
Poria Sclerotium	*Wolfiporia* extensa	3.0	Yeongcheon, Korea
Angelicae Dahuricae Radix	*Angelica dahurica* (Hoffm.) Benth. & Hook.f. ex Franch. & Sav	2.6	Yeongcheon, Korea
Cnidii Rhizoma	*Ligusticum officinale* (Makino) Kitag	2.6	Yeongcheon, Korea
Pinelliae Tuber	*Pinellia ternata* (Thunb.) Ten. ex Breitenb	2.6	China
Cinnamomi Cortex	*Cinnamomum cassia* (L.) J. Presl	2.6	Vietnam
Glycyrrhizae Radix et Rhizoma	*Glycyrrhiza uralensis* Fisch	2.2	China
Zingiberis Rhizoma recens	*Zingiber officinale* Roscoe	3.7	Hanam, Korea
Allii Fistulosi Bulbus	*Allium fistulosum* L	3.7	Hanam, Korea

2. Material and Methods

2.1. High-Performance Liquid Chromatography (HPLC) Analysis of OJS

Chemical marker compounds in an OJS sample were analyzed using a Shimadzu Prominence LC-20A series (Shimadzu Co., Kyoto, Japan) equipped with a solvent delivery unit (LC-20AT), an online degasser (DGU-20A3), a column oven (CTO-20A), an auto sample injector (SIL-20AC), and a photodiode array (PDA) detector (SPD-M20A). The chromatographic data were acquired and processed using LC solution software (Version 1.24, SP1, Kyoto, Japan). All marker compounds were separated on a Phenomenex (Phenomenex, Torrance, CA, USA) Gemini C18 (250 × 4.6 mm, 5 μm), and the column oven was maintained at 40 °C. The mobile phases consisted of distilled water (A) and acetonitrile (J.T. Baker, Phillipsburg, NJ, USA) (B), both with 1.0% (*v*/*v*) acetic acid (Sigma-Aldrich, St. Louis, MO, USA). The gradient elution conditions were as follows: 15–25% B (0–20 min), 25–55% B (20–40 min), 55–100% B (40–45 min), 100% B (45–50 min), and 10–15% B (50–55 min). The re-equilibrium time was 15 min. The flow rate was maintained at 1.0 mL/min, and the injection volume was 10 mL.

2.2. Experimental Animals

Six-week-old male apolipoprotein-E gene-deficient mice (ApoE −/−) and normal C57BL6 mice were obtained from Saeronbio. Inc. (Uiwang, Korea) and then housed in cages with automatic temperature, humidity (22 ± 2 °C, 50–60%), and lighting (12 h light/dark cycle) conditions. They were fed a pelletized commercial chow diet for acclimatization for 2 weeks on arrival. After acclimatization, the animals were randomly divided into five groups: (1) the control (C57BL6 mice + regular diet + Distilled Water (DW), n = 15); (2) ApoE −/− (ApoE −/− + Western diet + DW, n = 13); (3) telmisartan (ApoE −/− + Western diet + telmisartan 1 mg/kg/day, n = 13); (4) OJS low (ApoE −/− + Western diet + OJS 50 mg/kg/day, n = 14); and (5) OJS high groups (ApoE −/− + Western diet + OJS 200 mg/kg/day, n = 14). The angiotensin receptor blocker, telmisartan, an anti-atherosclerotic agent, was chosen as a positive control [21]. A Western diet was also carried out for 16 weeks to sufficiently induce atherosclerosis in the experimental animals [22]. The control group received a regular diet (RD) (D12450B) and ApoE −/− groups received a Western diet (WTD) (D12079B) (Table 2), respectively, for 16 weeks by oral intake. The RD and WTD were purchased from Saeronbio. Inc. (Uiwang, Korea). At the end of the experimental period, all mice were sacrificed after 12 h fasting, and blood samples were collected into 1 mg/mL ethylendiaminetetraacetic acid (EDTA)-coated tube after pulled out the eyeball. All procedures were approved by the animal Ethics Committee (WKU12-15) and conformed to the guidelines specified by the country.

Table 2. Diagrams of concerning composition in regular diets (RD) and Western diets (WTD) for experimental mice.

Product	D12450B		D12079B	
	gm %	kcal %	gm %	kcal %
Protein	19.2	20	20	17
Carbohydrate	67.3	70	50	43
Fat	4.3	10	21	40
Total		100		100
kcal/gm	3.85		4.7	
Ingredient	**gm**	**kcal**	**gm**	**kcal**
Casein, 80 Mesh	200		195	
DL-Methionine			3	
L-Cystine	3			
Corn Starch	315		50	
Maltodextrin 10	35		100	
Sucrose	350		341	
cellulose	50		50	
Milk Fat, Anhydrous			200	
Corn oil			10	
Soybean oil	25			
Lard	20			
Mineral Mix S10026	10		35	
Dicalcium Phosphate	13			
Calcium Carbonate	5.5		4	
Potassium Citrate, 1 H_2O	16.5			
Vitamin Mix V10001	10		10	
Choline Bitartrate	2		2	
Cholesterol, USP	0.05		1.5	
FD&C Yellow Dye #5				
Total	**1055.05**	**4057**	**1001.54**	**4686**

Unitied Statees Pharmacopeia (USP); Federal Food, Drug, and Cosmetic Act (FD&C).

2.3. *Cell Cultures*

Human Umbilical Vein Endothelial Cells (HUVECs) were purchased from American Type Culture Collection (ATCC) (CRL-2873; Manassas, VA, USA). HUVECs were cultured at a density of 5×10^5 cells/mL in Roswell Park Memorial Institute (RPMI) supplemented with 10% fetal bovine serum and 100 U/mL penicillin G and were then incubated at 37 °C in a humidified atmosphere containing 5% CO_2 and 95% air.

2.4. *Measurement of Systolic Blood Pressure*

Systolic blood pressure (SBP) was measured by using the noninvasive tail-cuff plethysmography method and was recorded by using an automatic sphygmomanometer (MK2000; Muromachi Kikai, Tokyo, Japan). The systolic blood pressure (SBP) was measured at Weeks 4, 8, 12, and 16. The blood pressure of 7 mice per group was measured. At least five measurements were obtained at every session, and the mean of the five values within 5 mmHg was taken as the SBP level. Values are presented as the mean $\pm$ SEM of five measurements.

2.5. *Plasma Biochemical Analysis*

Blood glucose was measured from tail vein samples of whole blood using the One-touch ultra-blood glucose meter and a test strip (Life Scan Inc., Milpitas, CA, USA) at every 4 weeks.

Approximately 500 μL of blood samples were collected from the periorbital vein for biochemical analysis per each mouse. Plasma glucose levels were measured using a commercial mouse ELISA kit (Abcam., Cambridge, MA, USA). Total cholesterol (T-cho), low-density lipoprotein-cholesterol (LDL-cho), very low-density lipoprotein-cholesterol (VLDL-cho), and high-density lipoprotein cholesterol (HDL-cho) levels in plasma were measured using commercially available kits (Abcam., Cambridge, MA, USA). Triglyceride (TG) level was measured using a commercial kit (AM157S-K, Asanpharm. Yeongcheon, Korea). The atherogenic index was calculated as follows: (Total cholesterol − HDL cholesterol)/HDL cholesterol [23].

2.6. Preparation of Carotid Artery Samples and Measurement of Vascular Reactivity

The carotid arteries of the mice were rapidly and carefully isolated and placed in cold Kreb's solution of the following composition (mM): NaCl 118, KCl 4.7, $MgSO_4$ 1.1, KH_2PO_4 1.2, $CaCl_2$ 1.5, $NaHCO_3$ 25, glucose 10, and pH 7.4 (Sigma-aldrich, Saint Louis, MO, USA). The carotid arteries were removed from connective tissue and fat and cut into rings of 3 mm lengths. The carotid artery rings were suspended by means of two L-shaped stainless-steel wires inserted into the lumen in a tissue bath containing Kreb's solution at 37 °C and aerated with 95% O_2 and 5% CO_2. The isometric forces of the rings were measured using a Grass FT 03 force displacement transducer connected to a Model 7E polygraph recording system (Grass Technologies, Quincy, MA, USA). In the carotid artery rings of mice, a passive stretch of 1 g was determined to be the optimal tension for maximal responsiveness to phenylephrine (10^{-6} M) (Sigma-aldrich, Saint Louis, MO, USA). The preparations were allowed to equilibrate for approximately 1 h with replacement of Kreb's solution every 10 min. The relaxant effects of acetylcholine (ACh, 10^{-10}–10^{-6} M) and sodium nitroprusside (SNP, 10^{-11}–10^{-7} M) were studied in carotid artery rings constricted with phenylephrine (PE, 10^{-7} M).

2.7. Histopathological Staining of Aorta

Aortic tissues were fixed by using 10% (*v*/*v*) formalin (Junsei Chemical, Tokyo, Japan) in 0.01 M phosphate-buffered saline (PBS) (Gibco, Carlsbad, CA, USA) for 2 days with change of formalin solution every day to remove traces of blood from tissue. The tissue samples were dehydrated and embedded in paraffin (Leica, Wetzlar, Germany), and thin sections (6 μm) of the aortic arch from each group were then cut and stained with hematoxylin and eosin (H&E) (Sigma-Aldrich, St. Louis, MO, USA). For quantitative histopathological comparisons, each section was evaluated by Axiovision 4 Imaging/Archiving software (Axiovision 4, Carl Zeiss, Jena, Germany). Images were analyzed using the ImageJ (NIH, Bethesda, MD, USA) program to select and quantify H&E-stained areas as a fold of the total area of each image.

2.8. Measurement of Atherosclerotic Lesions by Oil Red O Staining

The thoracic/abdominal aorta were stained with Oil Red O to visualize neutral lipid (cholesteryl ester and triglycerides) accumulation. The inner aortic surface was stained with Oil Red O After rinsing with 60% isopropyl alcohol (Amresco, Solon, OH, USA) and distilled water, and images of Oil Red O-stained aortas were obtained with Axiovision 4 Imaging/Archiving software (Axiovision 4, Carl Zeiss, Jena, Germany). Images were analyzed using the ImageJ (NIH, Bethesda, MD, USA) program to select and quantify H&E-stained areas as a fold of the total area of each image.

2.9. Immunofluorescence

Frozen sections for immunofluorescence staining were placed on poly-L-lysine-coated slides (Fisher scientific, Pittsburgh, PA, USA). The slides were incubated with primary antibodies for ICAM-1, VCAM-1, and E-selectin (1:500; Santa Cruz, CA, USA) in humidified chambers for 1 h at room temperature in PBS followed by heat-induced (pressure cooker) sodium citrate antigen retrieval and then exposure to a 1:500 dilution of Alexa Fluor 594 secondary antibody (Life technology, Carlsbad, CA, USA). Finally, the slides were washed three times with PBS and cover slips were mounted with Dako fluorescent mounting medium onto glass slides that were examined under a fluorescence microscope (Nikon Eclipse Ti, Tokyo, Japan).

2.10. *Western Blot Analysis*

Aortic tissue and cell homogenates (protein of 30–50 μg) were separated using 10% SDS-polyacrylamide gel electrophoresis (PAGE) and transferred onto nitrocellulose membranes. Blots were then blocked by 5% Bovine Serum Albumin (BSA) (GenDEPOT, Katy, TX, USA) powder in Tris-bufferd saline (TBS) for 1 h, and incubated with the antibodies against ICAM-1, VCAM-1, E-selectin, MMP-2, MMP-9, eNOS, p-eNOS, Akt, p-AKT, and GTPCH (Santa Cruz Biotechnology, INC, Dallas, TX, USA) (1:1000 dilution in 0.05%TBS-T (Tween 20)). Subsequently, the membrane was then incubated with a secondary antibody of goat anti rabbit IgG or goat anti mouse IgG conjugated to horseradish peroxidase (Enzo Life Sciences, Farmingdale, NY, USA) (1:5000 dilution in 0.05%TBS-T), and the bands were detected with EzWestLumi plus solution (Cat. no. WSE-7120, Atto Corporation) using a ChemiDoc (Bio-Rad Laboratories, Hercules, CA, USA). Densitometry analysis of protein bands was conducted with the ImageJ (NIH, Bethesda, MD, USA) program.

2.11. *RNA Preparation and Quantitative Real-Time Reverse Transcription-PCR (Real-Time RT-qPCR)*

Total RNA was extracted from the aorta using Ribozol reagent (Amresco, Solon, OH, USA) according to the manufacturer's instruction. The RNA quality was assessed by measuring the ratio of 260/280 nm light with a UV-spectrophotometer (Biophotometer plus, Eppendorf, Hambrug, Germany). The cDNA was synthesized from 500 ng mRNA via a 20 μL reverse transcription reaction incubated in the SimpliAmp Thermal Cycler (Life technology, Carlsbad, CA, USA). The sequences of primers and probes were as follows: ICAM-1 (forward: 5′-CTCACCCGTGTACTGGACTC-3′, reverse: 5′-CGCCGGAAAGCTGTAGATGG-3′), VCAM-1 (forward: 5′-ATGCCTGGGAAGATGGTCGTGA-3′, reverse: 5′-TGGAGCTGGTAGACCCTCGCTG-3′), E-selectin (forward: 5′-ATCATCCTGCAACTTCACC-3′, reverse: 5′-ACACCTCACCAAACCCTTC-3′), and Glyceraldehyde 3-phosphate dehydrogenase (GAPDH) (forward: 5′-CAAGGCTGAGAATGGGAAGC-3′, reverse: 5′-AGCATGTGGGAACTCAGATC-3′). The real-time RT-qPCR was carried out with an SYBR Green PCR Master Mix (Enzynomics, Inc., Daejeon, Korea) and performed at an initial denaturation step at 95 °C for 10 min, followed by 40 cycles at 95 °C for 15 s, and finally 60 °C for 60 s in the Step-One™ Real-Time PCR System (Applied Biosystems, Foster City, CA, USA). miR-10a and miR-126 3p were measured by using a hsa-mir-10a Real-Time RT-PCR detection kit (CPK1014) and a hsa-mir-126 3p Real-Time RT-PCR detection kit (CPK1083) (Cohesion Biosciences., London, UK).

2.12. *Measurement of NO Production Using Griess Reagent System*

NO production in the culture supernatant was spectrophotometrically evaluated by measuring nitrite content, an oxidative product of NO. Nitrite levels was determined with the Griess Reagent solution (Promega, Madison, WI, USA) and proceeded according to the description of the manufacturer. The fluorescent intensity was then measured using a spectrofluorometer (Infinite F200 pro, Tecan, Switzerland) at an excitation and emission wavelength of 485 and 535 nm.

2.13. *Fluorescence Microscopy*

To examine intracellular NO generation, the Diaminofluorescein-2 Diacetate (DAF-2DA) (Merck Biosciences, Schwalbach, Germany) was used. In brief, HUVECs were cultured at 6-well plate. The cells were serum-starved for 8 h before incubation with treatments OJS. The HUVECs were then incubated with OJS for 30 min. DAF-2DA was added for the final 30 min of incubation. Reactions were stopped and fixed the cells by using 2% paraformaldehyde for 30 min at room temperature. Coverslips were examined with a fluorescence microscope equipped with an excitation filter (485–535 nm).

2.14. Statistical Analysis

All experiments were repeated at least three times. Statistical analyses were performed using *t*-tests. The results are expressed as mean ± standard error (S.E.), and the data were analyzed using one-way analysis of variance followed by a Student's *t*-test to determine any significant differences. $p < 0.05$ indicated statistical significance.

3. Results

3.1. HPLC Analysis of OJS

The optimized HPLC–PDA method was applied for the simultaneous analysis of 11 marker ingredients in OJS. The 11 marker components were separated within 45 min. A representative three-dimensional HPLC chromatogram is shown in Figure 1. The retention times of albiflorin, paeoniflorin, liquiritin, ferulic acid, nodakenin, naringin, hesperidin, neohesperidin, cinnamaldehyde, glycyrrhizin, and 6-gingerol were 9.31, 10.65, 14.17, 14.96, 16.64, 18.86, 20.02, 21.74, 33.25, 41.42, and 42.34 min, respectively. The correlation coefficient of the calibration curves for the 11 compounds showed good linearity, ≥0.9997. The concentrations of the 11 compounds in lyophilized OJS sample were between 0.15 and 4.52 mg/g. Among these components, hesperidin, a marker compound of Citri unshii Pericarpium, was found to be the main compound in the OJS sample.

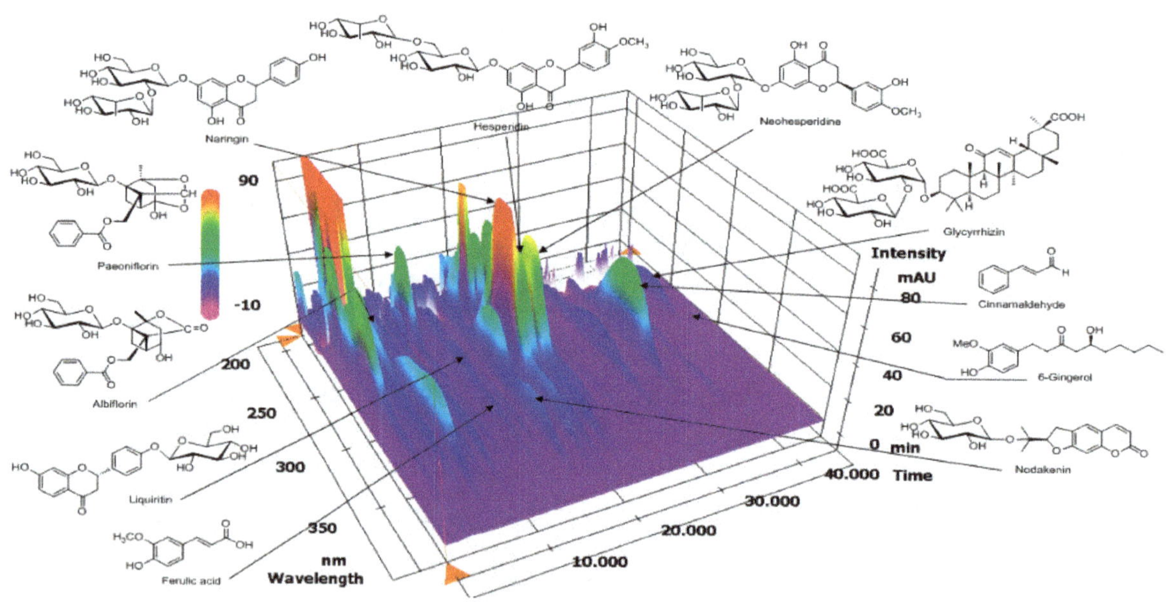

Figure 1. Three-dimensional chromatogram of OJS obtained using a high-performance liquid chromatography-photodiode array (HPLC-PDA).

3.2. The Effect of OJS on Food Intake and Body Weight

There was no significant change in food intake each group. Body weight was significantly increased in the ApoE −/− mice group compared with the control group. The OJS group showed significantly increased body weight compared with the ApoE −/− mice group (Table 3).

3.3. The Effect of OJS on Lipid Parameters in ApoE −/− Mice

ApoE −/− mice group fed a Western diet showed increased levels in plasma triglyceride, total cholesterol, LDL/VLDL-cholesterol levels, and atherogenic index. However, these levels were significantly suppressed by treatment of OJS. The plasma levels of HDL-cholesterol levels also increased compared to those in the disease group by OJS (Table 3).

Table 3. Effect of OJS treatment on plasma biomarker levels in Apolipoprotein-E gene knockout (ApoE −/−) mice.

	Food Intake (g)	Body Weight (g)	T-Cho (mg/dL)	TG (mg/dL)	LDL/VLDL-Cho (mg/dL)	HDL-Cho (mg/dL)	Atherogenic Index
Control	3.90 ± 0.12	29.26 ± 0.92	64.69 ± 2.89	78.71 ± 1.25	27.51 ± 3.31	46.91 ± 1.04	0.38 ± 0.06
ApoE −/−	3.82 ± 0.42	33.62 ± 1.32 **	271.78 ± 9.79 **	122.30 ± 1.90 **	128.58 ± 5.03 **	20.02 ± 1.10 **	12.69 ± 1.12 **
Telmisartan	4.14 ± 0.46	35.68 ± 0.86	100.52 ± 1.12 ##	90.28 ± 1.38 ##	87.20 ± 1.26 ##	32.96 ± 1.82 ##	2.07 ± 1.12 ##
OJS low	3.97 ± 0.07	37.14 ± 0.41	179.55 ± 2.42 ##	104.28 ± 0.76 ##	107.20 ± 0.82 #	22.62 ± 1.70	7.01 ± 0.54 ##
OJS high	3.72 ± 0.23	35.48 ± 1.25 #	122.73 ± 4.84 ##	90.06 ± 1.46 ##	79.43 ± 2.88 ##	30.21 ± 2.23 #	3.11 ± 0.33 ##

The control group (C57BL6 mice + regular diet + Distilled Water (DW)), ApoE −/− group (ApoE −/− + Western diet + DW), telmisartan group (ApoE −/− + Western diet + telmisartan 1 mg/kg/day), OJS low group (ApoE −/− + Western diet + OJS 50 mg/kg/day), OJS high group (ApoE −/− + Western diet + OJS 200 mg/kg/day). ApoE −/−, apolipoprotein E knockout; T-Cho, total cholesterol; TG, triglyceride; LDL/VLDL-Cho, low-density lipoprotein/very low-density lipoprotein-cholesterol; HDL-Cho, high-density lipoprotein-cholesterol. Data are mean ± S.E. values ($n = 12$). (** $p < 0.01$ vs. control and # $p < 0.05$, ## $p < 0.01$ vs. ApoE −/−).

3.4. *Effect of OJS on Vascular Dysfunction in ApoE −/− Mice*

The levels of SBP from all experimental groups were approximately 85–95 mmHg at the starting point of study. After four weeks, systolic blood pressure in the ApoE −/− group was significantly increased relative to that of the control ($p < 0.05$). After 8 weeks, systolic blood pressure in the ApoE −/− group was further increased ($p < 0.01$). However, in the OJS group, blood pressure was significantly decreased relative to that of the ApoE −/− group (Figure 2A). Vascular responses to ACh, an endothelium-dependent vasodilator (10^{-10}–10^{-6} M), and SNP, an endothelium-independent vasodilator (SNP, 10^{-11}–10^{-7} M), were measured in the carotid artery. Responses to ACh-induced relaxation of carotid artery rings were significantly decreased in the disease group compared to that in the control group. However, the impairment in vasorelaxation was remarkably decreased by treatment with OJS. (Figure 2B).

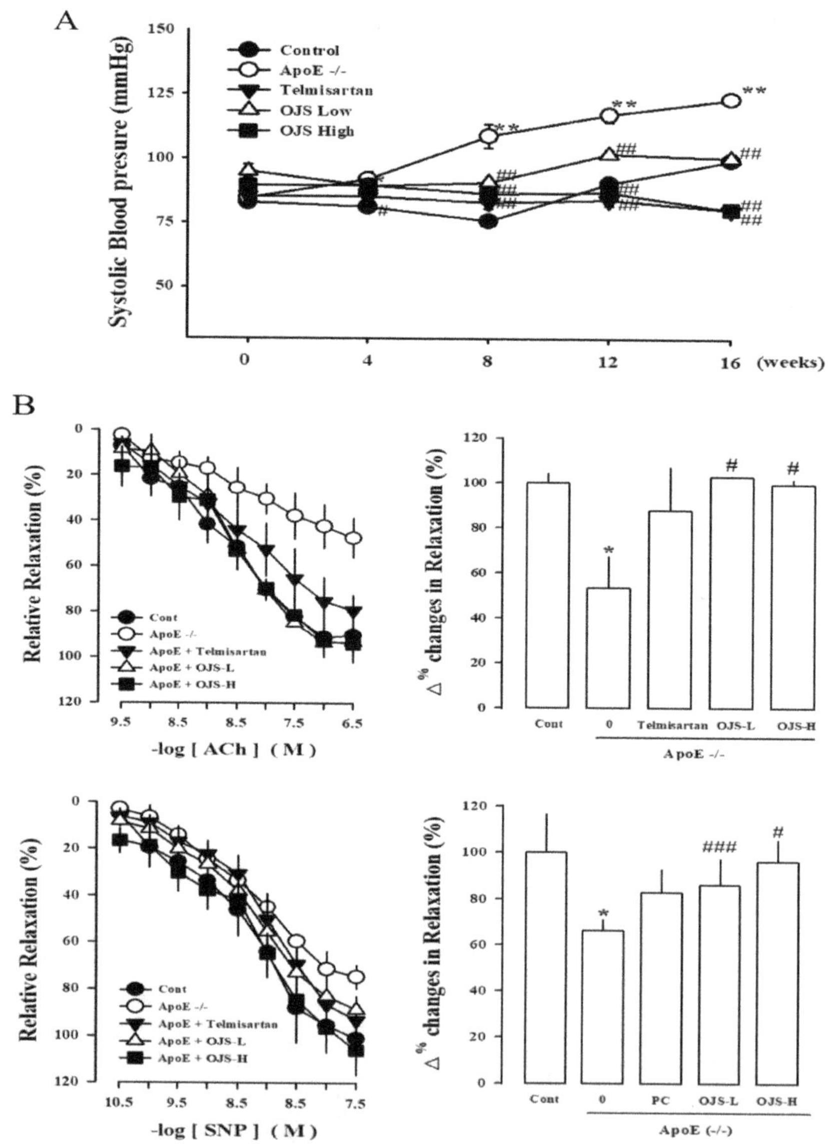

Figure 2. Effect of OJS on vasodilation in Apolipoprotein-E gene knockout (ApoE −/−) mice. The effect of OJS on systolic blood pressure in ApoE −/− mice (**A**). Cumulative concentration–response curves to acetylcholine (ACh) and the endothelium-dependent vasodilator, sodiumnitroprusside (SNP), in the arteries from experiment mice (**B**). PC, positive control; Values are expressed as mean ± S.E. (Standard Error) (n = 5). * $p < 0.05$, ** $p < 0.01$ vs. control group; # $p < 0.05$, ## $p < 0.01$, ### $p < 0.001$ vs. the ApoE −/− group.

3.5. *Effect of OJS on Atherosclerotic Lesions in ApoE −/− Mice*

To investigate the effect of OJS on the morphology of the aorta, histological changes were observed by staining with H&E. Morphological staining showed that aortas of the ApoE −/− group increased in layer thickness, plaques, and inflammatory lesions compared to those of the control group (400×) (Figure 3A). However, OJS decreased the intima-media thickness in aortic sections and the plaque area. In addition, to confirm the inhibitory effects of OJS on lipid accumulation, Oil Red O staining was performed. In the control group, no atherosclerotic lesion in the aorta was detected. In the disease group, most of the lesions, identified as areas that stained red, were found at the aortic sinus; Oil Red O staining analysis demonstrated that aortic atherosclerotic lesions significantly increased in the ApoE −/− group compared with the control group. However, consistent with the change in the lipid profile, treatment with positive control (telmisartan) and OJS significantly inhibited the development of atherosclerosis (Figure 3B).

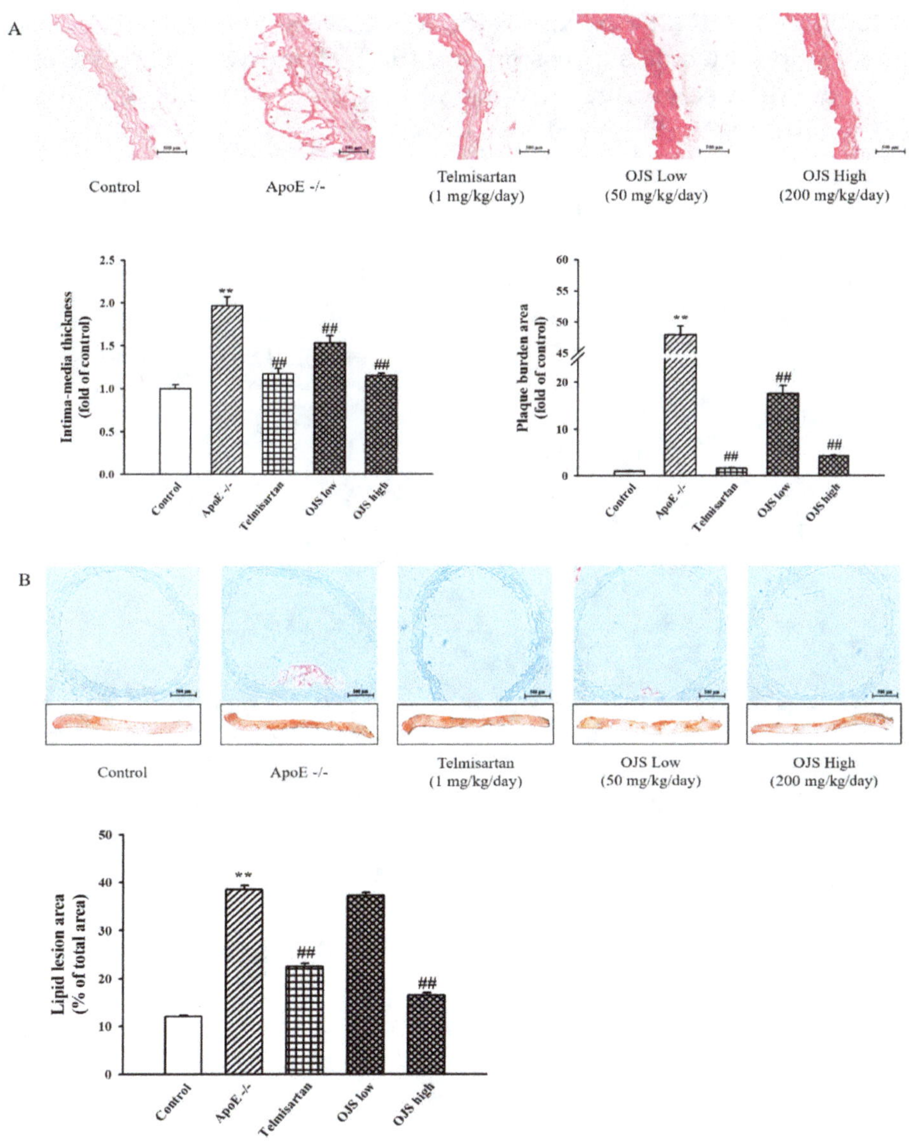

Figure 3. Effect of OJS on atherosclerotic lesion in ApoE −/− mice. Microscopic photographs of the aorta stained with hematoxylin and eosin (H&E) (**A**). Lipid lesion area staining in the aorta (100×). Thoracic and abdominal aorta from the indicated genotype were cut open with the luminal surface facing upward, and the inner aortic surface was stained with Oil Red O (**B**). Data are presented as means ± S.E. ** $p < 0.01$ vs. control group; ## $p < 0.01$ vs. ApoE −/− group.

3.6. *Effect of OJS on Vascular Inflammation in ApoE −/− Mice*

Immunofluorescence was performed to determine the direct expression of adhesion molecules in the aortic wall. Expression of adhesion molecules such as ICAM-1, VCAM-1, and E-selectin increased in the disease group compared to that of the control. However, treatment with OJS significantly decreased the expression levels of ICAM-1, VCAM-1, and E-selectin (Figure 4A). The OJS group had significantly decreased levels of ICAM-1, VCAM-1, and E-selectin proteins compared to those of the ApoE −/− group (Figure 4B). The expression of MMP-2/-9 was increased in the ApoE −/− group (Figure 5A). Treatment with OJS also significantly decreased the expression levels of MMPs. Protein levels of MMP2/9 were increased in the disease group compared to those in the control group. Treatment with OJS significantly decreased the expression levels of MMP proteins compared to those in the disease group (Figure 5B). In Figure 6A, mRNA expression levels of ICAM-1, VCAM-1, and E-selectin were increased in the ApoE −/− group compared to the control group. OJS significantly suppressed mRNA expression levels. To confirm the effect of OJS on the mRNA expression of adhesion molecules in greater detail, miR10a and miR126-3p expression levels were determined. These microRNAs are known to regulate adhesion molecule expression and the IκB pathway. The expression levels for the miRNAs decreased in the disease group. However, treatment with OJS significantly increased the expression levels of these miRNAs (Figure 6B).

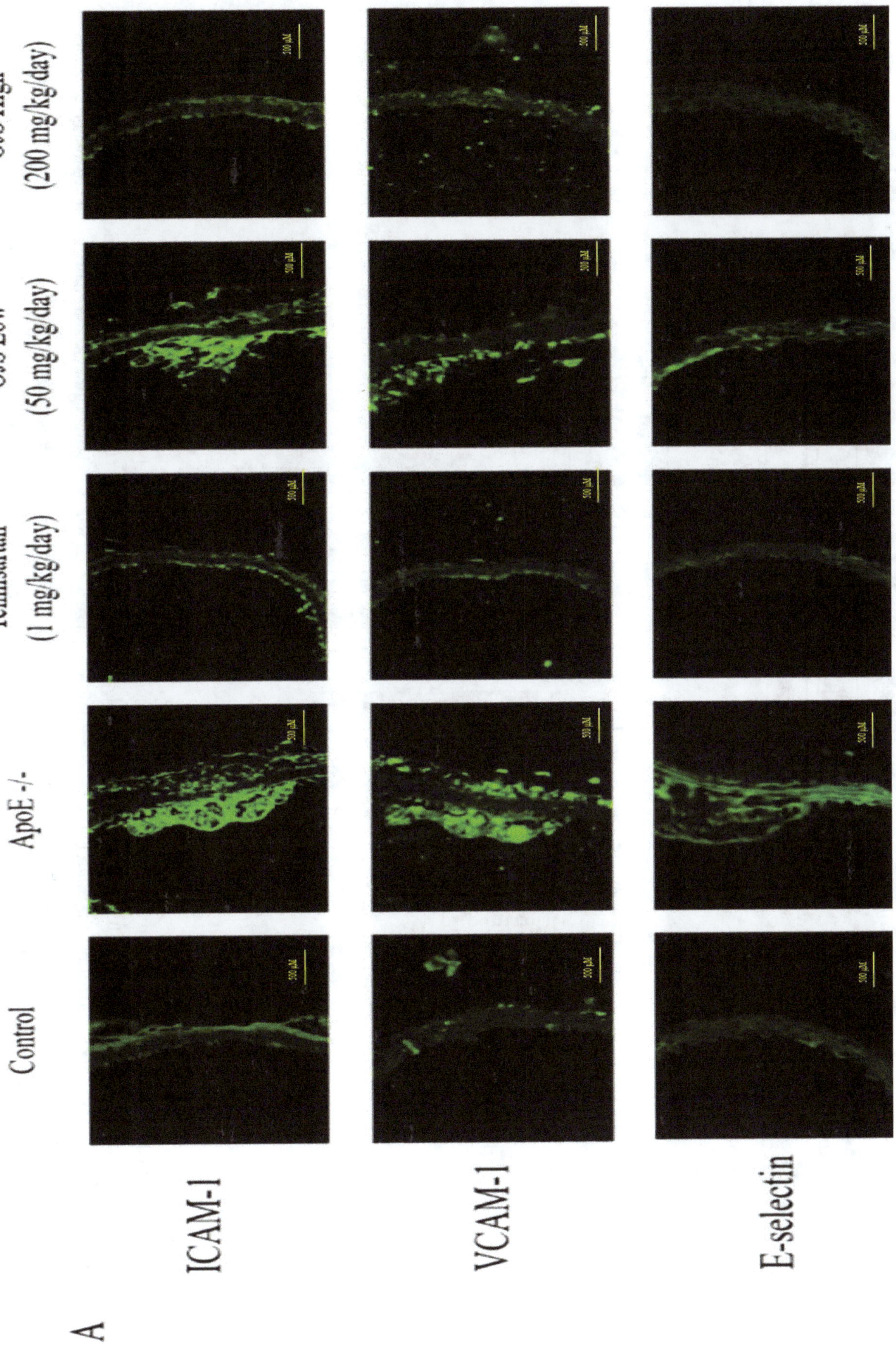

Figure 4. *Cont.*

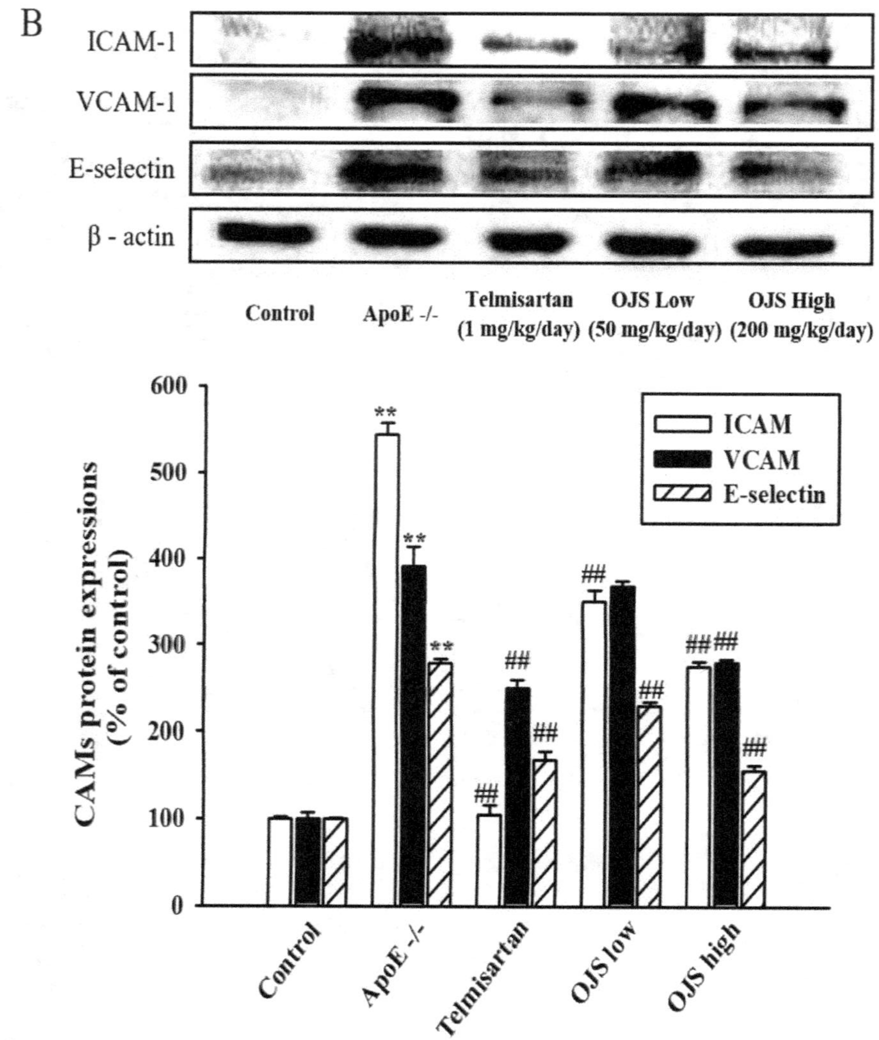

Figure 4. Effects of OJS on intracellular adhesion molecule-1 (ICAM-1), vascular cell adhesion molecule-1 (VCAM-1), and endothelial cell selectin (E-selectin) expression in the aortas of ApoE −/− mice (**A**). ICAM-1, VCAM-1, and E-selectin immunofluorescence in the aortas of ApoE −/− mice. Immunofluorescence staining of adhesion molecules in the aortas from the control, ApoE −/−, ApoE −/− mice treated with telmisartan groups, and ApoE −/− mice treated with OJS at low or high concentrations. Protein levels of the adhesion molecules determined by Western blot analysis (**B**). Data are presented as means ± S.E. ** $p < 0.01$ vs. control group; ## $p < 0.01$ vs. ApoE −/− group.

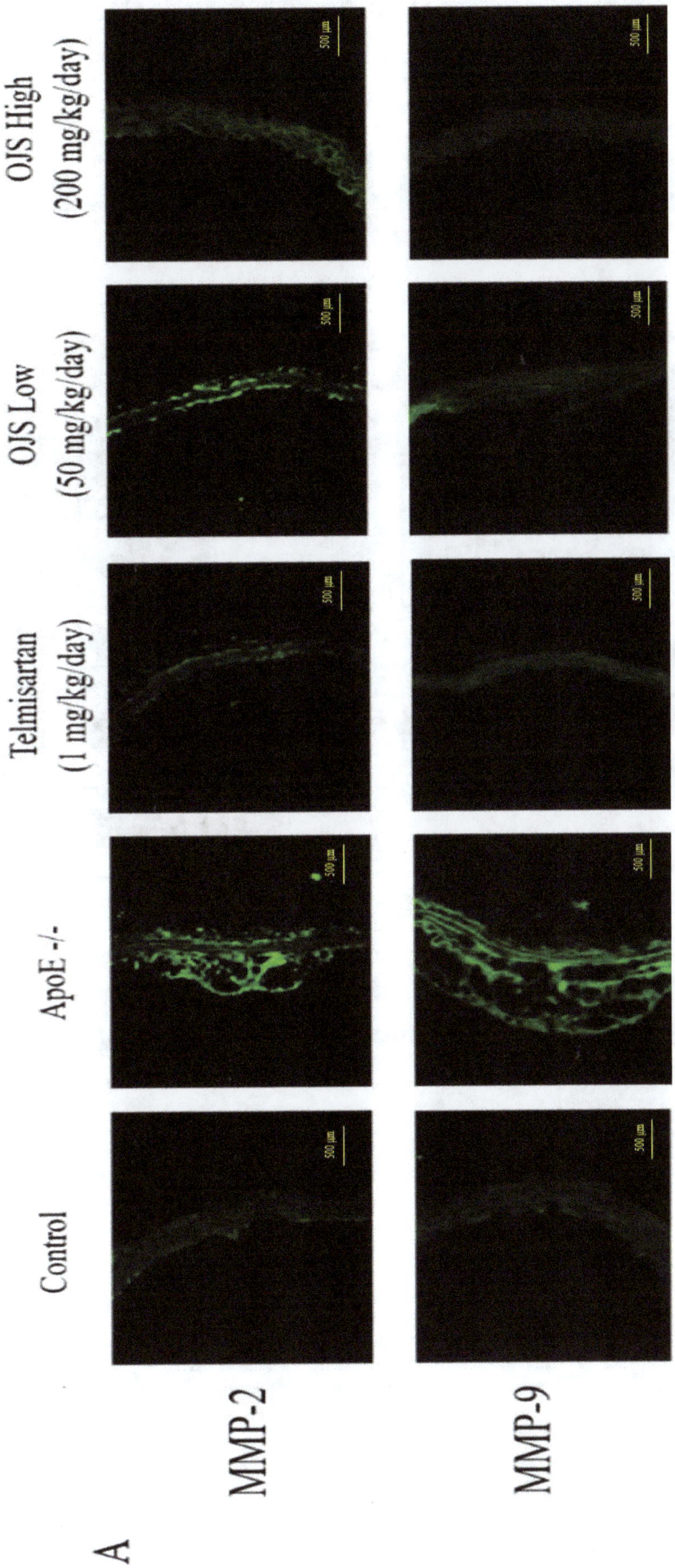

Figure 5. *Cont.*

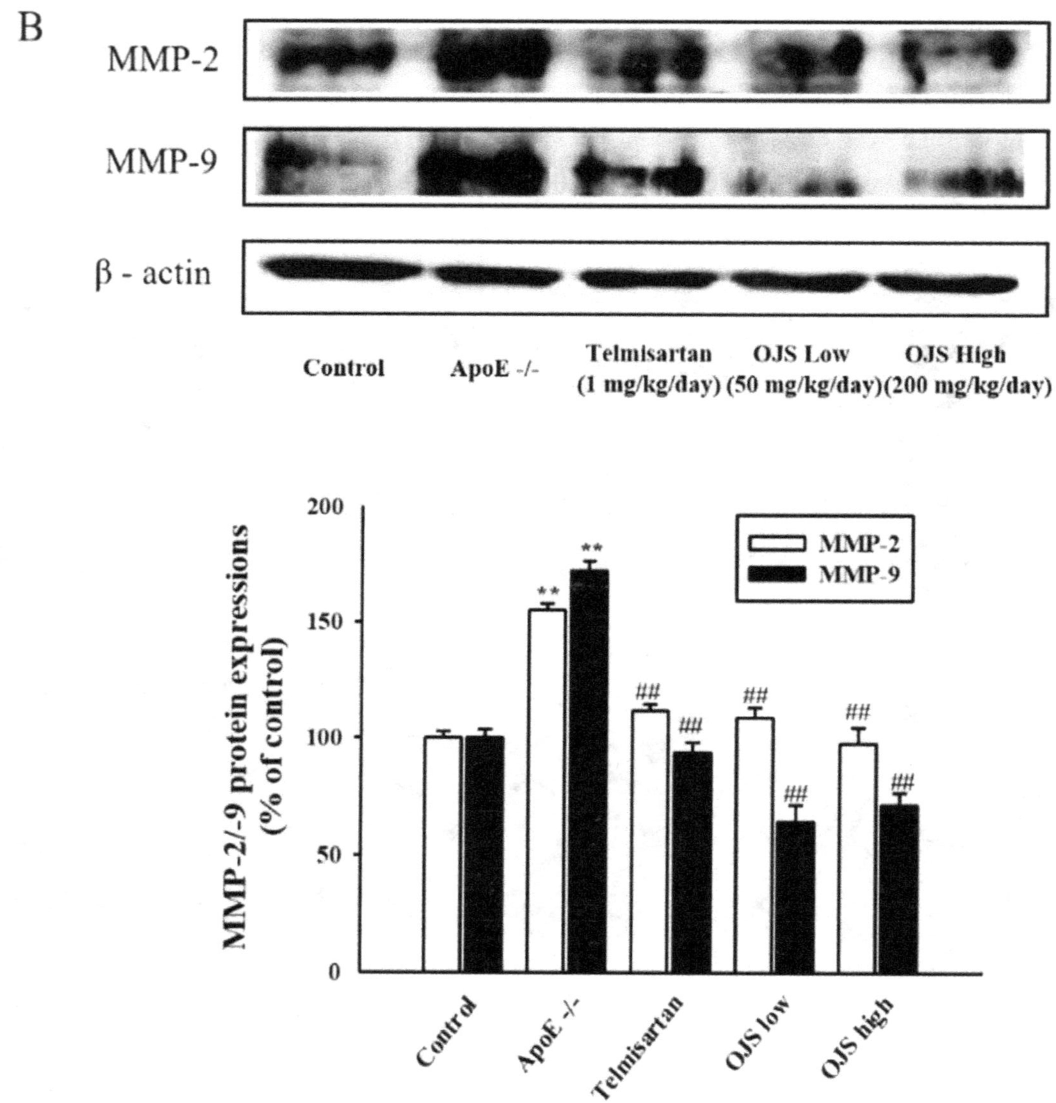

Figure 5. Effects of OJS on matrix metalloproteinases (MMP)-2/-9 expression in the aorta of ApoE −/− mice. MMP2, and MMP-9 immunofluorescence in the aorta of ApoE −/− mice (**A**). Immunofluorescence staining of MMP-2/-9 in the aorta from the control, ApoE −/−, and ApoE −/− mice treated with telmisartan groups and ApoE −/− mice treated with OJS at low or high concentrations. Protein levels of MMPs determined by Western blot analysis (**B**). Data are presented as means ± S.E. ** $p < 0.01$ vs. control group; ## $p < 0.01$ vs. ApoE −/− group.

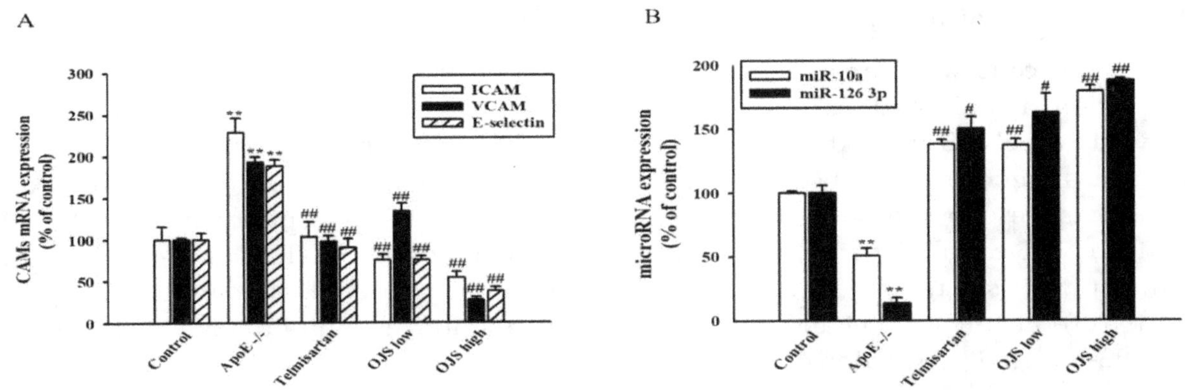

Figure 6. Effects of OJS on miR-10a and miR-126 3p expression in the aorta of ApoE −/− mice. mRNA expression of adhesion molecules determined by real-time Reverse Transcription-PCR (RT-qPCR) analysis (**A**). Levels of miRNA determined by real-time RT-qPCR (**B**). Data are presented as means ± S.E. ** $p < 0.01$ vs. control group; # $p < 0.05$, ## $p < 0.01$ vs. ApoE −/− group.

3.7. *Effects of OJS on TNF-α-Induced Adhesion Molecules and MMPs Expression in HUVECs*

Treatment of OJS significantly inhibited the TNF-α-induced expression of ICAM-1, VCAM-1, and E-selectin ($p < 0.05$) (Figure 7A). Western blot analysis of cell lysates was used to confirm the effect of OJS on the expression of MMP-2/9 proteins in HUVECs. Pretreatment with OJS inhibited TNF-α-induced MMP2/9 protein expression (Figure 7B).

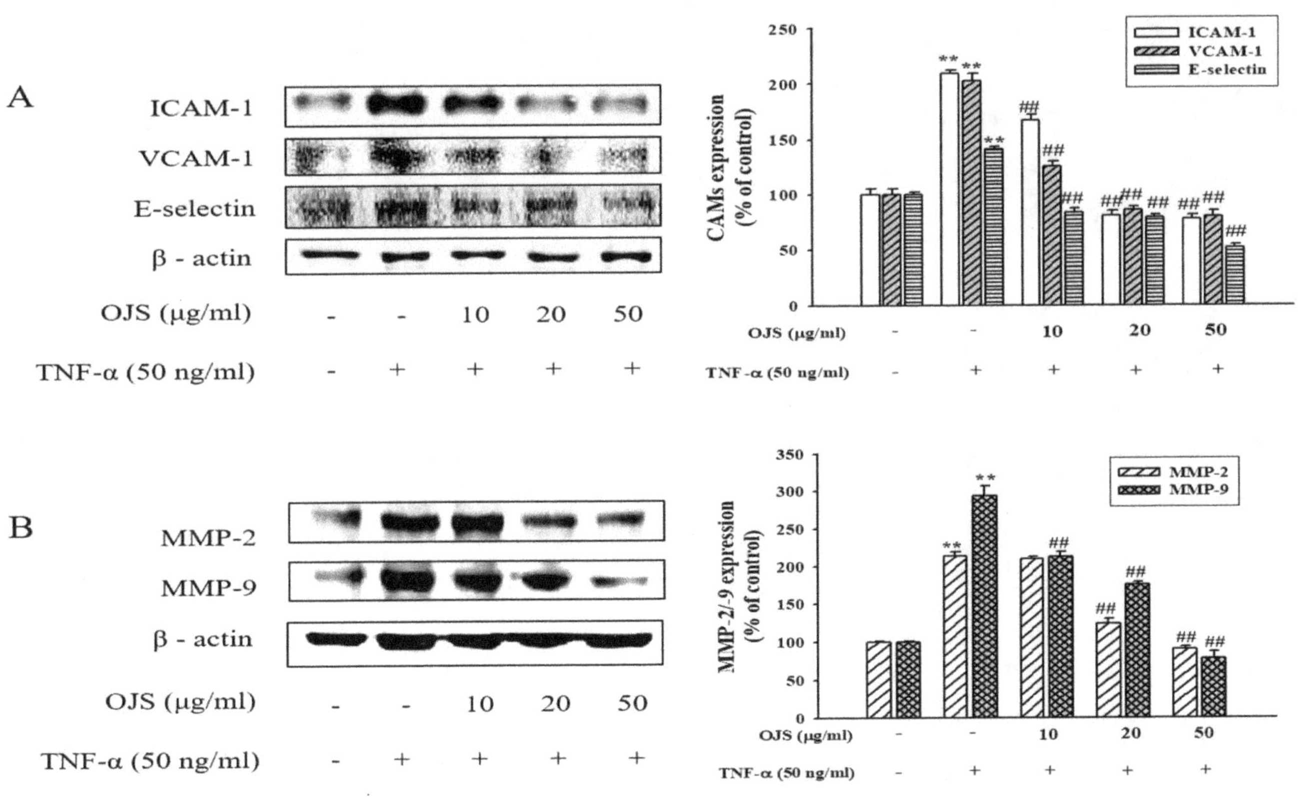

Figure 7. Effects of OJS on TNF-α-induced protein expressions of cell adhesion molecule and MMPs expression. Western blot analysis of ICAM-1, VCAM-1, and E-selectin expression. The blots are representative of three independent experiments and densitometric quantification of ICAM-1, VCAM-1, and E-selectin (**A**). Western blot analysis of MMP-2/-9 whole protein (**B**). Data are presented as means ± S.E. ** $p < 0.01$ vs. control; ## $p < 0.01$ vs. TNF-α alone.

3.8. OJS Regulates the Akt/eNOS-NO Pathway in HUVECs

Endothelial cells were treated with different doses of OJS for 30 min, and the degree of phosphorylation of eNOS and Akt was determined by Western blot analysis. As shown in Figure 8A, phosphorylation of eNOS and Akt increased following treatment with OJS in a dose-dependent manner. There were no significant differences in eNOS and Akt expression. OJS also increased the expression of GTPCH. These results suggest that OJS stimulates eNOS and Akt phosphorylation in HUVECs and regulates the eNOS coupling pathway by increasing the expression of GTPCH. Figure 8B shows that OJS treatment increased the production of NO in HUVECs in a dose-dependent manner. In addition, L-NAME (N(ω)-nitro-L-arginine methyl ester) and wortmannin as inhibitors of eNOS and Akt each inhibited OJS-induced production of NO (Figure 8C).

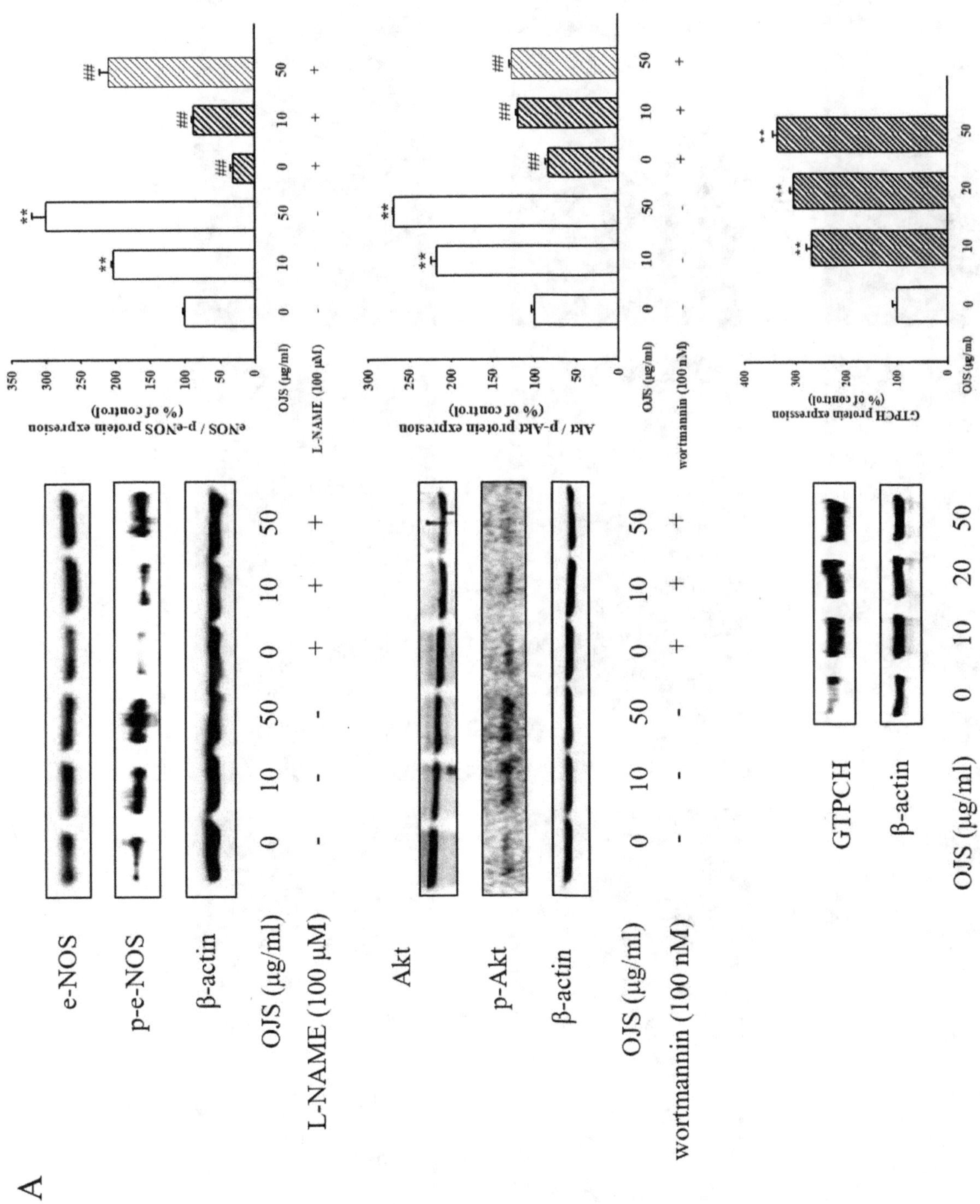

Figure 8. *Cont.*

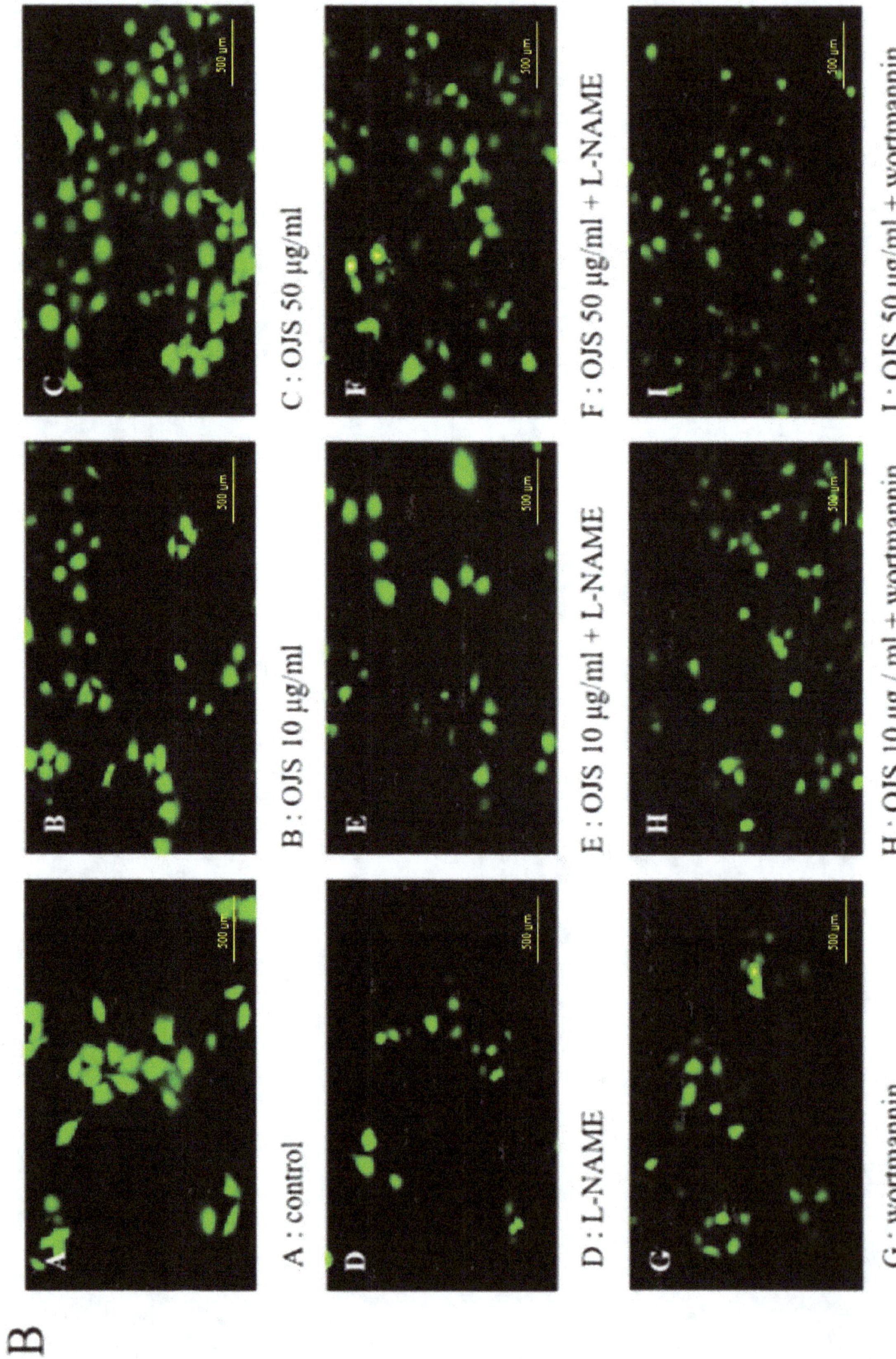

Figure 8. *Cont.*

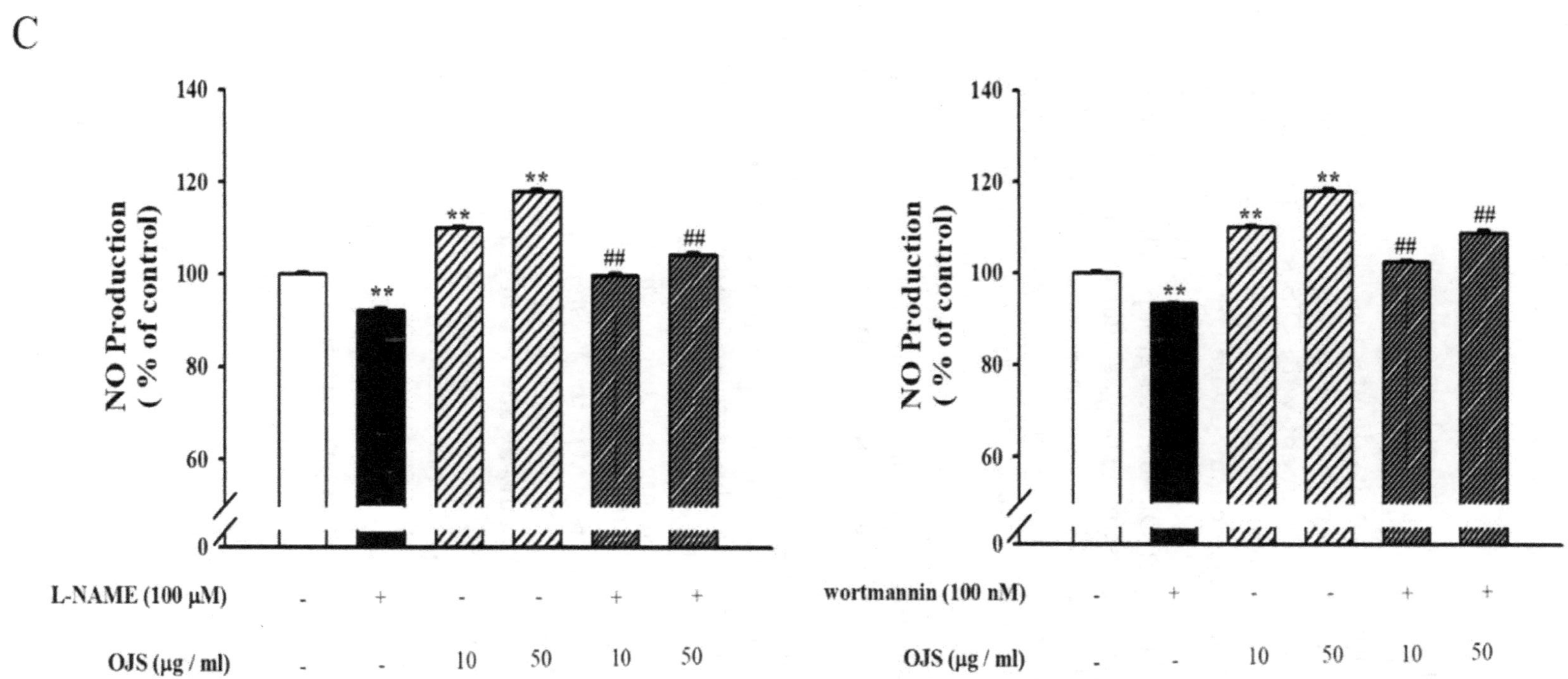

Figure 8. Effects of OJS on nitrite production. Protein expression of phosphorylated endothelial nitric oxide synthase (eNOS), phosphorylated protein kinase B (Akt), and GTP cyclohydrolase-1 (GTPCH) were analyzed by Western blotting (**A**). NO production was examined via fluorescence microscopy (original magnification ×100) (**B**). The effect of OJS on NO production was assayed as its stable reaction product nitrite by using the Griess reaction (**C**). Data are presented as means ± S.E. ** $p < 0.01$ vs. control, ## $p < 0.01$ vs. OJS treatment. L-NAME, N(G)-nitro-L-arginine methyl ester.

4. Discussion

OJS has been used to treat circulation disadvantage of qi (氣), blood (血), food (食), cold (寒), and congestion (痰). However, there are no reports regarding the protective effect of OJS against blood circulation disorders such as cardiovascular diseases. Here, we are the first to provide evidence indicating that OJS has an anti-atherogenic effect, improving vascular dysfunction in endothelial cells and Western-diet-fed ApoE −/− mice.

OJS has an effect on plasma HDL-cholesterol levels, which is related to cardiovascular disease. HDL can remove cholesterol from macrophage foam cells and suppresses atherosclerotic lesions [24]. Triglycerides are an important biomarker of cardiovascular disease. In this study, blood glucose, systolic blood pressure, and lipid parameter levels were measured, and these levels were increased in Western-diet-fed ApoE −/− mice. Treatment with OJS significantly reversed these changes. These findings demonstrate that OJS may elicit a protective role against the initiation and development of atherosclerosis by improving lipid metabolism. Overall, the ApoE −/− groups (WTD-fed group) were found to weigh more than the control group (RD-fed group). However, it is confirmed that there is no change in the body weight of OJS-treated group. The endothelium can sense changes or abnormalities in blood flow and pressure. The vascular endothelium also plays an important role in the modulation of vascular tone [25]. From these results, it is clear that the mean SBP was higher in the ApoE −/− group. However, treatment with telmisartan, both low and high dosages of OJS, significantly decreased mean SBP. This study also evaluated the effects of OJS on histological changes by examining the aorta using oil red O and H&E staining. Our results indicate that OJS administration significantly resolved atherosclerotic plaque formation in the aorta. In addition, the ApoE −/− group also showed endothelial dysfunction, as evidenced by decreases in ACh- and SNP-induced vascular tone. These findings suggest that the hypotensive effect of OJS is mediated by an endothelium-dependent NO/cGMP pathway.

The present study revealed that OJS can regulate the early and advanced stages of atherosclerotic process, which are linked closely the inflammatory response of blood vessels to injury caused by atherosclerotic plaques, which can lead to cardiovascular diseases [26]. miR-126 has been reported to reduce the expression of ICAM-1, VCAM-1, and E-selectin by directly targeting the 3′ untranslated region (3′UTR) of these genes [6,7]. miR-10a targeted two proteins MAP3K7 (TAK1) that regulate IκB degradation [8]. Therefore, the expression of miR-10a and miR-126 3p were investigated. The results showed that the expression levels were decreased in the Western-diet-fed ApoE −/− mice. However, OJS increased the expression of these miRNAs. Therefore, these results suggest that OJS has an inhibitory effect on the adhesion molecule pathway and IκB degradation by regulating the expression of miRNA. MMPs also damage the vascular extracellular matrix, resulting in weakening and dilatation of the aortic wall, which is a hallmark of vascular inflammation [27]. Therefore, the inhibition of MMP2/9 could be beneficial in the treatment of atherosclerosis. The results of immunofluorescence and Western blot analysis revealed that pretreatment with OJS suppressed the expression of MMP2/9. These results indicate that OJS has an inhibitory effect on MMP-2 and MMP-9 expression levels in ApoE −/− mice.

Cytokines-induced adhesion molecules such as ICAM-1, VCAM-1, and E-selectin are well known inflammatory markers [28]. Therefore, the present study was examined whether OJS has an inhibitory effect on TNF-α-stimulated HUVECs by inhibiting the protein expression of adhesion molecules. The results suggested that OJS has an inhibitory effect on TNF-α-induced vascular inflammation in endothelial cells by suppressing the expression of those adhesion molecules. Endothelial dysfunction, characterized by decreased production of NO, is an early and key mediator that links obesity and cardiovascular diseases [29]. Akt downstream of PI3K, is also thought to be an important factor for cell survival. In endothelial cells, Akt activation has been reported to promote cell survival [14]. Importantly, several clinical studies have demonstrated the beneficial effects of BH4, which is a required cofactor for the synthesis of NO, in patients with cardiovascular risk factors, such as hypercholesterolemia, smoking, hypertension, and diabetes or coronary artery disease [30].

Furthermore, endothelial cell BH4 synthesis by GTPCH is necessary for physiological eNOS function, and previous studies of BH4 biosynthesis have used systemic pharmacological inhibitors of GTPCH [31]. Data from the current study indicate that OJS promoted NO production. This study also examined the role of the PI3K/Akt pathway and phosphorylation of eNOS in the anti-inflammatory effect of OJS. eNOS and Akt phosphorylation were also increased by OJS. These results provide strong evidence that OJS elicits an anti-inflammatory effect via the PI3K/Akt-dependent eNOS pathway. In addition, eNOS coupling is a well-known defense mechanism against vascular disease via regulation of NO production [32]. The expression of the principal factor that regulates eNOS coupling, GTPCH, was increased by OJS. This result indicates that OJS plays a protective role in vascular dysfunction by regulating eNOS coupling. Therefore, further studies on the effect of OJS on expression of BH4 in HUVEC should be performed. There is a previous study to confirm the improvement of OJS in liver inflammation [19], and the present study similarly confirmed the improvement of atherosclerosis in OJS by suppressing the expression of atherogenic and inflammatory factors. Therefore, further studies to determine which of the 17 components in OJS have the effect of relieving atherosclerosis are also needed.

5. Conclusions

OJS treatment markedly lowered vascular dysfunction and inflammatory processes. OJS treatment not only ameliorated impairment of vascular dysfunction and metabolic abnormalities but also markedly lowered blood pressure, as well as vascular inflammatory processes in ApoE KO mice and HUVECs (Figure 9). To the best of our knowledge, these findings provide the first evidence to support the therapeutic efficacy of OJS in preventing the development of both early and advanced atherosclerosis.

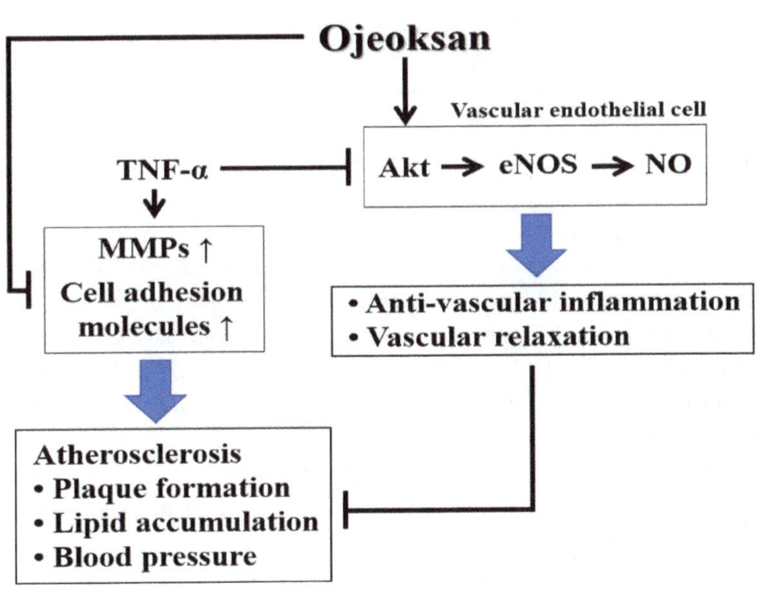

Figure 9. Schematic diagram of the effects of OJS in atherosclerosis.

Author Contributions: B.H.H. and Y.J.L. conceived and planned the experiments. C.S.S. and H.K.S. contributed to sample validation. J.J.Y., H.Y.K., Y.M.A., S.Y.E., M.H.H., and J.G.L. performed the experiments. H.S.L. and D.G.K. contributed interpreted the results. All the authors discussed the results and contributed to the final version of the manuscript.

Acknowledgments: This study was supported by a National Research Foundation of Korea (NRF) Grant funded by the Korean government (MSIP) (2017R1A5A2015805) (2017R1D1A3B03029089).

References

1. Tedgui, A.; Mallat, Z. Cytokines in atherosclerosis: Pathogenic and regulatory pathways. *Physiol. Rev.* **2006**, *86*, 515–581. [CrossRef] [PubMed]
2. Libby, P. Inflammation in atherosclerosis. *Arterioscler. Thrombosi Vasc. Biol.* **2012**, *32*, 2045–2051. [CrossRef] [PubMed]
3. Egan, B.E.; Greene, L.; Goodfriend, T.L. Insulin resistance and ardiovascular disease. *Am. J. Hypertens.* **2001**, *14*, 116–125. [CrossRef]
4. Blankenberg, S.; Barbaux, S.; Tiret, L. Adhesion molecules and atherosclerosis. *Atherosclerosis* **2003**, *170*, 191–203. [CrossRef]
5. Sana, T.R.; Janatpour, M.J.; Sathe, M.; McEvoy, L.M.; McClanahan, T.K. Microarray analysis of primary endothelial cells challenged with different inflammatory and immune cytokines. *Cytokine* **2005**, *29*, 256–269. [CrossRef] [PubMed]
6. Suarez, Y.; Wang, C.; Manes, T.D.; Pober, J.S. Cutting edge: TNF-induced micrornas regulate TNF-induced expression of e-selectin and intercellular adhesion molecule-1 on human endothelial cells: Feedback control of inflammation. *J. Immunol.* **2010**, *184*, 21–25. [CrossRef] [PubMed]
7. Harris, T.A.; Yamakuchi, M.; Ferlito, M.; Mendell, J.T.; Lowenstein, C.J. Microrna-126 regulates endothelial expression of vascular cell adhesion molecule 1. *Proc. Natl. Acad. Sci. USA* **2008**, *105*, 1516–1521. [CrossRef] [PubMed]
8. Fang, Y.; Shi, C.; Manduchi, E.; Civelek, M.; Davies, P.F. Microrna-10a regulation of proinflammatory phenotype in athero-susceptible endothelium in vivo and in vitro. *Proc. Natl. Acad. Sci. USA* **2010**, *107*, 13450–13455. [CrossRef] [PubMed]
9. Brownlee, M. Biochemistry and molecular cell biology of diabetic complications. *Nature* **2001**, *65*, 813–820. [CrossRef] [PubMed]
10. Ho, F.M.; Liu, S.H.; Lin, W.W.; Liau, C.S. Opposite effects of high glucose on MMP-2 and TMIP-2 in human endothelial cells. *J. Cell. Biochem.* **2007**, *101*, 442–450. [CrossRef] [PubMed]
11. Thomas, P.V.; Shahnaz, R.; Diana, N.; Shipeng, Y.; Srikanth, G.; Suresh, C.T. Matrix metalloproteinases in atherosclerosis: Role of nitric oxide, hydrogen sulfide, homocysteine, and polymorphisms. *Vasc. Health Risk Manag.* **2015**, *11*, 173–183.
12. Mariotto, S.; Menegazzi, M.; Suzuki, H. Biochemical aspects of nitric oxide. *Curr. Pharm. Des.* **2004**, *10*, 1627–1645. [CrossRef] [PubMed]
13. Colasanti, M.; Persichini, T. Nitric oside: An inhibitor of NF-kappaB/rel system in glial cells. *Brain Res. Bull.* **2000**, *10*, 1627–1645.
14. Susanne, K.; Philip, W.; Ari, W.; Thomas, M.; Andreas, D. eNOS uncoupling in cardiovascular disease–the role of oxidative stress and inflammation. *Curr. Pharm. Des.* **2014**, *20*, 3576–3594.
15. Mark, J.C.; Ashley, B.H.; Keith, M.C. Dihydrofolate reductase protects endothelial nitric oxide synthase from uncoupling in tetrahydrobiopterin deficiency. *Free Radic. Biol. Med.* **2011**, *50*, 1639–1646.
16. Fulton, D.; Gratton, J.P.; McCabe, T.J.; Fontana, J.; Fujio, Y.; Walsh, K.; Franke, T.F.; Papapetropoulos, A.; Sessa, W.C. Regulation of endothelium-derived nitric oxide production by the protein kinase Akt. *Nature* **1999**, *399*, 597–601. [CrossRef] [PubMed]
17. Emmanouil, C.; Elisabeth, D.; Corinna, H.; Ulrich, F.M.; Andreas, M.Z.; Stefanie, D. Oxidized LDL Inhibits Vascular Endothelial Growth Factor–Induced Endothelial Cell Migration by an Inhibitory Effect on the Akt/Endothelial Nitric Oxide Synthase Pathway. *Circulation* **2001**, *103*, 2102–2107.
18. National Health Insurance Corporation, Health Insurance Review & Assessment Service. *2010 National Health Insurance Statistical Yearbook*; National Health Insurance Corporation, Health Insurance Review & Assessment Service: Seoul, Korea, 2011; pp. 300–301.
19. Lee, S.Y.; Park, W.H.; Cha, Y.Y.; Lee, E. Effects of Ojeoksangamibang Extract on the Recovery of Liver Function in CCl4-exposed Rats. *J. Korean Med. Rehabil.* **2013**, *23*, 45–53.
20. Nakashima, Y.; Plump, A.S.; Raines, E.W.; Breslow, J.L.; Ross, R. ApoE-deficient mice develop lesions of all phases of atherosclerosis throughout the arterial tree. *Arterioscler. Thrombosi Vasc. Biol.* **1994**, *14*, 133–140. [CrossRef]

21. Fukuda, D.; Enomoto, S.; Hirata, Y.; Nagai, R.; Sata, M. The angiotensin receptor blocker, telmisartan, reduces and stabilizes atherosclerosis in ApoE and AT1aR double deficient mice. *Biomed. Pharmacother.* **2010**, *64*, 712–717. [CrossRef] [PubMed]
22. Angeli, V.; Llodra, J.; Rong, J.X.; Satoh, K.; Ishii, S.; Shimizu, T.; Fisher, E.A.; Randolph, G.J. Dyslipidemia associated with atherosclerotic disease systemically alters dendritic cell mobilization. *Immunity* **2004**, *21*, 561–574. [CrossRef] [PubMed]
23. Lauer, R.M.; Lee, J.; Clarke, W.R. Factors Affecting the Relationship between Childhood and Adult Cholesterol Levels: The Muscatine Study. *Pediatrics* **1988**, *8*, 309–321.
24. Tall, A.R. Cholesterol efflux pathways and other potential mechanisms involved in the athero-protective effect of high density lipoproteins. *J. Intern. Med.* **2008**, *263*, 256–273. [CrossRef] [PubMed]
25. Voelkel, N.F.; Tuder, R.M. Hypoxia-induced pulmonary vascular remodeling: A model for what human disease. *J. Clin. Investig.* **2000**, *106*, 733–738. [CrossRef] [PubMed]
26. Choi, J.H.; Jeong, T.S.; Kim, D.Y.; Kim, Y.M.; Na, H.J.; Nam, K.H.; Lee, S.B.; Kim, H.C.; Oh, S.R.; Choi, Y.K.; et al. Hematein inhibits atherosclerosis by inhibition of reactive oxygen generation and NF-κB-dependent inflammatory mediators in hyperlipidemic mice. *J. Cardiovasc. Pharmacol.* **2003**, *42*, 287–295. [CrossRef] [PubMed]
27. Kaneko, H.; Anzai, T.; Morisawa, M. Resveratrol prevents the development of abdominal aortic aneurysm through attenuation of inflammation, oxidative stress, and neovascularization. *Atherosclerosis* **2011**, *217*, 350–357. [CrossRef] [PubMed]
28. Tuttolomondo, A.; Pecoraro, R.; Pinto, A. Studies of selective TNF inhibitors in the treatment of brain injury from stroke and trauma: A review of the evidence to date. *Drug Des. Dev. Ther.* **2014**, *7*, 2221–2238. [CrossRef] [PubMed]
29. Diamant, M.; Tushuizen, M.E. The metabolic syndrome and endothelial dysfunction: Common highway to type 2 diabetes and CVD. *Curr. Diab. Rep.* **2006**, *6*, 279–286. [CrossRef] [PubMed]
30. Stroes, E.; Kastelein, J.; Cosentino, F. Tetrahydrobiopterin restores endothelial function in hypercholesterolemia. *J. Clin. Investig.* **1997**, *99*, 41–46. [CrossRef] [PubMed]
31. Chuaiphichai, S.; McNeill, E.; Douglas, G.; Crabtree, J.M.; Bendall, K.J.; Hale, A.B.; Alp, J.N.; Channon, M.K. Cell autonomous role of endothelial GTP Cyclohydrolase 1 and tetrahydrobiopterin in blood pressure regulation. *Hypertension* **2014**, *64*, 530–540. [CrossRef] [PubMed]
32. Mark, J.C.; Amy, L.T.; Yasir, A.; Nicholas, W.; Ashley, B.H.; Shijie, C.; Keith, M.C.; Nicholas, J.A. Quantitative regulation of intracellular indothelial nitric-oxide synthase (eNOS) coupling by both tetrahydrobiopterin-eNOS stoichiometry and biopterin redox status insights from cells with the-regulated GTP cyclohydrolase I expression. *J. Biol. Chem.* **2008**, *284*, 1134–1144.

6

The Effect of Electrolytes on Blood Pressure

Sehar Iqbal, Norbert Klammer and Cem Ekmekcioglu *

Department of Environmental Health, Center for Public Health, Medical University Vienna, Kinderspitalgasse 15, 1090 Vienna, Austria; n1637166@students.meduniwien.ac.at (S.I.); norbert.klammer@meduniwien.ac.at (N.K.)

* Correspondence: cem.ekmekcioglu@meduniwien.ac.at

Abstract: Nutrition is known to exert an undeniable impact on blood pressure with especially salt (sodium chloride), but also potassium, playing a prominent role. The aim of this review was to summarize meta-analyses studying the effect of different electrolytes on blood pressure or risk for hypertension, respectively. Overall, 32 meta-analyses evaluating the effect of sodium, potassium, calcium and magnesium on human blood pressure or hypertension risk were included after literature search. Most of the meta-analyses showed beneficial blood pressure lowering effects with the extent of systolic blood pressure reduction ranging between −0.7 (95% confidence interval: −2.6 to 1.2) to −8.9 (−14.1 to −3.7) mmHg for sodium/salt reduction, −3.5 (−5.2 to −1.8) to −9.5 (−10.8 to −8.1) mmHg for potassium, and −0.2 (−0.4 to −0.03) to −18.7 (−22.5 to −15.0) mmHg for magnesium. The range for diastolic blood pressure reduction was 0.03 (−0.4 to 0.4) to −5.9 (−9.7 to −2.1) mmHg for sodium/salt reduction, −2 (−3.1 to −0.9) to −6.4 (−7.3 to −5.6) mmHg for potassium, and −0.3 (−0.5 to −0.03) to −10.9 (−13.1 to −8.7) mmHg for magnesium. Moreover, sufficient calcium intake was found to reduce the risk of gestational hypertension.

Keywords: sodium; potassium; calcium; magnesium; electrolytes; blood pressure; hypertension; meta-analysis

---

1. Introduction

Hypertension is the major leading risk factor for atherosclerosis and several diseases, especially renal and cardiovascular disorders, including myocardial infarction, stroke, and heart failure [1]. Blood pressure is influenced by various genetic and lifestyle factors including nutrition [2]. In this regard, sodium is an important mineral which, besides its functions in fluid balance, action potential generation, digestive secretions and absorption of many nutrients, also plays an important role in blood pressure regulation with a reduced sodium intake being associated with a reduction in systolic and diastolic blood pressure [3]. Therefore, independent of body weight, sex and age, too much dietary salt (sodium chloride) is regarded as an established risk factor for hypertension [4]. Concomitant to sodium reduction, higher potassium intake or supplementation has also been repeatedly shown to reduce the blood pressure of especially hypertensive persons (reviewed in [5]). Therefore, the American Heart Association recently proposed a dietary potassium intake of 3500–5000 mg/day, in addition to the well-known advice to reduce the consumption of dietary sodium (<1500 mg/day or at least 1000 mg/day decrement) for adults with normal and elevated blood pressure [6]. In addition, the WHO recommends that sodium consumption should be less than 2000 mg (5 g of salt) and potassium intake at least 3510 mg for adults per day [7].

In addition to the blood pressure lowering effects of sodium reduction or higher potassium intake also in several studies and meta-analyses calcium supplementation has been shown to exert beneficial effects on the risk for gestational hypertension [8,9], especially in women with low dietary calcium intake.

Furthermore, from the electrolytes, magnesium is also effective in reducing blood pressure, especially by acting as a natural calcium channel blocker, increasing nitric oxide levels and improving endothelial dysfunction [10,11].

Early studies from the 1980s suggest that also chloride has an independent effect on blood pressure (reviewed in [12]). In these studies it was shown that replacing chloride with bicarbonate, citrate or phosphate as the anion for sodium did not lead to increases in blood pressure in rats or humans compared to sodium chloride [13–15]. On the other hand, interestingly, lower serum chloride levels were associated with higher cardiovascular and all-cause mortality risk in epidemiological studies [16].

Sulphur enters the body primarily as a component of the amino acids cysteine and methionine, and, as a part of the gaseous signaling molecule hydrogen sulfide (H_2S), it exerts antihypertensive effects in experimental models [17]. Also garlic, which contains several functional sulfur-containing components, has been consistently shown to exert blood pressure-lowering effects with an average of 8–9 mmHg in systolic blood pressure (SBP) and 6–7 mmHg in diastolic blood pressure (DBP) in hypertensive patients [18].

Dietary phosphorus has also been shown to be related to blood pressure [19]. For example, in the International Study of Macro and Micro-Nutrients and Blood Pressure (INTERMAP) it was shown that dietary phosphorus was inversely associated with blood pressure in a multiple regression model [20]. Also in 13,444 participants from the Atherosclerosis Risk in Communities cohort and the Multi-Ethnic Study of Atherosclerosis cohorts compared with individuals in the lowest quintile of phosphorus intake at baseline, those with the highest phosphorus intake showed lower systolic and diastolic blood pressures after adjustment for dietary and non-dietary confounders [21].

Hypertension remains a serious public health issue and found as one amongst the major risk factors, also including smoking, high blood glucose, and high body-mass index, all responsible for approximately 29 million deaths globally [22]. According to the World Heart Federation, hypertension is the most important risk factor for stroke which causes about 50% of ischaemic strokes [23]. Nutrition has an important impact on blood pressure with salt playing a prominent role. However, also especially potassium, in addition probably magnesium, and calcium, and possibly also chloride, sulphur and phosphorus exert at least some effects on blood pressure. Therefore, the objective of this review was to summarize meta-analyses studying the effect and associations of these electrolytes as supplements or diets on human blood pressure or risk for hypertension throughout the last years.

2. Materials and Methods

This review summarizes meta-analyses of publications studying the effect or association between electrolytes and blood pressure. In this regard, we conducted a search in PubMed, Scopus, and Google scholar databases by entering the search terms "(hypertension or blood pressure) and (sodium or potassium or calcium or magnesium or chloride or sulphur or sulphate or phosphorus or phosphate or salt) and (meta-analysis or metaanalysis)". The literature search was conducted in June 2018 with a 10-year publication restriction in order to ensure more recent studies. Search results were limited to English language articles.

2.1. Eligibility Criteria

Meta-analyses of randomized controlled trials or observational studies were included in this review. The availability of (mean) blood pressure reductions and/or relative risk estimates e.g., risk ratios, odds ratios, weighted mean difference and confidence intervals were a prerequisite for the inclusion of the meta-analyses. Reviews and summaries of meta-analyses, meta-analysis not including the primary outcome, (e.g., blood pressure reduction or hypertension risk), or meta-analysis with combined effects of two minerals were excluded.

The initial search revealed a total of 2182 articles (Figure 1). After screening irrelevant, duplicate and other studies not meeting the inclusion criteria 32 meta-analyses were included in this review [8,11,24–53].

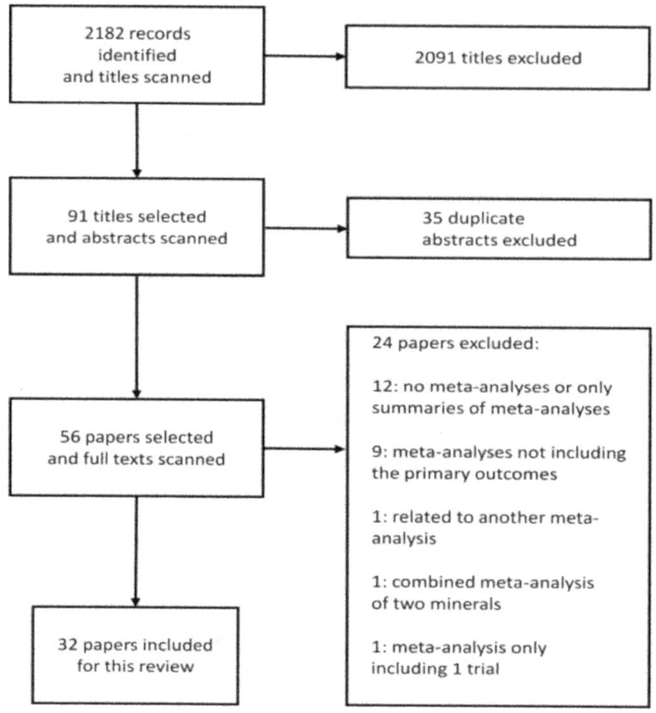

Figure 1. Flow chart of literature search to identify meta-analyses evaluating the effect of electrolytes on blood pressure or hypertension risk.

2.2. Data Extraction

Two reviewers (C.E and N.K) independently extracted the information from the papers. A third reviewer (S.I) rechecked the data and discrepancies were resolved through consensus. Study outcomes with defined number of trials/participants, study type/aims, patient characteristics, average study duration, minerals dosage (diet/supplements) and dietary modification were extracted from the selected meta-analyses. Also (mean) change in systolic and diastolic blood pressure (SBP and DBP), or relative risks (RR), odds ratios or effect sizes with 95% CI were extracted as main outcomes measures from the papers.

3. Results

We identified meta-analyses for sodium, potassium, calcium and magnesium. No meta-analyses were found for the electrolytes chloride, sulphur and phosphorus.

3.1. Effect of Dietary Sodium/Salt Intake/Reduction on Blood Pressure

Overall, fourteen meta-analyses of randomized control trials and observational studies analyzing the effect of sodium modification/reduction on blood pressure were selected [24–37].

The meta-analyses of randomized controlled studies (n = 12) included 5–177 numbers of trials with 12 to 23,858 participants (Table 1). The duration of trials varied between 4 days to 71 months with sodium intake being reduced from 1.2 to 5.7 g/day (52–250 mmol/day) and salt reduction was 2 to 9.6 g/day (34–164 mmol/day). The results showed that blood pressure lowering effects ranged from −0.7 (95% confidence interval: −2.6 to 1.2) mmHg for lowest and −8.9 (−14.1 to −3.7) mmHg for highest SBP reduction, respectively, while lowest to highest reduction for DBP was between 0.03 (−0.4 to 0.4) to −5.9 (−9.7 to −2.1) mmHg.

Moreover, two meta-analyses included observational studies, including 10–18 trials with 8093–134,916 participants. The observational study of Talukder et al. [36] observed a mean difference in blood pressure of 0.1 (−0.2 to 0.3) mmHg for SBP and 0.2 (0.1 to 0.4) mmHg for DBP with exposure of 4–405 mg/L water sodium levels. Subasinghe et al. [37] showed effect sizes of 1.36 (1.24 to 1.48) and

1.28 (1.13 to 1.45) for high salt exposure (6.9 to 42.3 g/day) on hypertension risk in rural and urban populations of low-and-middle income countries, respectively.

3.2. *Effect of Potassium Supplementation on Blood Pressure*

Five meta-analyses of randomized controlled trials evaluated the effect of oral potassium supplements on blood pressure [38–42]. The meta-analyses included 10–33 trials and 556–1892 participants (Table 2). Oral potassium dosages in the supplements were between 6 and 250 mmol/day (0.23–9.7 g/day) with study durations of 4–52 weeks. The lowest to highest reduction in blood pressure was between –3.5 (95% confidence interval: −5.2 to −1.8) to −9.5 (−10.8 to −8.1) mmHg for SBP and −2 (−3.1 to −0.9) to −6.4 (−7.3 to −5.6) mmHg for DBP. In addition, potassium was found to be especially effective in in reducing blood pressure of high sodium consumers.

3.3. *Calcium Intake in Form of Supplements or Diets and Risk for Gestational Hypertension or Blood Pressure Lowering*

We identified six meta-analyses which evaluated the association of dietary calcium intake on the risk for gestational hypertension [8,43–45] or the effect on blood pressure [46,47]. Five meta-analyses of randomized controlled trials with a range of 4–16 trials and 2947–36,806 participants were included. The follow up intervention period was between 8 weeks to 7 years and the calcium intake was found to be between 0.5 g/day to 2 g/day. The results showed RR ranging from 0.55 to 0.91 for gestational hypertension while, the meta-analysis of Cormick et al., [47] found a mean difference of −1.4 (95% confidence interval: −2.2 to −0.7) mmHg for SBP and −1 (−1.5 to −0.5) mmHg for DBP reduction in normotensive people.

Furthermore, we found one meta-analysis including 16 observational trials of 757–41,214 pregnant women showing a lower OR for gestational hypertension [OR: 0.63 (95% CI = 0.41–0.97)] for highest versus lowest category of calcium intake [45].

Most of the meta-analyses showed that calcium supplements were associated with a reduced risk of gestational hypertension (Table 3). Besides, based on the results from the meta-analysis of Wu and Sun [46] calcium plus vitamin D supplementation non-significantly slightly increased SBP with no effects on DBP.

3.4. *Effect of Magnesium on Blood Pressure or Hypertension Risk*

Eight meta-analyses of randomized control trials ($n = 5$) and observational studies ($n = 3$) were included to summarize the effects of magnesium on blood pressure or association with hypertension risk, respectively [11,45,48–53] The randomized control trials included 7–28 number trials with 135–1694 of participants with the trial durations varying between 3–24 weeks. Magnesium intake ranged between 120–1006 mg/day. The summary showed SBP reductions in the range of −0.2 (95% confidence interval: −0.4 to −0.03) mmHg and −18.7 (−22.5 to −15.0) mmHg, and DBP reductions between −0.3 (−0.5 to −0.03) and −10.9 (−13.1 to −8.7) mmHg (Table 4). However, the meta-analysis of Rosanoff and Plesset (2013) [51], which showed the largest effects, only included a small sample of treated hypertensive patients, which probably responded highly to magnesium. When omitting this meta-analysis, the blood pressure lowering effects of magnesium would switch to a rather low to moderate level.

Moreover, observational studies showed a lower risk for hypertension with increasing magnesium intake [52] or higher circulating magnesium levels [53], respectively.

Table 1. Effect of dietary sodium/salt reduction on blood pressure: A summary of meta-analyses of randomized (controlled) trials or observational studies.

Author/Year	No. of Trials	Study Characteristics	No. of Participants	Patient Characteristics	Duration of Trials	Sodium/Salt Intake or Reduction	Blood Pressure Lowering in mmHg (95% CI)	Further Remarks/Summary
Aburto et al., 2013a [24]	36	Randomized controlled trials	6736	2273 (hypertensive)	Most studies (n = 31) <3 months	Different reductions in sodium intake Relative sodium reduction in the intervention group: ≥1/3 of control	SBP: −3.4 (−4.3 to −2.5) DBP: −1.5 (−2.1 to −1.0)	Reduced sodium intake decreases blood pressure in people both with and without hypertension. The reduction in blood pressure was greater in those with hypertension.
Adler et al., 2014 [25]	6 (SBP) 5 (DBP)	Randomized controlled trials	3362 (SBP) 2754 (DBP)	SBP (end of trial): (normotensive) 2079 (hypertensive) 1283 DBP (end of trial): (normotensive) 2079 (hypertensive) 675	7–36 months	Sodium intake: 70 to >100 mmol/day	Normotensive: SBP: −1.2 (−2.3 to 0.02) DBP: −0.8 (−1.4 to −0.2) Hypertensive: SBP: −4.1 (−5.8 to −2.4) DBP: −3.7 (−8.4 to 0.9)	Normotensive persons: small blood pressure reduction. Hypertensive patients: greater reduction in SBP, no difference in DBP.
Graudal et al., 2015 [26]	15	Randomized controlled trials	12–114	"time to maximal efficacy" analysis 7 studies with hypertensive patients 7 studies with normotensive persons 1 study hypertensive + normotensive	1 to 6 weeks	Sodium reduction range: 55–118 mmol/day	No significant differences in SBP or DBP after initiation of salt reduction between week 1 and subsequent weeks.	Time dependent effects of salt reduction on blood pressure. The effect of salt reduction on blood pressure appears to reach maximal efficacy at 1 week and remain stable over subsequent time intervals.
Graudal and Jürgens 2015 [27]	92	Randomized controlled trials	661 Asians 561 Blacks 3782 Whites	9 Asian/9 Black/74 White population	7–365 days	Sodium reduction: 63–103 mmol	SBP: −3.2 (−4.0 to −2.5) (in Whites) −4.7 (−7.1 to −2.3) (in Blacks) −3.8 (−6.4 to −1.3) (in Asians) DBP:−1.5 (−2.1 to −1.0) (in Whites) −3.0 (−4.0 to −2.0) (in Blacks) −2.0 (−3.0 to −0.9) (in Asians)	SBP: no differences in ethnic groups. DBP: small differences between black and white people.
Gay et al., 2016 [28]	24	Randomized controlled trials	23,858	11 to 2570 participants (median: 129) participants >19 years old	Trial durations ranged from 6 to 48 months of follow−up (median: 12 months)	Dietary interventions (including low sodium diets)	Overall pooled net effect of diets: SBP: −3.1 (−3.9 to −2.3) DBP: −1.8 (−2.2 to −1.4)	This meta-analysis shows that dietary interventions (including low sodium diets) provide clinically significant net blood pressure reductions, and that some dietary patterns may be more effective than others.

Table 1. *Cont.*

Author/Year	No. of Trials	Study Characteristics	No. of Participants	Patient Characteristics	Duration of Trials	Sodium/Salt Intake or Reduction	Blood Pressure Lowering in mmHg (95% CI)	Further Remarks/Summary
Graudal et al., 2017 [29]	177	Randomized controlled trials	12,210	White people with hypertension. (84 studies; 5925 participants in SBP; 85 studies; 6001 participants in DBP) Black people with hypertension. (8 studies; 619 participants in SBP and DBP) Asian people with hypertension. (8 studies; 501 participants in SBP and DBP) White people with normotension. (89 studies, 8569 participants in SBP; 90 studies, 8833 participants in DBP) Black people with normotension. (7 studies, 506 participants in SBP and DBP) Asian people with normotension. (3 studies, 393 participants in SBP and DBP)	4–1100 days	Mean sodium reduction: 135 mmol/day range; <100 to ≥250 mmol/day	Hypertensive (White): SBP: −5.5 (−6.5 to −4.6) DBP: −2.9 (−3.4 to −2.3) Hypertensive (Black): SBP: −6.6 (−9.0 to −4.2) DBP: −2.9 (−4.5 to −1.30) Hypertensive (Asian): SBP: −7.8 (−11.4 to −4.1) DBP: −2.7 (−4.2 to −1.2) Normotensive (White): SBP: −1.1 (−1.6 to −0.6) DBP: 0.03 (−0.4 to 0.4) Normotensive (Black) SBP: −4.0 (−7.4 to −0.7) DBP: −2.0 (−4.4 to 0.4) Normotensive (Asian): SBP: −0.7 (−3.9 to 2.4) DBP: −1.6 (−3.4 to 0.1)	High-quality evidence for White people; moderate-quality evidence for Black/Asian people
He et al., 2013 [30]	34	Randomized trials	3230	990 (of 22 trials) hypertensive 2240 (of 12 trials) normotensive	Median duration: 5 weeks in hypertensive people, 4 weeks in normotensive people	Salt reduction: 75 mmol/day (4.4 g/day). Reduction of urinary sodium: 40–120 mmol/day (2.3–7.0 g/day).	Total SBP: −4.2 (−5.2 to −3.2) DBP: −2.1 (−2.7 to −1.5) Hypertensive: SBP: −5.4 (−6.6 to −4.2) DBP: −2.8 (−3.5 to −2.1) Normotensive: SBP: −2.4 (−3.6 to −1.3) DBP: −1.0 (−1.9 to −0.2)	Reduction in SBP was significant in both black and white people and in women and men. Significant effects on blood pressure were seen in hypertensives and normotensives. Dose-response relation: the greater the reduction in salt intake, the greater the fall in blood pressure.

Table 1. *Cont.*

Author/Year	No. of Trials	Study Characteristics	No. of Participants	Patient Characteristics	Duration of Trials	Sodium/Salt Intake or Reduction	Blood Pressure Lowering in mmHg (95% CI)	Further Remarks/Summary
He and MacGregor 2011 [31]	6	Outcome trials	6250	3 trials in normotensive participants 3 trials in hypertensive patients	6–36 months	Salt reduction: 2–2.3 g/day	Normotensive: SBP: −1.1 (−0.1 to 2.3) DBP: −0.8 (0.2 to 1.4) Hypertensive: SBP: −4.1 (2.4 to 5.8) DBP: −3.7 (−0.9 to 8.4)	Significant reduction in cardiovascular events
Kelly et al., 2016 [32]	5	Randomized and non-randomized controlled trials	1214	Normotensive participants (≥18 years) with SBP ≤140 mmHg	4 weeks to 48 months	Salt reduction: −75 mmol/day (range; −37 to −136 mmol).	SBP: −0.7 (−2.6 to 1.2) DBP: −0.6 (−1.3 to 0.1)	No significant change in SBP or DBP following reduction of dietary sodium over the period of 4 weeks to 36 months
Peng et al., 2014 [33]	5	Randomized controlled trials	1974	Hypertensive and normotensive participants	6 months to 2 years	Different salt substitutes vs. common salt (NaCl).	SBP: −4.9 (−7.3 to −2.5) DBP: −1.5 (−2.7 to −0.3)	Salt substitutes significantly reduced both SBP and DBP
Taylor et al., 2011 [34]	7	Randomized controlled trials	3 trials normotensive (3518), 2 trials hypertensive (758), 1 trial mixed pop. (1981), 1 trial with heart failure (234)	Adults ≥18 years, irrespective of gender/ethnicity. Studies of children/pregnant women were excluded.	Trials follow-up ranged 6 to 71 months	Salt reduction; <70–100 mmol/ day. Urinary 24-h sodium excretion: Normotensive (mean diff.): 34.2 mmol/24 h (18.8–49.6), Hypertensive (mean diff.): 39.1 mmol/24 h (31.1–47.1)	Normotensives (mean difference) SBP:−1.1 (−2.3 to 0.1) DBP:−0.8 (−1.4 to −0.2) Hypertensives SBP: −4.1 (−5.8 to −2.4) DBP: −3.7 (−8.4 to 0.9)	Significant reduction of SBP in hypertensive patients
Wang et al., 2015 [35]	6	Interventional studies	3153	Chinese adults aged ≥35 years	At most 1 week	Salt level reduced in hypertensive patients: 9.6 g/day (163.0 mmol/day sodium).	Normotensive + hypertensive: SBP: −6.3 (−7.2 to −5.4) DBP: −3.2 (−3.7 to −2.7) Hypertensive: SBP: −8.9 (−14.1 to −3.7) DBP: −5.9 (−9.7 to −2.1)	Salt restriction lowers mean BP in Chinese adults, with the strongest effect among hypertensive participants.
Observational Studies								
Talukder et al., 2017 [36]	10	Observational studies	8093	7 studies (12 datasets) with 3747 participants with low/high water sodium exposure groups		4–405 mg/L water sodium level	Standardized mean difference: SBP: 0.1 (−0.2 to 0.3) DBP: 0.2 (0.1 to 0.4)	An (inconclusive) association between water sodium and human blood pressure is suggested, more consistently for DBP.

Table 1. *Cont.*

Author/Year	No. of Trials	Study Characteristics	No. of Participants	Patient Characteristics	Duration of Trials	Sodium/Salt Intake or Reduction	Blood Pressure Lowering in mmHg (95% CI)	Further Remarks/Summary
Observational Studies								
Subasinghe et al., 2016 [37]	18	Observational studies	134,916	Participants in urban and rural areas in low-and-middle income countries (LMICs). Age: 24–65.		Daily salt intake range: 6.9 to 42.3 g/day	Effect size (ES) of hypertension ES 1.36 (1.24 to 1.48) ES 1.28 (1.13 to 1.45)	Excessive salt intake has a greater impact on the prevalence of hypertension in urban than rural regions.

SBP = Systolic blood pressure; DBP = Diastolic blood pressure.

Table 2. Effect of potassium supplementation on blood pressure: A summary of meta-analyses of randomized controlled trials.

Author/Year	No. of trials	Study Characteristic	No. of Participants	Patient Characteristics	Duration of Trials	Potassium Dosage (Supplements)	Blood Pressure Lowering in mmHg (95%CI)	Further Remarks/Summary
Aburto et al., 2013b [38]	21	Randomized controlled trials	1892/1857	Hypertensive 818(SBP)/828(DBP)	<2 to >4 months	<90 mmol/day to >155 mmol/day in the intervention group	SBP: −3.5 (−5.2 to −1.8) DBP: −2.0 (−3.1 to −0.9)	Effect seen in people with hypertension but not in those without hypertension. Intake above 120 mmol/day did not seem to have any additional benefit. Potassium may be more effective in reducing blood pressure at higher levels of sodium consumption.
Binia et al., 2015 [39]	15	Randomized controlled trials	917	400 hypertensives 329 normotensives 188 hypertensive or normotensive persons (mixed population)	4–24 weeks	<40–120 mmol/day	All: SBP: −4.7 (−7.0 to −2.4) DBP: −3.5 (−5.7 to −1.3) Hypertensive patients: SBP: −6.8 (−9.3 to −4.3) DBP: −4.7 (−7.5 to −1.8)	Potassium supplementation is associated with reduction of blood pressure in patients who are not on antihypertensive medication, and the effect is significant in hypertensive patients.
Filippini et al., 2017 [40]	33	Randomized controlled trials	1829	1163 (studies ≥4 weeks overall)	<4 to ≥12 weeks	25–250 mmol/day	SBP: −4.5 (−5.9 to −3.1) DBP: −3.0 (−4.8 to −1.1)	Potassium supplementation in hypertensives was generally associated with decreased blood pressure, particularly in high sodium consumers.
Poorolajal et al., 2017 [41]	23	Randomized controlled trials	1213	Primary hypertension: 732 (SBP) 695 (DBP)	4–52 weeks	6–200 mmol/day	SBP: −4.3 (−6.0 to −2.5) DBP: −2.5 (−4.1 to −1.0)	Potassium supplementation has a modest but significant impact on blood pressure.
Bommel and Cleophas 2012 [42]	10	Crossover and parallel design studies	556	High salt intake, >170 mmol/24h	Follow up 8–16 weeks	Not available	SBP: −9.5 (−10.8 to −8.1) DBP: −6.4 (−7.3 to −5.6)	Potassium treatment reduces considerably the blood pressure of hypertensive patients on salt rich diets.

SBP = Systolic blood pressure; DBP = Diastolic blood pressure.

Table 3. Calcium intake in form of diets or supplements and risk for gestational hypertension or effect on blood pressure: a summary of meta-analyses of randomized controlled trials or observational studies.

Author/Year	No. of Trials	Study Characteristic	No. of Participants	Study Aims	Duration of Trials	Calcium Dosage (Diet or Supplement)	Blood Pressure Lowering in mmHg or RR/OR for Gestational Hypertension (95% CI)	Further Remarks/Summary
Imdad et al., 2011 [8]	6	Randomized controlled trials	Calcium-group: 4919 Control group: 4942	Effect of calcium supplementation on gestational hypertensive disorders in studies from developing countries	Calcium supplements in all the included studies were before 20–32 weeks of gestation and continued till delivery.	0.5–2 g/day	RR: 0.55 (0.36 to 0.85)	Calcium supplementation during pregnancy was associated with a significant reduced risk of acquiring gestational hypertension.
Hofmeyr et al., 2014 [43]	12 trials	Randomized controlled trials	15,470 women	Assessing the effects of calcium supplementation during pregnancy on hypertensive disorders of pregnancy and related maternal and child outcomes	Calcium supplementation started at the latest from 34 weeks of pregnancy.	High-dose calcium supplementation (≥1 g/day)	RR: 0.65 (0.53 to 0.81)	Average risk of high blood pressure was reduced with calcium supplementation compared with placebo. There was also a reduction in hypertension with low-dose calcium supplementation (<1 g/day).
An et al., 2015 [44]	4	Randomized controlled trials	Gestational hypertension: 7252 Control group: 7272 Severe gestational hypertension: 6673 Control group: 6684	Assessing the effectiveness of calcium supplementation during pregnancy on reducing the risk of hypertensive disorders of pregnancy and related problems.	From ~11–24 weeks of pregnancy to delivery	Supplementation with calcium (at least >1 g/day)	Gestational hypertension: RR: 0.91 (0.84 to 0.99) Severe gestational hypertension: RR: 0.81 (0.60 to 1.09)	Calcium supplementation appears to reduce the risk of hypertension in pregnancy. No significant reduction in the risk of severe gestational hypertension.
Wu and Sun 2017 [46]	8	Randomized controlled trials	36,806	Evaluation the effect of calcium plus vitamin-D (CaD) supplements on the changes in BP from baseline to the longest follow-up time point in male and female participants.	8 weeks to 7 years	Intervention dose of calcium (≤1000 mg/day, 5 trials or >1000 mg/day, 3 trials)	Mean differences in SBP: 0.6 (−1 to 2.20) Mean differences in DBP: −0.2 (−0.9 to 0.5)	Calcium plus vitamin D supplementation slightly increased SBP, but the difference was not statistically significant. Calcium plus vitamin D supplementation did not significantly affected DBP reduction.

Table 3. *Cont.*

Author/Year	No. of Trials	Study Characteristic	No. of Participants	Study Aims	Duration of Trials	Calcium Dosage (Diet or Supplement)	Blood Pressure Lowering in mmHg or RR/OR for Gestational Hypertension (95% CI)	Further Remarks/Summary
Cormick et al., 2015 [47]	16	Randomized controlled trials	SBP: 3048 (16 studies) DBP: 2947 (15 studies)	Assessing the efficacy and safety of calcium supplementation versus placebo or control for reducing blood pressure in normotensive people	Median follow up intervention period of 3.5 months	For most studies the intervention was 1000 mg to 2000 mg of elemental calcium per day	Mean difference: SBP: −1.4 (−2.2 to −0.7) DBP: −1 (−1.5 to −0.5)	The quality of evidence was high for doses of calcium of 1000 to 1500 mg/day and was moderate for lower or higher doses. Calcium intake slightly reduced both SBP and DBP in normotensive people.
Observational studies								
Schoenaker et al., 2014 [45]	16	Observational studies	Case-control studies: 757 pregnant women Cohort studies: 41,214 pregnant women, 908 gestational hypertension	Assessing the effect of dietary factors on hypertensive disorders during pregnancy (gestational hypertension and pre-eclampsia)		Highest group >1600 mg/day versus lowest group <1000 mg/day	Gestational hypertension (comparing highest to lowest): OR: 0.63 (0.41 to 0.97)	Results from case–control studies consistently showed lower reported calcium intake for pregnant women with hypertensive disorders (gestational hypertension and preeclampsia)

SBP = Systolic blood pressure; DBP = Diastolic blood pressure.

Table 4. Effect magnesium on blood pressure or association with hypertension risk: A summary of meta-analyses of randomized controlled trials and observational studies.

Author-Year	No. of Trials	Study Characteristics	No. Participants	Study Aims	Duration of Trials	Magnesium Dosage (Diet or Supplement)	Blood Pressure Lowering in mmHg or RR (95% CI)	Further Remarks/Summary
Zhang et al., 2016 [11]	27	Randomized controlled trials	Magnesium group: 822 Placebo group: 800	Effect of magnesium supplementation in normotensive and hypertensive adults (age 18–84 years).	3 weeks–6 months	Median dose of 368 mg/day (range: 238–960 mg/day)	SBP: −2 (−0.4 to −3.6) DBP: −1.8 (−0.7 to −2.8)	Magnesium supplementation at a median dose of 368 mg/day for a median duration of 3 months significantly reduced SBP and DBP. Magnesium supplementation at a dose of 300 mg/day or duration of 1 month is enough to elevate serum magnesium and reduce blood pressure. Serum magnesium was negatively associated with DBP but not SBP.
Dibaba et al., 2017 [48]	11	Randomized controlled trials	543	Assessing the pooled effect of magnesium supplementation on blood pressure in participants with preclinical or non–communicable diseases.	1 to 6 months (mean: 3.6 months)	365–450 mg/day	Standardized mean difference: SBP: −0.2 (−0.4 to −0.03) DBP: −0.3 (−0.5 to −0.03)	Magnesium supplementation lowers blood pressure in individuals with insulin resistance, prediabetes, or other noncommunicable chronic diseases.
Verma and Garg 2017 [49]	28	Randomized controlled trials	1694 (834 treatment arm, 860 placebo arm)	Evaluation the effect of magnesium supplementation on type 2 diabetes associated cardiovascular risk factors in both diabetic and nondiabetic individuals. Only four studies were carried out in hypertensive subjects.	4–24 weeks	Elemental magnesium: 300–1006 mg/day	Weighted mean difference: SBP: −3.06 (−5.51 to −0.60) DBP: −1.37 (−3.02 to 0.29)	A significant improvement was observed in SBP. Insignificant improvement or no improvement was observed in DBP
Kass et al., 2012 [50]	22	Interventional studies	1173	Assessing the effect of magnesium supplementation on blood pressure. Adults from 12 different countries were included.	3 to 24 weeks of follow-up	Elemental magnesium dosage: 120–973 mg/day	Overall effect size: SBP: 0.3 (0.2 to 0.4) DBP: 0.4 (0.3 to 0.4)	Summary of all trials show a decrease in SBP of 3–4 mmHg and DBP of 2–3 mmHg. Magnesium supplementation appears to achieve a small but clinically significant reduction in blood pressure.

Table 4. *Cont.*

Author-Year	No. of Trials	Study Characteristics	No. Participants	Study Aims	Duration of Trials	Magnesium Dosage (Diet or Supplement)	Blood Pressure Lowering in mmHg or RR (95% CI)	Further Remarks/Summary
Rosanoff and Plesset 2013 [51]	7	Interventional studies	135 treated hypertensive subjects	Evaluation of magnesium supplementation in hypertension. Initial SBP of the patients was >155 mmHg	6 to 17 weeks	10.5–18.5 mmol magnesium-salt/day	Mean change: SBP: −18.7 (−22.5 to −15.0) DBP: −10.9 (−13.1 to −8.7)	This uniform subset of seven studies showed a strong effect of magnesium in treated hypertensive patients.
Observational studies								
Schoenaker et al., 2014 [45]	3	Observational studies	6616 pregnant women, age range 20–40 years	Assessing the effect of dietary factors, including magnesium, on hypertensive disorders of pregnant women.	NA	Not indicated	Significantly lower mean magnesium intake of mean 7.69 mg/day for women with hypertensive disorders of pregnancy (gestational hypertension and pre-eclampsia)	Pooled results revealed statistically significantly lower mean magnesium intake for women with hypertensive disorders of pregnancy.
Han et al., 2017 [52]	10	Prospective cohort studies	180,566 participates	Assessing the relationship between dietary magnesium intake and serum magnesium concentrations on the risk of hypertension in adults. Adult population >18 years was included.	4–15 years	96–425 mg/day	RR: 0.95 (0.90 to 1.00) for a 100 mg/increment in magnesium intake. Comparing highest to lowest: RR: 0.91 (0.80 to 1.02)	Increase in magnesium intake was associated with a lower risk of hypertension in a linear dose-response pattern.
Wu J et al., 2017 [53]	3	Prospective cohort studies with four cohorts	14,876 participants (3149 cases)	Evaluation of circulating magnesium levels and incidence of coronary heart diseases, hypertension, and type 2 diabetes mellitus	Average of 6.7 years of follow-up	NA	Per 0.1 mmol/L increment in serum magnesium levels: RR: 0.96 (0.93 to 0.99)	A significant inverse linear association was observed between circulating magnesium levels and incidence of hypertension.

SBP = Systolic blood pressure; DBP = Diastolic blood pressure; NA = not applicable.

4. Discussion

The major findings of this review were especially that sodium (salt) reduction and a higher intake of potassium have convincing blood pressure lowering effects. In addition, higher magnesium intake is suggested to possibly reduce blood pressure, especially in patients with hypertension. Moreover, sufficient calcium intake confers a protective effect regarding the risk for gestational hypertension.

There are several mechanistical explanations for the association between high sodium intake and blood pressure like enhanced reabsorption and retention of filtered sodium through the renal tubules [54], or activation of the brain renin–angiotensin–aldosterone system (RAAS), which is suggested to increase blood pressure through angiotensin II and aldosterone promoting locally oxidative stress and activating the sympathetic nervous system [55]. Furthermore, based on the "vasodysfunction theory" of salt induced hypertension, salt loading results in subnormal decreases in systemic vascular resistance leading to an increase in blood pressure [56]. In this regard salt sensitivity, which varies among individuals, is suggested to play an important role [3,55].

In addition to blood pressure, in a recent systematic review and meta-analysis of randomized controlled trials it was analyzed that restriction of dietary sodium intake can reduce arterial stiffness, as expressed by carotid-femoral pulse wave velocity [57].

In addition to sodium modification, several studies and meta-analysis showed that potassium supplements reduce blood pressure and also the risk of hypertension [58]. Suggested mechanisms of the blood pressure lowering effects of potassium are (reviewed in [5]): improvement of endothelial function and NO release, vasodilatation by lowering cytosolic smooth muscle cell calcium, increasing natriuresis, and lowering the activity of the sympathetic nervous system. Furthermore the supportive blood pressure reducing effects of sodium modification in combination with potassium is well-documented [59].

Besides the interdependent effect of sodium and potassium, calcium and magnesium have also been implicated in the regulation of blood pressure [60]. Based on our results, magnesium showed a moderate blood pressure reducing effect in general, while the effects of calcium were primarily restricted to the prevention of gestational hypertension. The potential antihypertensive effects of magnesium are for example suggested to be related to calcium channel blockage, increases in nitric oxide, and better endothelial function [10]. In vascular smooth muscle cells, magnesium antagonizes Ca^{2+} by inhibiting transmembrane calcium transport and calcium entry with low magnesium levels causing an increase in intracellular free Ca^{2+} concentration and subsequently vascular contraction [61].

On the other hand, low dietary calcium intake is shown to be a risk factor for the development of hypertension especially for women with a history of gestational hypertension [62]. In this regard the World Health Organization recommends daily calcium supplementation of 1.5–2.0 g oral elemental calcium for pregnant women in populations with low dietary calcium intake to reduce the risk of pre-eclampsia and related complications [63].

Lifestyle modifications including weight loss, exercise, and healthy diets are proved to be important predictors to lower blood pressure or the risk for hypertension, respectively. For example, the Canadian hypertension education program guidelines (2016) proposed health behavior management for the prevention of hypertension such as physical exercise, weight management, limited alcohol consumption, stress management, reduce sodium intake and recommended dietary modification as the preferred method of increasing potassium intake (in patients who are not at risk of hyperkalemia) to get additional nutritional benefits of whole foods over prescribed supplements [64]. Similarly, the study findings of a systematic review and meta-analysis of randomized control trials showed that healthy dietary patterns including the dietary approaches to stop hypertension (DASH) diet, Nordic diet, and Mediterranean diet significantly lowered systolic and diastolic blood pressure [65].

5. Conclusions and Future Perspectives

Our brief exploration of meta-analyses showed that lowering sodium and increasing potassium intake would exert convincing blood pressure lowering effects, especially in hypertensive patients. The maximum extent of systolic blood pressure lowering was approximately in the order of 8 to

9 mmHg, which roughly equals a monotherapy with an antihypertensive drug [66]. This reflects the significant importance of healthy nutrition, in this case salt reduction and increase of dietary potassium intake, on blood pressure. Our summary of meta-analytic reviews also suggests that higher magnesium intake may exert beneficial effects on blood pressure, although the results were rather moderate. However, in some (treated) hypertensive patients ("high-responders") higher magnesium intake might result in larger effects. So, increasing/optimizing dietary magnesium intake could also be a helpful recommendation in patients with hypertension. Furthermore, there is convincing evidence that increasing/optimizing calcium intake can lower the risk for gestational hypertension, especially in women with initial low calcium intake.

We did not find any meta-analyses summarizing the effects of chloride, phosphorus and sulphur on blood pressure or hypertension risk. In general, few studies are available, which assessed the effect of these electrolytes on blood pressure. There are indications from observational studies that there might be some effects, however robust evidence is missing. For example, a very recent systematic review from McClure et al. (2019) did not detected a consistent association between total dietary phosphorus intake and blood pressure [67].

Relating to earlier studies replacing the chloride component of salt with other anions like bicarbonate or citrate might be a certain strategy, which could not only beneficially affect blood pressure but could show co-benefits regarding a (western) diet induced metabolic acid load [68]. Obviously, randomized (controlled) trials are necessary to study this assumption. Also, future clinical trials could determine the effect of different electrolytes on blood pressure by patients' self-assessment of blood pressure with new validated mHealth devices, like a previous study in obese individuals has shown [69].

Author Contributions: Conceptualization, C.E.; methodology, C.E., S.I.; literature search, N.K.; C.E.; validation, S.I.; original draft preparation, S.I.; review and editing, C.E.; supervision, C.E.

References

1. Rahimi, K.; Emdin, C.A.; Macmahon, S. The Epidemiology of Blood Pressure and Its Worldwide Management. *Circ. Res.* **2015**, *116*, 925–936. [CrossRef] [PubMed]
2. Zhao, D.; Qi, Y.; Zheng, Z.; Wang, Y.; Zhang, X.; Li, H.; Liu, H.; Zhang, X.-T.; Du, J.; Liu, J. Dietary factors associated with hypertension. *Nat. Rev. Cardiol.* **2011**, *8*, 456–465. [CrossRef] [PubMed]
3. Rust, P.; Ekmekcioglu, C. Impact of Salt Intake on the Pathogenesis and Treatment of Hypertension. *Adv. Exp. Med. Biol.* **2017**, *956*, 61–84. [PubMed]
4. Ekmekcioglu, C.; Blasche, G.; Dorner, T.E. Too much salt and how we can get rid of it. *Forsch. Komplementmed.* **2013**, *20*, 454–460. [CrossRef] [PubMed]
5. Ekmekcioglu, C.; Elmadfa, I.; Meyer, A.L.; Moeslinger, T. The role of dietary potassium in hypertension and diabetes. *J. Physiol. Biochem.* **2016**, *72*, 93–106. [CrossRef] [PubMed]
6. Flack, J.M.; Calhoun, D.; Schiffrin, E.L. The New ACC/AHA Hypertension Guidelines for the Prevention, Detection, Evaluation, and Management of High Blood Pressure in Adults. *Am. J. Hypertens.* **2018**, *31*, 133–135. [CrossRef] [PubMed]
7. World Health Organization. WHO Issues New Guidance on Dietary Salt and Potassium. Available online: https://www.who.int/mediacentre/news/notes/2013/salt_potassium_20130131/en/ (accessed on 14 June 2019).
8. Imdad, A.; Jabeen, A.; Bhutta, Z.A. Role of calcium supplementation during pregnancy in reducing risk of developing gestational hypertensive disorders: A meta-analysis of studies from developing countries. *BMC Public Health* **2011**, *11*, S18. [CrossRef] [PubMed]
9. Khanam, F.; Hossain, B.; Mistry, S.K.; Mitra, D.K.; Raza, W.A.; Rifat, M.; Afsana, K.; Rahman, M. The association between daily 500 mg calcium supplementation and lower pregnancy-induced hypertension risk in Bangladesh. *BMC Pregnancy Childbirth* **2018**, *18*, 406. [CrossRef] [PubMed]
10. Houston, M. The role of magnesium in hypertension and cardiovascular disease. *J. Clin. Hypertens.* **2011**, *13*, 843–847. [CrossRef]
11. Zhang, X.; Li, Y.; Del Gobbo, L.C.; Rosanoff, A.; Wang, J.; Zhang, W.; Song, Y. Effects of Magnesium

Supplementation on Blood Pressure: A Meta-Analysis of Randomized Double-Blind Placebo-Controlled Trials. *Hypertension* **2016**, *68*, 324–333. [CrossRef]

12. McCallum, L.; Lip, S.; Padmanabhan, S. The hidden hand of chloride in hypertension. *Pflugers Arch. Eur. J. Physiol.* **2015**, *467*, 595–603. [CrossRef] [PubMed]
13. Kurtz, T.W.; Morris, R.C. Dietary Chloride as a Determinant of "Sodium-Dependent" Hypertension. *Science* **1983**, *222*, 1139–1141. [CrossRef] [PubMed]
14. Kurtz, T.W.; Al-Bander, H.A.; Morris, R.C. "Salt-sensitive" essential hypertension in men. Is the sodium ion alone important? *N. Engl. J. Med.* **1987**, *317*, 1043–1048. [CrossRef] [PubMed]
15. Shore, A.C.; Markandu, N.D.; MacGregor, G.A. A randomized crossover study to compare the blood pressure response to sodium loading with and without chloride in patients with essential hypertension. *J. Hypertens.* **1988**, *6*, 613–617. [CrossRef] [PubMed]
16. De Bacquer, D.; De Backer, G.; De Buyzere, M.; Kornitzer, M. Is low serum chloride level a risk factor for cardiovascular mortality? *J. Cardiovasc. Risk* **1998**, *5*, 177–184. [CrossRef] [PubMed]
17. Van Goor, H.; Van Den Born, J.C.; Hillebrands, J.L.; Joles, J.A. Hydrogen sulfide in hypertension. *Curr. Opin. Nephrol. Hypertens.* **2016**, *25*, 107–113. [CrossRef] [PubMed]
18. Ried, K. Garlic Lowers Blood Pressure in Hypertensive Individuals, Regulates Serum Cholesterol, and Stimulates Immunity: An Updated Meta-analysis and Review. *J. Nutr.* **2016**, *146*, 389S–396S. [CrossRef] [PubMed]
19. Chan, Q.; Stamler, J.; Griep, L.M.O.; Daviglus, M.L.; Van Horn, L.; Elliott, P. An update on nutrients and blood pressure: Summary of INTERMAP Study findings. *J. Atheroscler. Thromb.* **2016**, *23*, 276–289. [CrossRef] [PubMed]
20. Elliott, P.; Kesteloot, H.; Appel, L.J.; Dyer, A.R.; Ueshima, H.; Chan, Q.; Brown, I.J.; Zhao, L.; Stamler, J. Dietary Phosphorus and Blood Pressure: International Study of Macro- and Micro-Nutrients and Blood Pressure. *Hypertension* **2008**, *51*, 669–675. [CrossRef]
21. Alonso, A.; Nettleton, J.A.; Ix, J.H.; de Boer, I.H.; Folsom, A.R.; Bidulescu, A.; Kestenbaum, B.R.; Chambless, L.E.; Jacobs, D.R. Dietary phosphorus, blood pressure and incidence of hypertension in the Atherosclerosis Risk in Communities (ARIC) Study and the Multi-Ethnic Study of Atherosclerosis (MESA). *Hypertension* **2010**, *55*, 776–784. [CrossRef]
22. The Lancet. GBD 2017: A fragile world. *Lancet* **2018**, *392*, 1683. [CrossRef]
23. World Heart Foundation. Fact Sheet: Cardiovascular Disease Risk Factors—World Heart Federation. Available online: https://www.world-heart-federation.org/resources/risk-factors/?cats=29 (accessed on 14 June 2019).
24. Aburto, N.J.; Ziolkovska, A.; Hooper, L.; Elliott, P.; Cappuccio, F.P.; Meerpohl, J.J. Effect of lower sodium intake on health: Systematic review and meta-analyses. *BMJ* **2013**, *346*, f1326. [CrossRef] [PubMed]
25. Adler, A.; Taylor, F.; Martin, N.; Gottlieb, S.; Taylor, R.; Ebrahim, S. Reduced dietary salt for the prevention of cardiovascular disease (Review). *Cochrane Database Syst. Rev.* **2014**, CD009217. [CrossRef]
26. Graudal, N.; Hubeck-Graudal, T.; Jürgens, G.; McCarron, D.A. The Significance of Duration and Amount of Sodium Reduction Intervention in Normotensive and Hypertensive Individuals: A Meta-Analysis. *Adv. Nutr.* **2015**, *6*, 169–177. [CrossRef] [PubMed]
27. Graudal, N.; Jürgens, G. The blood pressure sensitivity to changes in sodium intake is similar in Asians, Blacks and Whites. An analysis of 92 randomized controlled trials. *Front. Physiol.* **2015**, *6*, 157. [CrossRef] [PubMed]
28. Gay, H.C.; Rao, S.G.; Vaccarino, V.; Ali, M.K. Effects of Different Dietary Interventions on Blood Pressure; Systematic Review and Meta-Analysis of Randomized Controlled Trials. *Hypertension* **2016**, *67*, 733–739. [CrossRef] [PubMed]
29. Graudal, N.; Hubeck-Graudal, T.; Jurgens, G. Effects of low sodium diet versus high sodium diet on blood pressure, renin, aldosterone, catecholamines, cholesterol, and triglyceride (Review). *Cochrane Database Syst. Rev.* **2017**, *2017*, CD004022.
30. He, F.J.; Li, J.; MacGregor, G.A. Effect of longer term modest salt reduction on blood pressure: Cochrane systematic review and meta-analysis of randomised trials. *BMJ* **2013**, *346*, f1325. [CrossRef]
31. He, F.J.; MacGregor, G.A. Salt reduction lowers cardiovascular risk: Meta-analysis of outcome trials. *Lancet* **2011** *378*, 380–382. [CrossRef]

32. Kelly, J.; Khalesi, S.; Dickinson, K.; Hines, S.; Coombes, J.S.; Todd, A.S. The effect of dietary sodium modification on blood pressure in adults with systolic blood pressure less than 140 mmHg: A systematic review. *JBI Database Syst. Rev. Implement. Rep.* **2016**, *14*, 196–237. [CrossRef]
33. Peng, Y.; Li, W.; Wen, X.; Li, Y.; Hu, J.; Zhao, L. Effects of salt substitutes on blood pressure: A meta-analysis of randomized controlled trials. *Am. J. Clin. Nutr.* **2014**, *100*, 1448–1454. [CrossRef] [PubMed]
34. Taylor, R.S.; Ashton, K.E.; Moxham, T.; Hooper, L.; Ebrahim, S. Reduced dietary salt for the prevention of cardiovascular disease: A meta-analysis of randomized controlled trials (cochrane review). *Am. J. Hypertens.* **2011**, *24*, 843–853. [CrossRef] [PubMed]
35. Wang, M.; Moran, A.E.; Liu, J.; Qi, Y.; Xie, W.; Tzong, K.; Zhao, D. A Meta-Analysis of Effect of Dietary Salt Restriction on Blood Pressure in Chinese Adults. *Glob. Heart* **2015**, *10*, 291–299. [CrossRef] [PubMed]
36. Talukder, M.R.R.; Rutherford, S.; Huang, C.; Phung, D.; Islam, M.Z.; Chu, C. Drinking water salinity and risk of hypertension: A systematic review and meta-analysis. *Arch. Environ. Occup. Heal.* **2017**, *72*, 126–138. [CrossRef] [PubMed]
37. Subasinghe, A.K.; Arabshahi, S.; Busingye, D.; Evans, R.G.; Walker, K.Z.; Riddell, M.A.; Thrift, A.G. Association between salt and hypertension in rural and urban populations of low to middle income countries: A systematic review and meta-analysis of population based studies. *Asia Pac. J. Clin. Nutr.* **2016**, *25*, 402–413.
38. Aburto, N.J.; Hanson, S.; Gutierrez, H.; Hooper, L.; Elliott, P.; Cappuccio, F.P. Effect of increased potassium intake on cardiovascular risk factors and disease: Systematic review and meta-analyses. *BMJ* **2013**, *346*, f1378. [CrossRef] [PubMed]
39. Binia, A.; Jaeger, J.; Hu, Y.; Singh, A.; Zimmermann, D. Daily potassium intake and sodium-to-potassium ratio in the reduction of blood pressure: A meta-analysis of randomized controlled trials. *J. Hypertens.* **2015**, *33*, 1509–1520. [CrossRef]
40. Filippini, T.; Violi, F.; D'Amico, R.; Vinceti, M. The effect of potassium supplementation on blood pressure in hypertensive subjects: A systematic review and meta-analysis. *Int. J. Cardiol.* **2017**, *230*, 127–135. [CrossRef]
41. Poorolajal, J.; Zeraati, F.; Soltanian, A.R.; Sheikh, V.; Hooshmand, E.; Maleki, A. Oral potassium supplementation for management of essential hypertension: A meta-analysis of randomized controlled trials. *PLoS ONE* **2017**, *12*, e0174967. [CrossRef]
42. Bommel, E.V.; Cleophas, T. Potassium treatment for hypertension in patients with high salt intake: A meta-analysis. *Int. J. Clin. Pharmacol. Ther.* **2012**, *50*, 478–482. [CrossRef]
43. Hofmeyr, G.J.; Lawrie, T.A.; Atallah, Á.N.; Duley, L.; Torloni, M.R. Calcium supplementation during pregnancy for preventing hypertensive disorders and related problems (Review). *Cochrane Database Syst. Rev.* **2014**, CD001059. [CrossRef]
44. An, L.; Li, W.; Xie, T.; Peng, X.; Li, B.; Xie, S.; Xu, J.; Zhou, X.; Guo, S. Calcium supplementation reducing the risk of hypertensive disorders of pregnancy and related problems: A meta-analysis of multicentre randomized controlled trials. *Int. J. Nurs. Pract.* **2015**, *21*, 19–31. [CrossRef] [PubMed]
45. Schoenaker, D.A.J.M.; Soedamah-muthu, S.S.; Mishra, G.D. The association between dietary factors and gestational hypertension and pre-eclampsia: A systematic review and meta-analysis of observational studies. *BMC Med.* **2014**, *12*, 157. [CrossRef] [PubMed]
46. Wu, L.; Sun, D. Effects of calcium plus Vitamin D supplementation on blood pressure: A systematic review and meta-analysis of randomized controlled trials. *J. Hum. Hypertens.* **2017**, *31*, 547–554. [CrossRef] [PubMed]
47. Cormick, G.; Ciapponi, A.; Cafferata, M.L.; Belizán, J.M. Calcium supplementation for prevention of primary hypertension (Review). *Cochrane Database Syst. Rev.* **2015**, CD010037. [CrossRef]
48. Dibaba, D.T.; Xun, P.; Song, Y.; Rosanoff, A.; Shechter, M.; He, K. The effect of magnesium supplementation on blood pressure in individuals with insulin resistance, prediabetes, or noncommunicable chronic diseases: A meta-analysis of randomized controlled trials. *Am. J. Clin. Nutr.* **2017**, *106*, 921–929. [CrossRef] [PubMed]
49. Verma, H.; Garg, R. Effect of magnesium supplementation on type 2 diabetes associated cardiovascular risk factors: A systematic review and meta-analysis. *J. Hum. Nutr. Diet.* **2017**, *30*, 621–633. [CrossRef]
50. Kass, L.; Weekes, J.; Carpenter, L. Effect of magnesium supplementation on blood pressure: A meta-analysis. *Eur. J. Clin. Nutr.* **2012**, *66*, 411–418. [CrossRef]
51. Rosanoff, A.; Plesset, M.R. Oral magnesium supplements decrease high blood pressure (SBP > 155mmHg) in hypertensive subjects on anti-hypertensive medications: A targeted meta-analysis. *Magnes. Res.* **2013**, *26*, 93–99.

52. Han, H.; Fang, X.; Wei, X.; Liu, Y.; Jin, Z.; Chen, Q.; Fan, Z.; Aaseth, J.; Hiyoshi, A.; He, J.; et al. Dose-response relationship between dietary magnesium intake, serum magnesium concentration and risk of hypertension: A systematic review and meta-analysis of prospective cohort studies. *Nutr. J.* **2017**, *16*, 26. [CrossRef]
53. Wu, J.; Xun, P.; Tang, Q.; Cai, W.; He, K. Circulating magnesium levels and incidence of coronary heart diseases, hypertension, and type 2 diabetes mellitus: A meta-analysis of prospective cohort studies. *Nutr. J.* **2017**, *16*, 60. [CrossRef] [PubMed]
54. Adrogué, H.J.; Madias, N.E. Sodium and Potassium in the Pathogenesis of Hypertension. *N. Engl. J. Med.* **2007**, *356*, 1966–1978. [CrossRef] [PubMed]
55. Takahashi, H.; Yoshika, M.; Komiyama, Y.; Nishimura, M. The central mechanism underlying hypertension: A review of the roles of sodium ions, epithelial sodium channels, the renin-angiotensin-aldosterone system, oxidative stress and endogenous digitalis in the brain. *Hypertens. Res.* **2011**, *34*, 1147–1160. [CrossRef] [PubMed]
56. Morris, R.C.; Schmidlin, O.; Sebastian, A.; Tanaka, M.; Kurtz, T.W. Vasodysfunction That Involves Renal Vasodysfunction, Not Abnormally Increased Renal Retention of Sodium, Accounts for the Initiation of Salt-Induced Hypertension. *Circulation* **2016**, *133*, 881–893. [CrossRef] [PubMed]
57. D'Elia, L.; Galletti, F.; La Fata, E.; Sabino, P.; Strazzullo, P. Effect of dietary sodium restriction on arterial stiffness: Systematic review and meta-analysis of the randomized controlled trials. *J. Hypertens.* **2018**, *36*, 734–743. [CrossRef] [PubMed]
58. Houston, M.C. The Importance of potassium in managing hypertension. *Curr. Hypertens. Rep.* **2011**, *13*, 309–317. [CrossRef] [PubMed]
59. Murao, S.; Takata, Y.; Yasuda, M.; Osawa, H.; Kohi, F. The Influence of Sodium and Potassium Intake and Insulin Resistance on Blood Pressure in Normotensive Individuals Is More Evident in Women. *Am. J. Hypertens.* **2018**, *31*, 876–885. [CrossRef]
60. Feyh, A.; Bracero, L.; Lakhani, H.V.; Santhanam, P.; Shapiro, J.; Khitan, Z.; Sodhi, K. Role of Dietary Components in Modulating Hypertension. *J. Clin. Exp. Cardiol.* **2016**, *7*, 433. [CrossRef]
61. Sontia, B.; Touyz, R.M. Role of magnesium in hypertension. *Arch. Biochem. Biophys.* **2007**, *458*, 33–39. [CrossRef]
62. Egeland, G.M.; Skurtveit, S.; Sakshaug, S.; Daltveit, A.K.; Vikse, B.E.; Haugen, M. Low Calcium Intake in Midpregnancy Is Associated with Hypertension Development within 10 Years after Pregnancy: The Norwegian Mother and Child Cohort Study. *J. Nutr.* **2017**, *147*, 1757–1763. [CrossRef]
63. World Health Organization. WHO Recommendation: Calcium Supplementation during Pregnancy for the Prevention of Pre-eclampsia and Its Complications. Available online: https://apps.who.int/iris/bitstream/handle/10665/277235/9789241550451-eng.pdf?ua=1 (accessed on 14 June 2019).
64. Leung, A.A.; Nerenberg, K.; Daskalopoulou, S.S.; McBrien, K.; Zarnke, K.B.; Dasgupta, K.; Cloutier, L.; Gelfer, M.; Lamarre-Cliche, M.; Milot, A.; et al. Hypertension Canada's 2016 Canadian Hypertension Education Program Guidelines for Blood Pressure Measurement, Diagnosis, Assessment of Risk, Prevention, and Treatment of Hypertension. *Can. J. Cardiol.* **2016**, *32*, 569–588. [CrossRef] [PubMed]
65. Ndanuko, R.N.; Tapsell, L.C.; Charlton, K.E.; Neale, E.P.; Batterham, M.J. Dietary Patterns and Blood Pressure in Adults: A Systematic Review and Meta-Analysis of Randomized Controlled Trials. *Adv. Nutr.* **2016**, *7*, 76–89. [CrossRef] [PubMed]
66. Zhang, Y.; Agnoletti, D.; Safar, M.E.; Blacher, J. Effect of antihypertensive agents on blood pressure variability: The natrilix SR versus candesartan and amlodipine in the reduction of systolic blood pressure in hypertensive patients (X-CELLENT) study. *Hypertension* **2011**, *58*, 155–160. [CrossRef] [PubMed]
67. McClure, S.T.; Rebholz, C.M.; Medabalimi, S.; Hu, E.A.; Xu, Z.; Selvin, E.; Appel, L.J. Dietary phosphorus intake and blood pressure in adults: A systematic review of randomized trials and prospective observational studies. *Am. J. Clin. Nutr.* **2019** *109*, 1264–1272. [CrossRef] [PubMed]
68. Pizzorno, J.; Frassetto, L.A.; Katzinger, J. Diet-induced acidosis: Is it real and clinically relevant? *Br. J. Nutr.* **2010**, *103*, 1185–1194. [CrossRef] [PubMed]
69. Mazoteras-Pardo, V.; Becerro-De-Bengoa-Vallejo, R.; Losa-Iglesias, M.E.; López-López, D.; Palomo-López, P.; Rodríguez-Sanz, D.; Calvo-Lobo, C. The QardioArm Blood Pressure App for Self-Measurement in an Obese Population: Validation Study Using the European Society of Hypertension International Protocol Revision 2010. *JMIR Mhealth Uhealth* **2018**, *6*, e11632. [CrossRef] [PubMed]

7

Mechanisms Involved in the Relationship between Low Calcium Intake and High Blood Pressure

Cecilia Villa-Etchegoyen [1,*], Mercedes Lombarte [2], Natalia Matamoros [3], José M. Belizán [4] and Gabriela Cormick [4,5]

1 Laboratory of Cardiovascular Surveillance of Drugs, Department of Toxicology and Pharmacology, School of Medicine, Universidad de Buenos Aires, Ciudad Autonoma de Buenos Aires, Buenos Aires 1121, Argentina
2 Bone Biology Laboratory, School of Medicine, Rosario National University, Rosario, Santa Fe 3100, Argentina; mercedes_lombarte@yahoo.com.ar
3 Instituto de Desarrollo e Investigaciones Pediátricas "Prof. Dr. Fernando E. Viteri" Hospital de Niños "Sor María Ludovica de La Plata (IDIP), Ministerio de Salud/Comisión de Investigacines Científicas de la Provincia de Buenos Aires, La Plata, Buenos Aires 1900, Argentina; natymatamoros@gmail.com
4 Department of Mother and Child Health Research, Institute for Clinical Effectiveness and Health Policy (IECS-CONICET), Ciudad Autonoma de Buenos Aires, Buenos Aires 1414, Argentina; belizanj@gmail.com (J.M.B.); gabmick@yahoo.co.uk (G.C.)
5 Departamento de Salud, Universidad Nacional de La Matanza, Florencio Varela, San Justo 1903, Argentina
* Correspondence: c.villaetchegoyen@gmail.com

Abstract: There is increasing epidemiologic and animal evidence that a low calcium diet increases blood pressure. The aim of this review is to compile the information on the link between low calcium intake and blood pressure. Calcium intake may regulate blood pressure by modifying intracellular calcium in vascular smooth muscle cells and by varying vascular volume through the renin–angiotensin–aldosterone system. Low calcium intake produces a rise of parathyroid gland activity. The parathyroid hormone increases intracellular calcium in vascular smooth muscles resulting in vasoconstriction. Parathyroidectomized animals did not show an increase in blood pressure when fed a low calcium diet as did sham-operated animals. Low calcium intake also increases the synthesis of calcitriol in a direct manner or mediated by parathyroid hormone (PTH). Calcitriol increases intracellular calcium in vascular smooth muscle cells. Both low calcium intake and PTH may stimulate renin release and consequently angiotensin II and aldosterone synthesis. We are willing with this review to promote discussions and contributions to achieve a better understanding of these mechanisms, and if required, the design of future studies.

Keywords: calcium intake; blood pressure; parathyroid function; vitamin D; renin-angiotensin-aldosterone system

1. Introduction

The relationship between calcium intake and blood pressure has been widely studied since the 1980s [1–3]. Dietary calcium has been shown to have an effect on blood pressure in animal studies. Normotensive rats fed a free-calcium diet significantly increased their systolic blood pressure (SBP) between 15 to 35 mmHg in comparison with rats fed with normal calcium diet [4–6]. On the other hand, normotensive and hypertensive rats supplemented with calcium had significant lower values of SBP [7–10]. Systematic reviews of calcium supplementation randomized controlled trials in hypertensive and normotensive populations have shown a consistent decrease of blood pressure, with a mean difference in systolic blood pressure (SBP) of 2.5 mmHg (95% confidence interval (CI) = 0.6–4.5) in hypertensive subjects and of 1.4 mmHg (95% (CI) = 0.72–2.15) in normotensive subjects [11,12].

In humans, even such a small reduction in blood pressure was estimated to be associated with about 10% lower stroke mortality and about 7% lower mortality from ischemic heart disease [13].

The effect of calcium supplementation on SBP was higher in people aged less than 35 years (−2.11 mmHg) and with doses of calcium equal to or over 1500 mg/day (−2.79 mmHg). The higher impact on BP reduction observed in these cases seem to be diluted in the overall revision due to these studies only representing approximately 20% of the participants [11]. Also, the vast majority of the included trials were performed in high-income countries that usually have a higher basal dietary calcium intake.

Most importantly this effect on blood pressure has been studied during pregnancy for the prevention of preeclampsia [14]. A systematic review of randomized controlled trials of calcium supplementation on the prevention of preeclampsia shows a large effect (13 trials, 15,730 women: RR = 0.45, 95% CI = 0.31–0.65) [15]. This evidence was used to update WHO guidelines for the prevention of preeclampsia, which include the recommendation to supplement pregnant women from areas with low calcium intake with 1.5 to 2 g of calcium per day during the second half of pregnancy [16,17]. Moreover, the follow up of children whose mothers were supplemented during pregnancy show noticeable effects on preventing high blood pressure and dental caries in the progeny [18,19]. Recently, the preconceptional and early pregnancy effect of a low calcium supplementation dose was studied in a multi-country randomized placebo controlled trial showing the beneficial effect of calcium before conception and throughout pregnancy [20]. All these effects of calcium intake have also been replicated in animal models so as to gain insight on the mechanisms that link calcium intake and blood pressure regulation [1,2,4–6].

The aim of this literature review is to contribute to finding the mechanisms that could explain the relationship between calcium intake and blood pressure.

2. Calcium and Blood Pressure Regulation

Calcium intake may regulate blood pressure by increasing intracellular calcium in vascular smooth muscle cells leading to vasoconstriction, and by increasing vascular volume through the renin–angiotensin–aldosterone system (RAAS). We found three major mechanisms explaining the relationship between a low calcium intake and the increase in blood pressure: (a) parathyroid function, (b) vitamin D, and (c) the renin–angiotensin–aldosterone system (RAAS). These three mechanisms are described below (Figure 1).

2.1. *Calcium Intake and Parathyroid Function on Blood Pressure Regulation*

Calcium intake has a role in blood pressure regulation and the parathyroid glands play a role in calcium homeostasis, thus the link between calcium intake, parathyroid function, and blood pressure seems to be intuitively valid. However, few studies have evaluated the pathways linking calcium intake, parathyroid function, and blood pressure altogether. The following section accounts for the physiological bases of this relationship, focusing on the effects of the parathyroid hormone (PTH) and the not completely purified and characterized parathyroid hypertensive factor (PHF).

2.1.1. Mechanisms Mediated by Parathyroid Hormone (PTH)

Several studies have reported that calcium intake is inversely associated with blood pressure, both in humans [3,11,12,21–23] and in animals [2,5,6]. The inverse relationship between calcium intake and plasma PTH levels has also been widely studied at different ages and physiological stages in both humans and animals, in acute and long term studies [24–27]. Similarly, the direct relationship between plasma PTH and blood pressure both in healthy subjects and animals is also well documented [25,28–33]. The relationship between the reported parathyroid hormone serum levels and blood pressure measurements in normotensive and hypertensive subjects is shown in Table 1. Studies showing a correlation between blood pressure values and quartiles and quintiles of parathyroid hormone levels in human studies are shown in Table 2. Some studies in humans have shown low calcium intake, increased PTH levels, and increased blood pressure in the same subjects, although no description of mechanisms involved in this relationship were mentioned [34–36] (Table 3).

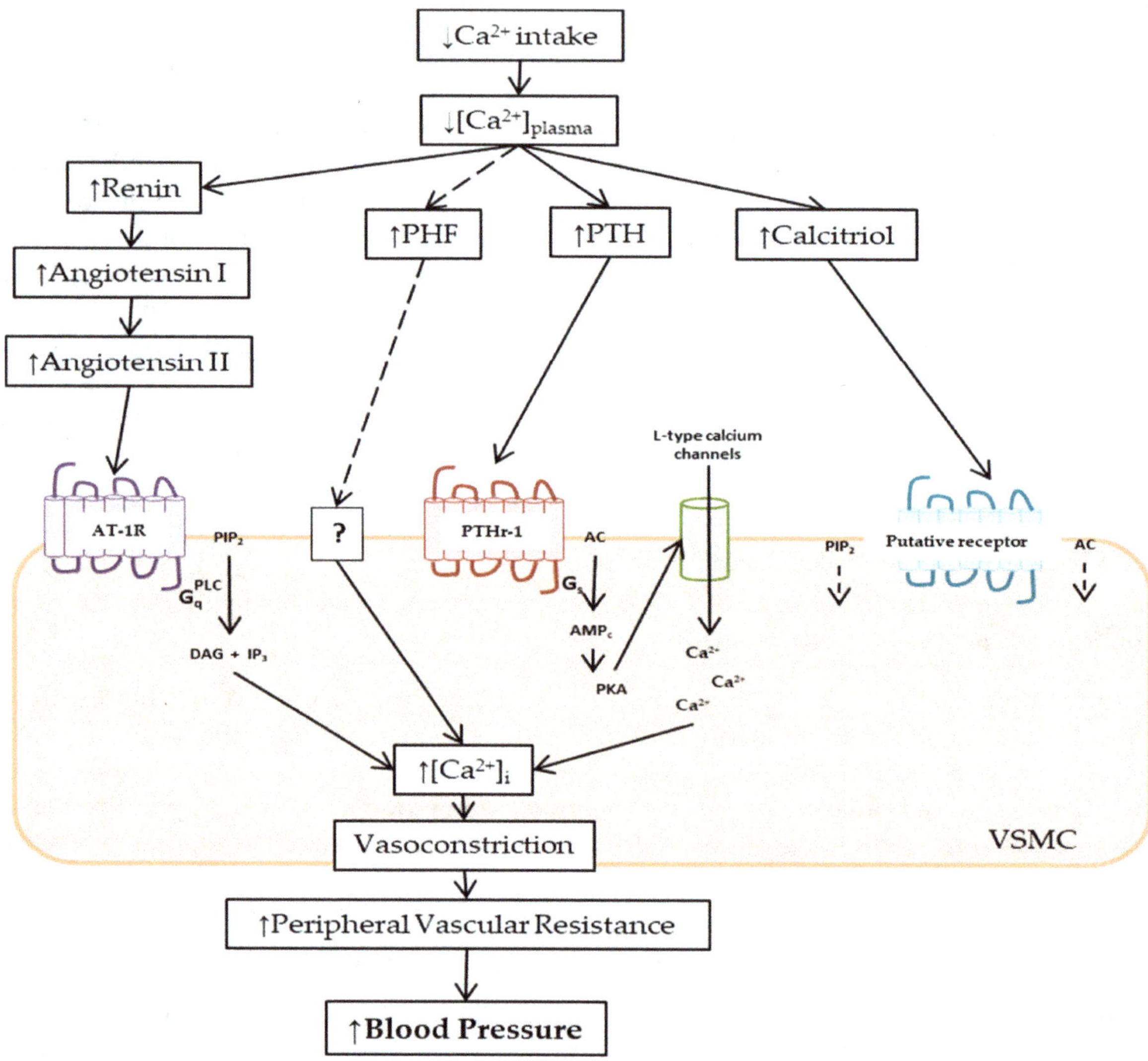

Figure 1. Scheme of the mechanisms involved in the rise of blood pressure in low calcium intake by an increase in peripheral vascular resistance. Low calcium intake decreases plasmatic calcium concentration ($[Ca^{2+}]_{plasma}$), stimulating the release of parathyroid hormone (PTH) and parathyroid hypertensive factor (PHF), the synthesis of calcitriol, and the activation of the renin–angiotensin–aldosterone system (RAAS). In vascular smooth muscle cells (VSMC), angiotensin II via the angiotensin II type I receptor (AT1R)/Gq/phospholipase C (PLC)/inositol trisphosphate (IP3) pathway, PTH via PTHr-1/Gs/3′,5′-cyclic adenosine monophosphate (cAMP)/protein kinase A (PKA), and calcitriol via adenylate cyclase (AC)/cAMP/PKA and PLC/IP3 signaling pathways increased the intracellular calcium concentration ($[Ca^{2+}]_i$). The rise of $[Ca^{2+}]_i$ leads to vasoconstriction, and hence increases in peripheral vascular resistance and blood pressure. The PHF mechanism of action remains unknown. See text for further details.

Table 1. Parathyroid hormone (PTH) serum levels and blood pressure (BP) values in normotensive and hypertensive subjects.

Reference (First Author)	Method	Country and Participants	PTH (pmol/L)	BP (SBP − DBP mmHg)
Young 1990 [28]	Cross-sectional	USA, 115 subjects, ≈45 years	NT = 4.5 ± 2.2 HT = 5.0 ± 2.4	NT = 120(±11) − 80(±8) HT = 138(±8) − 95(±5)
Brickman 1990 [29]	Cross-sectional	USA, 38 men, ≈56 years	NT = 20.8 ± 1.1 HT = 28.4 + 3.5	NT = 123(±2.8) − 78(±1.3) HT = 150(±3.9) − 97(±0.9)
Morfis 1997 [30]	Cross-sectional	Australia, 123 subjects, 63–88 years	NT = 2.7 ± 1.1	NT = 125(±12) − 71(±7)
			HT = 2.9 ± 1.3	HT =135(±14) − 73(±10)
Park 2015 [32]	Cross-sectional	Korea, 1664 postmenopausal women, >50 years	NT = 63.7 ± 23.4 HT = 68.3 ± 23.6	NT = 117.5(±12.4) − 73.3(±8.1) HT = 149.4(±11.4) − 86.0(±10.1)

NT = normotensive people; HT = hypertensive people, SBP = systolic blood pressure; DBP = diastolic blood pressure. Values are expressed as mean (±standard deviation).

Table 2. Blood pressure (BP) values by quartiles or quintiles of parathyroid hormone (PTH) levels in human studies.

Reference (First Author)	Method	Country and Participants	PTH (pmol/L)	BP (SBP − DBP mmHg)
Snijder 2007 [31]	Cross-sectional	The Netherlands, 1205 subjects, participants, 55–85 years	Q1: <2.45 Q2: 2.45–3.13 Q3: 3.14–4.25 Q4: >4.25	150.1(±26.1) − 82.5(±13.0) 151.7(±24.8) − 82.6(±13.4) 154.7(±24.6) − 84.3(±13.6) 156.2(±27.6) − 83.9(±13.0)
Chan 2011 [25]	Cross-sectional	China, 939 men, >65 years	Q1: <3.1 Q2: 3.2–4.1 Q3: 4.2–5.5 Q4: >5.5	135.8(±1.7) − 76.5(±0.8) 139.9(±1.6) − 76.5(±0.8) 141.4(±1.7) − 76.5(±0.8) 143.6(±1.8) − 79.9(±0.8)
Yao 2016 [33]	Cohort study	USA, 7504 subjects, 45–64 years	Q1: 3.2–28.8 Q2: 28.9–34.9 Q3: 35.0–41.5 Q4: 41.6–50.1 Q5: 50.2–162.6	112(±13) − 68.0(±8.2) 113(±12) − 68.4(±8.3) 114(±12) − 69.4(±8.5) 115(±12) − 69.9(±8.1) 115(±12) − 70.5(±8.2)

SBP = systolic blood pressure; DBP = diastolic blood pressure. Values are expressed as mean (±standard deviation) or mean [±standard error of the mean].

Table 3. Parathyroid hormone (PTH) and blood pressure (BP) and dietary calcium intake in human studies.

Reference (First Author)	Method	Country and Participants		Ca Intake (mg/day)	PTH (pmol/L)	BP (SBP − DBP mmHg)
Takagi 1991 [34]	Clinical trial	Japan, 9 HT, 65–86 years, CaSup (1 g) vs. diet Ca 500 mg, 8 weeks		1 g/day (CaSup)	27	−13.6 mmHg to −5.0 mmHg
				500 mg/day (diet)	33	−1.5 mmHg to +1.0 mmHg
Jorde 2000 [36]	Cohort study	Norway, 1113 subjects, 30–79 years		592.1(±459.6)	4.5(±1.2)	143.4(±19.9) − 84.3(±10.4)
				400.3(±227.3)	9.1(±2.4)	153.9(±27.1) − 89.7(±14.1)
Kamycheva 2004 [35]	Cross-sectional	Norway, 3570 subjects, >24 years	♂	499(±259) 476(±257) 443(±233) 430(±243)	Q1 <1.9 Q2 1.9–2.6 Q3 2.61–3.5 Q4 >3.5	136.9(±17.7) 140.1(±19.6) 142.0(±20.3) 145.2(±20.3)
			♀	478(±277) 428(±227) 431(±226) 408(±217)	Q1 <1.8 Q2 1.8–2.4 Q3 2.41–3.3 Q4 >3.3	133.2(±18.5) 135.5(±21.5) 141.9(±22.4) 146.5(±23.2)

NT = normotensive people; HT = hypertensive people, CaSup= calcium supplementation; SBP = systolic blood pressure; DBP = diastolic blood pressure. Values are expressed as mean (±standard deviation).

Several studies have shown that PTH levels can independently predict cardiovascular disease and mortality [35,37–39]. The prospective and multicenter Osteoporotic Fractures in Men (MrOS) study, including 1490 men older than 65 years and followed up for 7.3 years, shows that concentrations of PTH were associated with an increased risk of cardiovascular mortality (adjusted hazard ratio SD = 1.21, 95% CI = 1.00–1.45) and from all causes (adjusted HR per SD = 1.15, 95% CI = 1.03–1.29) [37]. The Multi-Ethnic Study of Atherosclerosis (MESA) cohort study in which 3002 men and women, aged 59 ± 9.7 years, without cardiovascular antecedents were followed up for 9.0 years found that higher PTH serum concentrations were associated with a greater risk of hypertension, even after adjusting for potential confounders (HR = 1.27, 95% CI = 1.01–1.59) [39]. The population-based, cross-sectional Tromsø study including 3570 men and women aged 25–79 years found a positive relationship between serum PTH and SBP with the highest quartile of serum PTH found to be an independent predictor of coronary heart disease in both sexes (OR = 1.70, 95% CI = 1.08–2.70 for males, OR = 1.73, 95% CI = 1.04–2.88 for females, $p < 0.05$).

PTH is an 84-amino-acid polypeptide (≈9.5 kilodalton (kDa)) secreted by the chief cells of the parathyroid gland. PTH acts on the cell membrane of its target tissues through a G-protein-coupled receptor, the parathyroid hormone receptor type 1 (PTHr-1). Expression of PTH receptors has been reported in many tissues, including vascular smooth muscle and endothelial cells [40]. The PTHr-1 couples to several signaling pathways, namely: the Gαs/adenylate cyclase (AC)/cAMP/protein kinase A (PKA), the Gαq/phospholipase C (PLC)β/inositol trisphosphate (IP3)/intracellular Ca/protein kinase C (PKC), the Gα12/13 phospholipase D/RhoA pathway, and the mitogen-activated protein kinase (extracellular signal regulated kinase [ERK1/2]) signaling cascade [41,42].

Several mechanisms have been proposed to explain the effect of PTH on blood pressure: (a) an increase in cytosolic free calcium concentration ($[Ca^{2+}]_i$) through the PTH receptor (PTHr-1) in vascular smooth muscle, (b) increase calcitriol concentration, and (c) a cross-talk with the renin–angiotensin–aldosterone system (RAAS). The last two will be described in its corresponding sections.

High $[Ca^{2+}]_i$ increases vascular reactivity, and therefore peripheral vascular resistance and responsiveness to the sympathetic and the RAAS, which all elevate blood pressure. Calcium channel blockers, such as nifedipine and verapamil, are valuable antihypertensive drugs as they inhibit Ca^{2+} entry to the cell and reduce $[Ca^{2+}]_i$. In the same way, calcium supplementation in subjects with low calcium intake has been described to decrease $[Ca^{2+}]_i$ [43,44], hence diminishing blood pressure. It has been shown that PTH increases calcium entry into a variety of mammalian tissues and cell lines, such as cardiomyocytes [45], enterocytes [46], kidney [47], liver [48], peripheral nerves [49], osteosarcoma cells [50], and osteoblastlike cells [51]. Significantly higher $[Ca^{2+}]_i$ was also found in human platelets and lymphocytes of hypertensive patients [29,52]. The activation of PTHr-1/Gq/PLC/IP3, PTHr-1/Gα12-13/phospholipase D/RhoA cascades, and of calcium channels are the signaling pathways by which PTH increases $[Ca^{2+}]_i$ and blood pressure [47].

A controversial effect is the vasodilator effect of acute PTH infusion, both in vivo and in vitro. In vascular smooth muscle cells, PTHr-1 couples primarily to Gαs, which increases cAMP and decreases $[Ca^{2+}]_i$ [53]. Nonetheless, the sustained activation of this cascade shows desensitization to PTH in a time- and concentration-dependent fashion [54–56]. The chronic infusion of PTH has been associated with arterial hypertension [57]. Long-standing high levels of PTH, such as in hyperparathyroidism, are frequently related to hypertension, whereas parathyroidectomy is associated with a decrease in $[Ca^{2+}]_i$ and blood pressure [58]. A rise of $[Ca^{2+}]_i$ through PTHr-1/Gαs/AC/cAMP via opening calcium channels in a cell line derived from fetal rat aorta was also described [59]. Therefore, the desensitization of the cAMP pathway to PTH, as well as the stimulation of other blood pressure mediators considered below, like the RAAS and calcitriol, may explain the long-term pressor effects of PTH.

2.1.2. Parathyroid Hypertensive Factor (PHF)

In the early 1990s, Lewanczuk et al. described that the infusion of plasma from hypertensive rats and from hypertensive subjects on normotensive rats increased the mean arterial pressure of those rats [60,61]. They attributed this effect to the presence of a novel hypertensive factor in the plasma of the hypertensive donors. The same group also reported the parathyroid origin of this factor by transplanting parathyroid glands from hypertensive rats into parathyroidectomized normotensive rats. An increase in blood pressure was shown in the rats after transplantation [60,62,63]. Due to this, the non-isolated substance was called parathyroid hypertensive factor (PHF) [60].

In spontaneously hypertensive rat strains, low calcium intake increases blood pressure that the authors explained was due to an increase of PFH [64]. These authors also proposed that PHF regulates blood pressure by modifying the concentration of $[Ca^{2+}]_i$ in vascular smooth muscle [60,65,66]. In isolated vascular smooth muscle cells from rat tail arteries, Shan et al. found that the infusion of semi-purified plasma from hypertensive rats enhanced the opening of the L-type calcium channel, an effect antagonized by the dihydropyridine calcium channel blocker nifedipine [67].

Although the effect of plasma from hypertensive rats has been well-documented, the purification and characterization of PHF is uncomplete. Benishin et al. showed the correlation of a UV spectrum of dialyzed plasma from hypertensive rats with a small (≈3 kDa), trypsin-inactivated and boiled-resistant peptide [68]. Years later, the same group proposed that the PHF structure has both peptide and lysophospholid motifs, critical for its biological activity [69]. Schlüter et al. also isolated a peptide-like vasopressor of low molecular weight (0.6–2.5 kDa) from parathyroid tissue of patients with tertiary hyperparathyroidism. The eluent was shown to be polar, hydrophilic, and protease-sensitive, but not heat-resistant. Schlüter's group also suggested that further purifications were needed as several substances were shown on the mass spectrometry [70].

Although the existence of PHF may explain the blood pressure changes induced by alterations in a calcium diet, there is still much to know about this mediator. First, the published results have been poorly replicated outside the group that described PHF [71]. On the other hand, after 30 years of being described, the definitive chemical structure of this mediator is still unknown and there have not been reports of new attempts to purify it. Nonetheless, the function of the parathyroid gland seems to play a key role in blood pressure regulation, as was reported both in humans and in normotensive and hypertensive animals.

In summary, the bulk of information of this section orients towards an increase of the parathyroid gland activity by low calcium intake leading to an increase of $[Ca^{2+}]_i$ in vascular smooth muscle cells and consequently a rise in blood pressure (Figure 1). In addition to the direct effect of PTH (or PHF) in smooth muscle, we will later discuss the effects of PTH mediated by calcitriol and RAAS. A demonstration of the effect of parathyroid activity in the regulation of blood pressure related to calcium intake is shown in a study of parathyroidectomized rats in comparison with sham operation rats. After 10 weeks on a calcium-free diet, the sham operation rats showed an increase in SBP of 3.44 (SE = 1.95) mmHg, while the parathyroidectomized rats showed a decrease in SBP of −9.67 (SE = 2.05) mmHg. A highly statistical significant difference of 13.11 mmHg was found between the two groups [2].

2.2. *Calcium Intake and Vitamin D in Blood Pressure Regulation*

Most systematic reviews of randomized controlled trials do not show an effect of vitamin D supplementation on blood pressure. A systematic review of 46 trials (4541 participants) found no effect of vitamin D supplementation on SBP (effect size = 0.0 [95% CI = −0.8 to 0.8] mmHg; $p = 0.97$; $I^2 = 21\%$) or diastolic blood pressure (DBP) (effect size = −0.1 [95% CI = −0.6 to 0.5] mmHg; $p = 0.84$; $I^2 = 20\%$) nor in subgroup analysis via basal vitamin D or blood pressure levels [72]. A systematic review in hypertensive subjects did not find evidence of vitamin D supplementation on blood pressure [73]. However, one systematic review found that in vitamin D deficient populations, supplementation has a small effect on peripheral DBP but not in central DBP nor in peripheral nor central SBP, though this evidence is weak as it mainly comes from one small trial on vitamin D deficient and hypertensive subjects [74,75]. However, in these systematic reviews some population groups, such as those with vitamin D deficiency, might be underrepresented. One randomized, double-blind, placebo-controlled clinical trial of oral calcitriol in African-Americans with low baseline calcitriol level reported a significant decrease in SBP but not DBP after a three-month follow up [76].

Vitamin D is a steroid hormone that can be synthesized in the skin under the influence of sunlight (cholecalciferol or vitamin D3) or be obtained from foods such as fish and vegetables (ergocalciferol or vitamin D2). Later, a two-step hydroxylation is required to procure its biological active form (1,25-OHVitD, calcitriol). Low calcium intake increases calcitriol concentration, both in human and in animals [77–79]. PTH stimulates the renal α-1 hydroxylase enzyme to produce the final activation. However, PTH is probably not the sole regulator of calcitriol synthesis as an increase in the efficiency of calcium absorption has been described with low calcium intake diets even after parathyroidectomy [79]. The renal α-1 hydroxylase activity seems to be directly modulated by calcium, as the addition of calcium ions in vitro produced an inhibitory effect of the enzyme activity [80]. In addition, α-1 hydroxylase activity was found in tissues other than kidney such as endothelial cells. Vitamin D receptor (VDR) expression was described in endothelial cells. These findings could orient towards an auto/paracrine action of calcitriol in endothelial cells [81].

The effects of calcitriol are mediated by both genomic and nongenomic mechanisms. Genomic responses are mediated by intracellular vitamin D receptor (VDR) functioning as transcription factors to modulate gene expression, whilst the short-term effects seem to be mediated by putative receptors [82].

Among the rapid nongenomic effects, it has been shown that calcitriol increases $[Ca^{2+}]_i$ by increasing calcium uptake in many types of cells, including rat vascular smooth muscle cells and aorta-derived cell lines [83–85]. The intraperitoneal administration of calcitriol on spontaneously hypertensive and normotensive rats enhanced the contractile response of isolated mesenteric resistance arteries, showing that the effect is not related to the hypertensive condition [86]. Furthermore, Shan et al. reported a significant increase in the calcium channel current of rat artery-derived smooth muscle cells after calcitriol infusion [87]. In skeletal muscle, calcitriol effects have been extensively studied showing that calcitriol: (a) stimulates L-type voltage-operated calcium channels by cAMP pathway, (b) activates AC/cAMP/PKA and PLC/IP3/PKC signaling cascades, and (c) boosts the calcium messenger system [88], all of which are responsible for the increase of $[Ca^{2+}]_i$ (Figure 1).

Calcitriol regulates RAAS via genomic mechanisms [89]. An inverse association between serum calcitriol levels and plasma renin activity, in both human and animals, has been described [90]. Studies in VDR knockout mice show that calcitriol negatively regulates the RAAS and blood pressure by a genomic calcium- and PTH-independent mechanism [91–93].

The mechanism by which calcitriol regulates blood pressure seems not to be the same with low calcium intake as it is with vitamin D deficiency. Whereas restrictive calcium diets may dominate the nongenomic short-term effects by increasing $[Ca^{2+}]_i$, vitamin D deficiency may preponderate the VDR mediated actions on the RAAS.

In summary, the mechanism by which calcitriol regulates blood pressure in low calcium diets may be mediated by the nongenomic short-term effects increasing $[Ca^{2+}]_i$ and consequently rising blood pressure.

2.3. *Calcium Intake and Renin–Angiotensin–Aldosterone System*

The renin–angiotensin–aldosterone system (RAAS) plays a key role in the physiologic regulation of blood pressure. As shown below, several interactions between calcium intake, calcium homeostatic hormones and the RAAS have been described.

2.3.1. Renin

Renin enzymatic activity consists in the hydrolysis of angiotensinogen to angiotensin I. The acute incubation or infusion of high concentrations of calcium has an inhibitory effect on renin secretion, both in isolated cells and animals [94–97]. Dietary calcium supplementation has shown to decrease but not to abolish the renin release [98]. It has been reported that acute activation of the calcium sensing receptor in juxtaglomerular cells by high extracellular calcium concentration decreases renin release and plasma renin activity, both in vivo and in vitro. Renin secretion is dependent on cAMP formation. Increased extracellular calcium concentration decreases renin release by diminishing AC and enhancing phosphodiesterase activities [95,99]. cAMP concentration could also be raised by PTH as PTHr-1 along the nephron, including the juxtaglomerular apparatus [100]. The stimulation of PTHr-1 increases cAMP and enhances renin release [101] (Figure 1).

2.3.2. Angiotensin II

Angiotensin II is the primary active product of the RAAS and a potent vasoconstrictor whose actions are mediated by the type I angiotensin II receptor (AT-1R). Low calcium diets have been shown to increase angiotensin II [6,102]. In animals fed low calcium diets, the binding of angiotensin II withAT-1R decreases in smooth muscle cells and increases in the adrenal cortex. These findings suggest that with low calcium intake, angiotensin II may raise blood pressure via increasing aldosterone synthesis or secretion [5].

It has also been described that the infusion of angiotensin II produced a significant dose-dependent increase in PTH serum levels [101]. Moreover, AT-1R has been isolated in the parathyroid glands, and although the intracellular pathway is still unknown, AT-1R inhibition lowered PTH levels [103]. These observations may explain the blood pressure elevation by angiotensin II in a low calcium diet (Figure 1).

2.3.3. Aldosterone

Aldosterone, a steroid hormone, is synthesized by the zona glomerulosa of the adrenal cortex (CZG) in the adrenal gland. Its primary effect is the regulation of blood pressure through the reabsorption of sodium and excretion of potassium in the distal tubules and the collecting ducts of the nephron [104], increasing apical membrane permeability for sodium, thus causing sodium and water reabsorption. This rise of extracellular fluid volume increased cardiac output, and hence blood pressure (Figure 2).

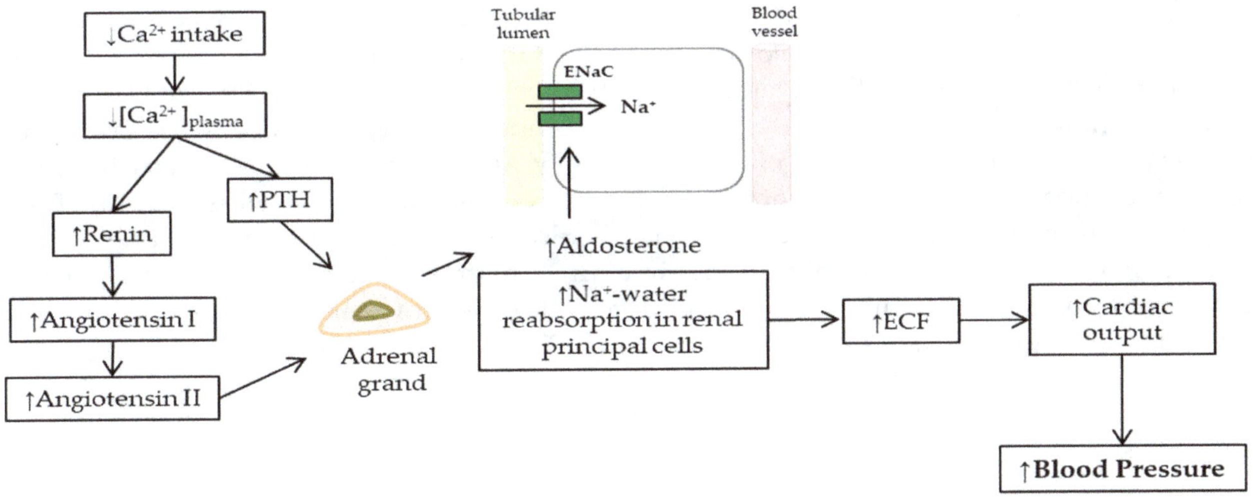

Figure 2. Scheme of the mechanisms involved in the rise of blood pressure in low calcium intake via an increase in cardiac output. Low calcium intake decreased the plasmatic calcium concentration ($[Ca^{2+}]_{plasma}$), stimulating PTH and the renin–angiotensin–aldosterone system (RAAS). Both angiotensin II and PTH were increased aldosterone secretion due to the adrenal gland. Aldosterone upregulates epithelial sodium channels (ENaC) in the principal cells of the collecting duct in the kidney, increasing apical membrane permeability for Na^+, thus Na^+ and water reabsorption. The rise of extracellular fluid volume (ECF) increased cardiac output and hence blood pressure.

Aldosterone synthesis is stimulated by angiotensin II and high extracellular potassium levels via the calcium messenger system that boosts the steroidogenic cascade within the mitochondria. The acute steroidogenic regulatory protein (StAR) is a key molecule that transports cholesterol through the inner mitochondrial membrane, a fundamental step for the synthesis of steroid hormones, such as aldosterone. StAR is activated by increases in $[Ca^{2+}]_i$. Angiotensin II, via AT-1R activating the PLC/IP3 cascades, and high extracellular potassium levels via depolarizing the plasma membrane of the cell activating calcium voltage-dependent channels, increase $[Ca^{2+}]_i$ and thus aldosterone synthesis [105].

A bidirectional stimulating relationship between PTH and aldosterone is reported. Patients with primary aldosteronism have high levels of PTH that return to physiological concentration after the adenoma removal or pharmacological treatment with aldosterone antagonists [106]. Similarly, hypertension associated with secondary aldosteronism due to hyperparathyroidism resolves after parathyroidectomy [107,108]. Studies in humans have also shown a rise in blood pressure and aldosterone after two weeks of an infusion of PTH [57], and this effect is antagonized by PTH-receptor blocking agents [109]. PTHr-1 has been found in the CZG of animals and humans [110], and mineralocorticoid receptors, for aldosterone, have been identified in the parathyroid gland [111].

It has been shown that PTHr-1 stimulates basal steroid secretion (aldosterone, cortisol) from adrenal cells through both AC/PKA- and PLC/PKC-dependent signaling mechanisms [109]. Adrenal cells incubated with PTH increase cAMP and IP3 production, with this effect being partially suppressed by inhibitors of both cascade. The activation of PKA, by increasing the concentration of cAMP, activates StAR. PTH can also indirectly favor steroidogenesis by increasing $[Ca^{2+}]_i$ [109].

In summary, it has been shown that both low calcium intake and PTH stimulate renin release, and consequently, angiotensin II and aldosterone synthesis.

3. Conclusions

In this manuscript, we reviewed the literature exploring the mechanisms involved in the relationship between calcium intake and blood pressure. It has been shown that, particularly in individuals with low calcium intake, an increase in calcium intake reduces blood pressure. We consider that in view of hypertension being a major factor involved in the global burden of disease, the study of interventions that could prevent the development of hypertension should be prioritized [112]. The link between calcium intake and blood pressure involves a connection between calciotropic hormones and blood pressure regulators. As was hypothesized many years ago, parathyroid activity increases the cytosolic concentration of calcium and increases vascular reactivity and blood pressure [113]. The effect of calcium intake on blood pressure is not shown in parathyroidectomized animal studies. Low calcium intake also increases the synthesis of calcitriol in a direct manner or is mediated by PTH. Calcitriol increases intracellular calcium in vascular smooth muscle cells. Low calcium intake stimulates renin release, and consequently, angiotensin II synthesis. PTH stimulates renin release, angiotensin II and aldosterone synthesis (Figure 3). We are willing with this review to promote discussions and contributions to achieve a better understanding of these mechanisms, and if required, the design of future studies.

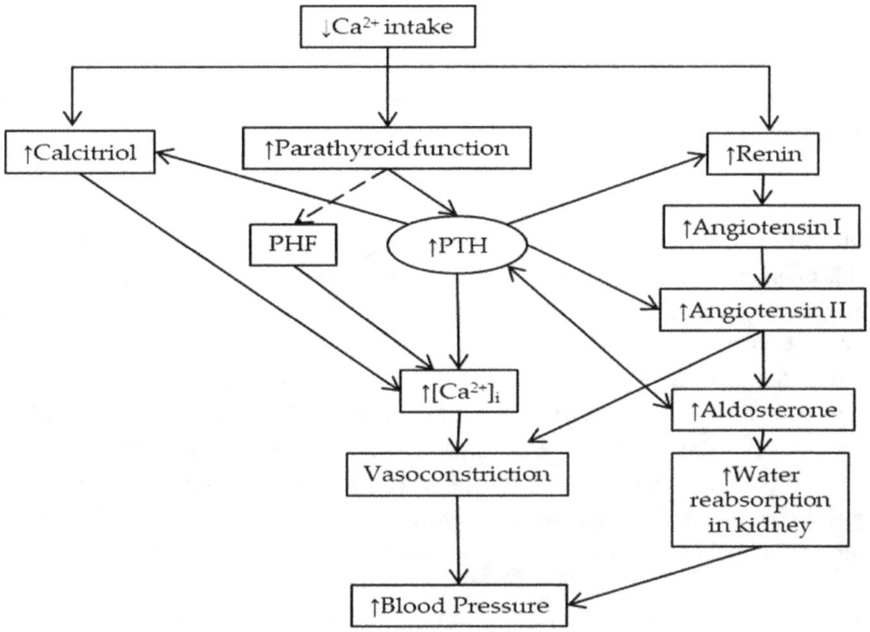

Figure 3. Scheme of the mechanisms involved in the rise of blood pressure due to low calcium intake, namely the link between calciotropic hormones and blood pressure regulators. Low calcium intake: (a) increases calcitriol serum levels, (b) stimulates parathyroid function, and (c) increases renin secretion. Calcitriol may increase cytosolic free calcium concentration ($[Ca^{2+}]_i$) via non-genomic short-term mechanisms. The parathyroid gland secretes parathyroid hormone (PTH) and possibly (dash arrow) the parathyroid hypertensive factor (PHF). Both mediators increase $[Ca^{2+}]_i$, leading to the contraction of the vascular smooth muscle cells (vasoconstriction). Renin release is stimulated both by low extracellular calcium and PTH, activating the renin–angiotensin–aldosterone system (RAAS). In addition, PTH increases angiotensin II and aldosterone synthesis, which also leads to vasoconstriction and increases renal water reabsorption, increasing blood pressure. Aldosterone also increases PTH serum levels (double-headed arrow). See text for further details.

Author Contributions: Conceptualization, project administration and funding acquisition J.M.B. and G.C.; investigation and writing—original draft preparation C.V.-E.; writing—review & editing, M.L., N.M., J.M.B. and G.C.

Abbreviations

$[Ca^{2+}]_i$	cytosolic free calcium/intracellular calcium concentration
ACAT-1R	adenylate cyclasetype I angiotensin II receptor
cAMP	3′,5′-cyclic adenosine monophosphate
CZG	zona glomerulosa of the adrenal cortex of the adrenal gland
DBP	diastolic blood pressure
IP3	inositol trisphosphate
PHF	parathyroid hypertensive factor
PKA	protein kinase A
PKC	protein kinase C
PLC	phospholipase C
PRA	plasma renin activity
PTH	parathyroid hormone
PTHr-1	PTH receptor
RAAS	the renin–angiotensin-aldosterone system
StAR	acute steroidogenic regulatory protein
SBP	systolic blood pressure
VDR	Vitamin D intracellular receptor

References

1. Belizan, J.M.; Villar, J. The relationship between calcium intake and edema-, proteinuria-, and hypertension-gestosis: An hypothesis. *Am. J. Clin. Nutr.* **1980**, *33*, 2202–2210. [CrossRef]
2. Belizán, J.M.; Villar, J.; Self, S.; Pineda, O.; González, I.; Sainz, E. The mediating role of the parathyroid gland in the effect of low calcium intake on blood pressure in the rat. *Arch. Latinoam. Nutr.* **1984**, *34*, 666–675. [PubMed]
3. Belizan, J.M.; Villar, J.; Pineda, O.; Gonzalez, A.E.; Sainz, E.; Garrera, G.; Sibrian, R. Reduction of blood pressure with calcium supplementation in young adults. *J. Am. Med. Assoc.* **1983**, *249*, 1161–1165. [CrossRef]
4. Belizan, J.M.; Pineda, O.; Sainz, E.; Menendez, L.A.; Villar, J. Rise of blood pressure in calcium-deprived pregnant rats. *Am. J. Obstet. Gynecol.* **1981**, *141*, 163–169. [CrossRef]
5. Baksi, S.N.; Abhold, R.H.; Speth, R.C. Low-calcium diet increases blood pressure and alters peripheral but not central angiotensin II binding sites in rats. *J. Hypertens.* **1989**, *7*, 423–427. [CrossRef] [PubMed]
6. Takahashi, N.; Yuasa, S.; Shoji, T.; Miki, S.; Fujioka, H.; Uchida, K.; Sumikura, T.; Takamitsu, Y.; Yura, T.; Matsuo, H. Effect of Low Dietary Calcium Intake on Blood Pressure and Pressure Natriuresis Response in Rats: A Possible Role of the Renin-Angiotensin System. *Blood Press.* **1996**, *5*, 121–127.
7. McCarron, D. Blood pressure and calcium balance in the Wistar-Kyoto rat. *Life Sci.* **1982**, *30*, 683–689. [CrossRef]
8. Furspan, P.B.; Rinaldi, G.J.; Hoffman, K.; Bohr, D.F. Dietary calcium and cell membrane abnormality in genetic hypertension. *Hypertension* **1989**, *13*, 727–730. [CrossRef] [PubMed]
9. Hatton, D.C.; Scrogin, K.E.; Levine, D.; Feller, D.; Mccarron, D.A. Dietary calcium modulates blood pressure through alpha 1-adrenergic receptors. *Am. J. Physiol.* **1993**, *264*, 234–238. [CrossRef]
10. Arvola, P.; Ruskoaho, H.; Pörsti, I. Effects of high calcium diet on arterial smooth muscle function and electrolyte balance in mineralocorticoid-salt hypertensive rats. *Br. J. Pharmacol.* **1993**, *108*, 948–958. [CrossRef]
11. Cormick, G.; Ciapponi, A.; Cafferata, M.L.; Belizán, J.M. Calcium supplementation for prevention of primary hypertension. *Cochrane Database Syst. Rev.* **2015**, *30*, CD010037. [CrossRef]
12. Dickinson, H.O.; Nicolson, D.J.; Cook, J.V.; Campbell, F.; Beyer, F.R.; Ford, G.A.; Mason, J. Calcium supplementation for the management of primary hypertension in adults. *Cochrane Database Syst. Rev.* **2006**, *19*, CD004639. [CrossRef] [PubMed]
13. Whelton, P.K.; He, J.; Appel, L.J.; Cutler, J.A.; Havas, S.; Kotchen, T.A.; Roccella, E.J.; Stout, R.; Vallbona, C.; Winston, M.C.; et al. Primary prevention of hypertension: Clinical and public health advisory from The National High Blood Pressure Education Program. *JAMA J. Am. Med. Assoc.* **2002**, *288*, 1882–1888. [CrossRef]
14. Belizán, J.M.; Villar, J.; Gonzalez, L.; Campodonico, L.; Bergel, E. Calcium supplementation to prevent hypertensive disorders of pregnancy. *N. Engl. J. Med.* **1991**, *325*, 1399–1405. [CrossRef] [PubMed]
15. Hofmeyr, G.J.; Lawrie, T.A.; Atallah, A.N.; Duley, L.; Torloni, M.R. Calcium supplementation during pregnancy for preventing hypertensive disorders and related problems. *Cochrane Database Syst. Rev.* **2014**, *24*, CD001059. [CrossRef]
16. Hofmeyr, G.J.; Betrán, A.P.; Singata-Madliki, M.; Cormick, G.; Munjanja, S.P.; Fawcus, S.; Mose, S.; Hall, D.; Ciganda, A.; Seuc, A.H.; et al. Prepregnancy and early pregnancy calcium supplementation among women at high risk of pre-eclampsia: A multicentre, double-blind, randomised, placebo-controlled trial. *Lancet* **2019**, *393*, 330–339. [CrossRef]
17. World Health Organization (WHO). *Guideline: Calcium Supplementation in Pregnant Women*; WHO: Geneva, Switzerland, 2013; pp. 1–35.
18. Belizan, J.M.; Villar, J.; Bergel, E.; del Pino, A.; Di Fulvio, S.; Galliano, S.V.; Kattan, C. Long-term effect of calcium supplementation during pregnancy on the blood pressure of offspring: Follow up of a randomised controlled trial. *BMJ* **1997**, *315*, 281–285. [CrossRef]
19. Bergel, E.; Gibbons, L.; Rasines, M.G.; Luetich, A.; Belizán, J.M. Maternal calcium supplementation during pregnancy and dental caries of children at 12 years of age: Follow-up of a randomized controlled trial. *Acta Obstet. Gynecol. Scand.* **2010**, *89*, 1396–1402. [CrossRef]
20. Hofmeyr, G. Protocol 11PRT/4028: Long term calcium supplementation in women at high risk of pre-eclampsia: A randomised, placebo-controlled trial. *Lancet* **2011**. Available online: https://www.thelancet.com/protocol-reviews/11PRT-4028 (accessed on 17 May 2019).

21. McCarron, D.A.; Morris, C.D.; Henry, H.J.; Stanton, J.L. Blood pressure and nutrient intake in the United States. *Nutr. Today* **1984**, *19*, 14–23. [CrossRef]
22. Skowrońska-Jóźwiak, E.; Jaworski, M.; Lorenc, R.; Karbownik-Lewińska, M.; Lewiński, A. Low dairy calcium intake is associated with overweight and elevated blood pressure in Polish adults, notably in premenopausal women. *Public Health Nutr.* **2016**, *20*, 630–637. [CrossRef] [PubMed]
23. Schröder, H.; Schmelz, E.; Marrugat, J. Relationship between diet and blood pressure in a representative Mediterranean population. *Eur. J. Nutr.* **2002**, *41*, 161–167. [CrossRef]
24. Grubenmann, W.; Binswanger, U.; Hunziker, W.; Fischer, J.A. Effects of calcium intake and renal function on plasma immunoreactive parathyroid hormone levels in rats. *Horm. Metab. Res.* **1978**, *10*, 438–443. [CrossRef]
25. Chan, R.; Woo, J.; Chan, D.; Mellström, D.; Leung, P.; Ohlsson, C.; Kwok, T. Serum 25-hydroxyvitamin D and parathyroid hormone levels in relation to blood pressure in a cross-sectional study in older Chinese men. *J. Hum. Hypertens.* **2011**, *26*, 20–27. [CrossRef]
26. Schoenmakers, I.; Jarjou, L.M.A.; Goldberg, G.R.; Tsoi, K.; Harnpanich, D.; Prentice, A. Acute response to oral calcium loading in pregnant and lactating women with a low calcium intake: A pilot study. *Osteoporos. Int.* **2013**, *24*, 2301–2308. [CrossRef]
27. Sadideen, H.; Swaminathan, R. Effect of acute oral calcium load on serum PTH and bone resorption in young healthy subjects: An overnight study. *Eur. J. Clin. Nutr.* **2004**, *58*, 1661–1665. [CrossRef]
28. Young, E.W.; McCarron, D.A.; Morris, C.D. Calcium regulating hormones in essential hypertension. Importance of gender. *Am. J. Hypertens.* **1990**, *3*, 161S–166S. [CrossRef]
29. Brickman, A.S.; Nyby, M.D.; Von Hungen, K.; Eggena, P.; Tuck, M.L. Calcitropic hormones, platelet calcium, and blood pressure in essential hypertension. *Hypertension* **1990**, *16*, 515–522. [CrossRef]
30. Morfis, L.; Smerdely, P.; Howes, L.G. Relationship between serum parathyroid hormone levels in the elderly and 24 h ambulatory blood pressures. *J. Hypertens.* **1997**, *15*, 1271–1276. [CrossRef]
31. Snijder, M.B.; Lips, P.; Seidell, J.C.; Visser, M.; Deeg, D.J.H.; Dekker, J.M.; Van Dam, R.M. Vitamin D status and parathyroid hormone levels in relation to blood pressure: A population-based study in older men and women. *J. Intern. Med.* **2007**, *261*, 558–565. [CrossRef]
32. Park, J.S.; Choi, S.B.; Rhee, Y.; Chung, J.W.; Choi, E.Y.; Kim, D.W. Parathyroid Hormone, Calcium, and Sodium Bridging Between Osteoporosis and Hypertension in Postmenopausal Korean Women. *Calcif. Tissue Int.* **2015**, *96*, 417–429. [CrossRef]
33. Yao, L.; Folsom, A.R.; Pankow, J.S.; Selvin, E.; Michos, E.D.; Alonso, A.; Tang, W.; Lutsey, P.L. Parathyroid hormone and the risk of incident hypertension: The Atherosclerosis Risk in Communities study. *J. Hypertens.* **2016**, *34*, 196–203. [CrossRef] [PubMed]
34. Takagi, Y.; Fukase, M.; Takata, S.; Fujimi, T.; Fujita, T. Calcium Treatment of Essential Hypertension in Elderly Patients Evaluated by 24 H Monitoring. *Am. J. Hypertens.* **1991**, *4*, 836–839. [CrossRef] [PubMed]
35. Kamycheva, E.; Sundsfjord, J.; Jorde, R. Serum parathyroid hormone levels predict coronary heart disease: The Tromsø Study. *Eur. J. Prev. Cardiol.* **2004**, *11*, 69–74. [CrossRef]
36. Jorde, R.; Sundsfjord, J.; Haug, E.; Bønaa, K.H. Relation between low calcium intake, parathyroid. hormone, and blood pressure. *Blood Press.* **2000**, *35*, 1154–1159. [CrossRef]
37. Cawthon, P.M.; Parimi, N.; Barrett-Connor, E.; Laughlin, G.A.; Ensrud, K.E.; Hoffman, A.R.; Shikany, J.M.; Cauley, J.A.; Lane, N.E.; Bauer, D.C.; et al. Serum 25-hydroxyvitamin D, parathyroid hormone, and mortality in older men. *J. Clin. Endocrinol. Metab.* **2010**, *95*, 4625–4634. [CrossRef]
38. Grandi, N.C.; Breitling, L.P.; Hahmann, H.; Wüsten, B.; März, W.; Rothenbacher, D.; Brenner, H. Serum parathyroid hormone and risk of adverse outcomes in patients with stable coronary heart disease. *Heart* **2011**, *97*, 1215–1221. [CrossRef]
39. Van Ballegooijen, A.J.; Kestenbaum, B.; Sachs, M.C.; de Boer, I.H.; Siscovick, D.S.; Hoofnagle, A.N.; Ix, J.H.; Visser, M.; Brouwer, I.A. Association of 25-Hydroxyvitamin D and Parathyroid Hormone with Incident Hypertension. *J. Am. Coll. Cardiol.* **2014**, *63*, 1214–1222. [CrossRef] [PubMed]
40. Jiang, B.; Morimoto, S.; Yang, J.; Niinoabu, T.; Fukuo, K.; Ogihara, T. Expression of parathyroid hormone/parathyroid hormone-related protein receptor in vascular endothelial cells. *J. Cardiovasc. Pharmacol.* **1998**, *31*, S142–S144. [CrossRef]
41. Vilardaga, J.P.; Romero, G.; Friedman, P.A.; Gardella, T.J. Molecular basis of parathyroid hormone receptor signaling and trafficking: A family B GPCR paradigm. *Cell. Mol. Life Sci.* **2011**, *68*, 1–13. [CrossRef]

42. Gardella, T.J.; Vilardaga, J.P. International Union of Basic and Clinical Pharmacology. XCIII. The Parathyroid Hormone Receptors—Family B G Protein-Coupled Receptors. *Pharmacol. Rev.* **2015**, *67*, 310–337. [CrossRef]
43. Hilpert, K.F.; West, S.G.; Bagshaw, D.M.; Fishell, V.; Barnhart, L.; Lefevre, M.; Most, M.M.; Zemel, M.B.; Chow, M.; Hinderliter, A.L.; et al. Effects of Dairy Products on Intracellular Calcium and Blood Pressure in Adults with Essential Hypertension. *J. Am. Coll. Nutr.* **2009**, *28*, 142–149. [CrossRef] [PubMed]
44. Sánchez, M.; de la Sierra, A.; Coca, A.; Poch, E.; Giner, V.; Urbano-Márquez, A. Oral Calcium Supplementation Reduces Intraplatelet Free Calcium Concentration and Insulin Resistance in Essential Hypertensive Patients. *Hypertension* **1997**, *29*, 531–536. [CrossRef] [PubMed]
45. Bogin, E.; Massry, S.G.; Harary, I. Effect of parathyroid hormone on rat heart cells. *J. Clin. Investig.* **1981**, *67*, 1215–1227. [CrossRef] [PubMed]
46. Picotto, G. Rapid effects of calciotropic hormones on female rat enterocytes: Combined actions of 1,25(OH)2-vitamin D3, PTH and 17β-estradiol on intracellular CA2+ regulation. *Horm. Metab. Res.* **2001**, *33*, 733–738. [CrossRef] [PubMed]
47. Tanaka, H.; Smogorzewski, M.; Koss, M.; Massry, S.G. Pathways involved in PTH-induced rise in cytosolic Ca2+ concentration of rat renal proximal tubule. *Am. J. Physiol. Physiol.* **1995**, *268*, F330–F337. [CrossRef] [PubMed]
48. Chausmer, A.B.; Sherman, B.S.; Wallach, S. The eflfect of parathyroid hormone on hepatic cell transport of calcium. *Endocrinology* **1972**, *90*, 663–672. [CrossRef] [PubMed]
49. Goldstein, D.A.; Chui, L.A.; Massry, S.G. Effect of parathyroid hormone and uremia on peripheral nerve calcium and motor nerve conduction velocity. *J. Clin. Investig.* **1978**, *62*, 88–93. [CrossRef]
50. Yamaguchi, D.T.; Hahn, T.J.; Iida-Klein, A.; Kleeman, C.R.; Muallem, S. Parathyroid hormone-activated calcium channels in an osteoblast-like clonal osteosarcoma cell line. cAMP-dependent and cAMP-independent calcium channels. *J. Biol. Chem.* **1987**, *262*, 7711–7718. [PubMed]
51. Reid, I.R.; Civitelli, R.; Halstead, L.R.; Avioli, L.V.; Hruska, K.A. Parathyroid hormone acutely elevates intracellular calcium in osteoblastlike cells. *Am. J. Physiol. Metab.* **1987**, *253*, E45–E51. [CrossRef]
52. Fardella, C.; Rodriguez-Portales, J.A. Intracellular calcium and blood pressure: Comparison between primary hyperparathyroidism and essential hypertension. *J. Endocrinol. Investig.* **1995**, *18*, 827–832. [CrossRef]
53. Song, G.J.; Fiaschi-Taesch, N.; Bisello, A. Endogenous Parathyroid Hormone-Related Protein Regulates the Expression of PTH Type 1 Receptor and Proliferation of Vascular Smooth Muscle Cells. *Mol. Endocrinol.* **2009**, *23*, 1681–1690. [CrossRef] [PubMed]
54. Hanson, A.S.; Linas, S.L. Parathyroid hormone/adenylate cyclase coupling in vascular smooth muscle cells. *Hypertension* **1994**, *23*, 468–475. [CrossRef] [PubMed]
55. Bergmann, C.; Schoefer, P.; Stoclet, J.C.; Gairard, A. Effect of parathyroid hormone and antagonist on aortic cAMP levels. *Can. J. Physiol. Pharmacol.* **1987**, *65*, 2349–2353. [CrossRef]
56. Nickols, G.A.; Metz, M.A.; Cline, W.H. Endothelium-independent linkage of parathyroid hormone receptors of rat vascular tissue with increased adenosine 3′,5′-monophosphate and relaxation of vascular smooth muscle. *Endocrinology* **1986**, *119*, 349–356. [CrossRef]
57. Hulter, H.N.; Melby, J.C.; Peterson, J.C.; Cooke, C.R. Chronic continuous PTH infusion results in hypertension in normal subjects. *J. Clin. Hypertens.* **1986**, *2*, 360–370.
58. Oshima, T.; Schleiffer, R.; Young, E.W.; McCarron, D.A.; Bukoski, R.D. Parathyroidectomy lowers blood pressure independently of changes in platelet free calcium. *J. Hypertens.* **1991**, *9*, 155–158. [CrossRef] [PubMed]
59. Kawashima, H. Parathyroid hormone causes a transient rise in intracellular ionized calcium in vascular smooth muscle cells. *Biochem. Biophys. Res. Commun.* **1990**, *166*, 709–714. [CrossRef]
60. Lewanczuk, R.Z.; Wang, J.; Zhang, Z.R.; Pang, P.K.T. Effects of Spontaneously Hypertensive Rat Plasma on Blood Pressure and Tail Artery Calcium Uptake in Normotensive Rats. *Am. J. Hypertens.* **1989**, *2*, 26–31.
61. Lewanczuk, R.Z.; Resnick, L.M.; Blumenfeld, J.D.; Laragh, J.H.; Pang, P.K. A new circulating hypertensive factor in the plasma of essential hypertensive subjects. *J. Hypertens.* **1990**, *8*, 105–108. [CrossRef]
62. Pernot, F.; Burkhard, C.; Gairard, A. Parathyroid cross-transplantation and development of high blood pressure in rats. *J. Cardiovasc. Pharmacol.* **1994**, *23*, S18–S22. [CrossRef]
63. Neuser, D.; Schulte-Brinkmann, R.; Kazda, S. Development of hypertension in WKY rats after transplantation of parathyroid glands from SHR/SP. *J. Cardiovasc. Pharmacol.* **1990**, *16*, 971–974. [CrossRef] [PubMed]

64. Pang, P.K.Y.; Benishin, C.G.; Lewanczuk, R.Z. Combined effect of dietary calcium and calcium antagonists on blood pressure reduction in spontaneously hypertensive rats. *J. Cardiovasc. Pharmacol.* **1992**, *19*, 442–446. [CrossRef] [PubMed]
65. Lewanczuk, R.Z. In vivo potentiation of vasopressors by spontaneously hypertensive rat plasma correlation with blood pressure and calcium uptake. *Clin. Exp. Hypertens. A* **1989**, *11*, 1471–1485. [CrossRef] [PubMed]
66. Lewanczuk, R.Z.; Pang, P.K.T. Vascular and calcemic effects of plasma of spontaneously hypertensive rats. *Am. J. Hypertens.* **1990**, *3*, 189S–194S. [CrossRef]
67. Shan, J.; Benishin, C.G.; Lewanczuk, R.Z.; Pang, P.K. Mechanism of the vascular action of parathyroid hypertensive factor. *J. Cardiovasc. Pharmacol.* **1994**, *23*, S1–S8. [CrossRef] [PubMed]
68. Pang, P.K.T.; Benishin, C.G.; Lewanczuk, R.Z. Parathyroid hypertensive factor, a circulating factor in animal and human hypertension. *Am. J. Hypertens.* **1991**, *4*, 472–477. [CrossRef] [PubMed]
69. Benishin, C.G.; Lewanczuk, R.Z.; Shan, J.; Pang, P.K. Purification and structural characterization of parathyroid hypertensive factor.pdf. *J. Cardiovasc. Pharmacol.* **1994**, *23*, S9–S13. [CrossRef]
70. Schlüter, H.; Quante, C.; Buchholz, B.; Dietl, K.H.; Spieker, C.; Karas, M.; Zidek, W. A vasopressor factor partially purified from human parathyroid glands. *Biochem. Biophys. Res. Commun.* **1992**, *188*, 323–329. [CrossRef]
71. Mangos, G.J.; Brown, M.A.; Whitworth, J.A. Difficulties in detecting parathyroid hypertensive factor in the rat. *Clin. Exp. Pharmacol. Physiol.* **1998**, *25*, 936–938. [CrossRef]
72. Beveridge, L.A.; Struthers, A.D.; Khan, F.; Jorde, R.; Scragg, R.; Macdonald, H.M.; Alvarez, J.A.; Boxer, R.S.; Dalbeni, A.; Gepner, A.D.; et al. Effect of vitamin D supplementation on blood pressure a systematic review and meta-analysis incorporating individual patient data. *JAMA Intern. Med.* **2015**, *175*, 745–754. [CrossRef]
73. Lennon, S.L.; DellaValle, D.M.; Rodder, S.G.; Prest, M.; Sinley, R.C.; Hoy, M.K.; Papoutsakis, C. 2015 Evidence Analysis Library Evidence-Based Nutrition Practice Guideline for the Management of Hypertension in Adults. *J. Acad. Nutr. Diet.* **2017**, *117*, 1445–1458. [CrossRef]
74. Mozaffari-Khosravi, H.; Loloei, S.; Mirjalili, M.R.; Barzegar, K. The effect of vitamin D supplementation on blood pressure in patients with elevated blood pressure and vitamin D deficiency: A randomized, double-blind, placebo-controlled trial. *Blood Press. Monit.* **2015**, *20*, 83–89. [CrossRef] [PubMed]
75. Shu, L.; Huang, K. Effect of vitamin D supplementation on blood pressure parameters in patients with vitamin D deficiency: A systematic review and meta-analysis. *J. Am. Soc. Hypertens.* **2018**, *12*, 488–496. [CrossRef] [PubMed]
76. Forman, J.P.; Scott, J.B.; Ng, K.; Drake, B.F.; Suarez, E.G.; Hayden, D.L.; Bennett, G.G.; Chandler, P.D.; Hollis, B.W.; Emmons, K.M.; et al. Effect of vitamin D supplementation on blood pressure in blacks. *Hypertension* **2013**, *61*, 779–785. [CrossRef] [PubMed]
77. Areco, V.; Rivoira, M.A.; Rodriguez, V.; Marchionatti, A.M.; Carpentieri, A.; De Talamoni, N.T. Dietary and pharmacological compounds altering intestinal calcium absorption in humans and animals. *Nutr. Res. Rev.* **2015**, *28*, 83–99. [CrossRef] [PubMed]
78. Centeno, V.; Díaz De Barboza, G.; Marchionatti, A.; Rodríguez, V.; Tolosa De Talamoni, N. Molecular mechanisms triggered by low-calcium diets. *Nutr. Res. Rev.* **2009**, *22*, 163–174. [CrossRef] [PubMed]
79. Favus, M.J.; Walling, M.W.; Kimberg, D.V. Effects of dietary calcium restriction and chronic thyroparathyroidectomy on the metabolism of [3H]25 hydroxyvitamin D3 and the active transport of calcium by rat intestine. *J. Clin. Investig.* **1974**, *53*, 1139–1148. [CrossRef]
80. Colston, K.W.; Evans, I.M.A.; Galante, L.; MacIntyre, I.; Moss, D.W. Regulation of vitamin D metabolism: Factors influencing the rate of formation of 1,25-dihydroxycholecalciferol by kidney homogenates (Short Communication). *Biochem. J.* **2015**, *134*, 817–820. [CrossRef]
81. Zehnder, D.; Bland, R.; Chana, R.S.; Wheeler, D.C.; Howie, A.J.; Williams, M.C.; Stewart, P.M.; Hewison, M. Synthesis of 1,25-dihydroxyvitamin D(3) by human endothelial cells is regulated by inflammatory cytokines: A novel autocrine determinant of vascular cell adhesion. *J. Am. Soc. Nephrol.* **2002**, *13*, 621–629.
82. Norman, A.W.; Okamura, W.H.; Bishop, J.E.; Henry, H.L. Update on biological actions of 1α,25(OH)2-vitamin D3 (rapid effects) and 24R,25(OH)2-vitamin D3. *Mol. Cell. Endocrinol.* **2002**, *197*, 1–13. [CrossRef]
83. Bukoski, R.D.; Xue, H.; McCarron, D.A. Effect of 1,25(OH)2 vitamin D3 and ionized Ca2+ on 45Ca uptake by primary cultures of aortic myocytes of spontaneously hypertensive and Wistar Kyoto normotensive rats. *Biochem. Biophys. Res. Commun.* **1987**, *146*, 1330–1335. [CrossRef]

84. Inoue, T.; Kawashima, H. 1,25-Dihydroxyvitamin D3 stimulates 45Ca2+-uptake by cultured vascular smooth muscle cells derived from rat aorta. *Biochem. Biophys. Res. Commun.* **1988**, *152*, 1388–1394. [CrossRef]
85. Xue, H.; Mccarron, D.A.; Bukoski, R.D. 1,25 (OH)2 vitamin D3-induced 45CA uptake in vascular myocytes cultured from spontaneously hypertensive and normotensive rats. *Life Sci.* **1991**, *49*, 651–659. [CrossRef]
86. Bukoski, R.D.; Wang, D.; Wagman, D.W. Injection of 1,25-(OH)2 vitamin D3 enhances resistance artery contractile properties. *Hypertension* **1990**, *16*, 523–531. [CrossRef] [PubMed]
87. Shan, J.; Resnick, L.M.; Lewanczuk, R.Z.; Karpinski, E.; Li, B.; Pang, P.K.T. 1,25-dihydroxyvitamin D as a cardiovascular hormone. Effects on calcium current and cytosolic free calcium in vascular smooth muscle cells. *Am. J. Hypertens* **1993**, *6*, 983–988. [CrossRef]
88. Boland, R.; Buitrago, C.; de Boland, A.R. Modulation of tyrosine phosphorylation signalling pathways by 1α,25(OH)2-vitamin D3. *Trends Endocrinol. Metab.* **2005**, *16*, 280–287. [CrossRef] [PubMed]
89. Li, Y.C. Vitamin D regulation of the renin-angiotensin system. *J. Cell. Biochem.* **2003**, *88*, 327–331. [CrossRef] [PubMed]
90. Resnick, L.M.; Müller, F.B.; Laragh, J.H. Calcium-regulating hormones in essential hypertension: Relation to plasma renin activity and sodium metabolism. *Ann. Intern. Med.* **1986**, *105*, 649–654. [CrossRef]
91. Li, Y.C.; Kong, J.; Wei, M.; Chen, Z.F.; Liu, S.Q.; Cao, L.P. 1,25-Dihydroxyvitamin D 3 is a negative endocrine regulator of the renin-angiotensin system. *J. Clin. Investig.* **2002**, *110*, 229–238. [CrossRef] [PubMed]
92. Zhou, C.; Lu, F.; Cao, K.; Xu, D.; Goltzman, D.; Miao, D. Calcium-independent and 1,25(OH)2D3-dependent regulation of the renin-angiotensin system in 1α-hydroxylase knockout mice. *Kidney Int.* **2008**, *74*, 170–179. [CrossRef]
93. Kong, J.; Qiao, G.; Zhang, Z.; Liu, S.Q.; Li, Y.C. Targeted vitamin D receptor expression in juxtaglomerular cells suppresses renin expression independent of parathyroid hormone and calcium. *Kidney Int.* **2008**, *74*, 1577–1581. [CrossRef] [PubMed]
94. Grünberger, C.; Kurtz, A.; Klar, J.; Obermayer, B.; Schweda, F. The Calcium Paradoxon of Renin Release. *Circ. Res.* **2006**, *99*, 1197–1206. [CrossRef] [PubMed]
95. Ortiz-Capisano, M.C.; Ortiz, P.A.; Garvin, J.L.; Harding, P.; Beierwaltes, W.H. Expression and function of the calcium-sensing receptor in juxtaglomerular cells. *Hypertension* **2007**, *50*, 737–743. [CrossRef] [PubMed]
96. Watkins, B.E.; Davis, J.O.; Lohmeier, T.E.; Freeman, R.H. Intrarenal site of action of calcium on renin secretion in dogs. *Circ. Res.* **1976**, *36*, 847–853. [CrossRef]
97. Helwig, J.J.; Musso, M.J.; Judes, C.; Nickols, G.A. Parathyroid hormone and calcium: Interactions in the control of renin secretion in the isolated, nonfiltering rat kidney. *Endocrinology* **1991**, *129*, 1233–1242. [CrossRef]
98. Kotchen, T.A.; Maull, K.I.; Luke, R. Effect of acute and chronic calcium administration on plasma renin. *J. Clin. Investig.* **1974**, *54*, 1279–1286. [CrossRef]
99. Atchison, D.K.; Harding, P.; Beierwaltes, W.H. Hypercalcemia reduces plasma renin via parathyroid hormone, renal interstitial calcium, and the calcium-sensing receptor. *Hypertension* **2011**, *58*, 604–610. [CrossRef]
100. Riccardi, D.; Lee, W.S.; Lee, K.; Segre, G.V.; Brown, E.M.; Hebert, S.C. Localization of the extracellular Ca(2+)-sensing receptor and PTH/PTHrP receptor in rat kidney. *Am. J. Physiol. Physiol.* **1996**, *271*, F951–F956. [CrossRef]
101. Grant, F.D.; Mandel, S.J.; Brown, E.M.; Williams, G.H.; Seely, E.W. Interrelationships between the renin-angiotensin-aldosterone and calcium homeostatic systems. *J. Clin. Endocrinol. Metab.* **1992**, *75*, 988–992.
102. Doris, P.A. Plasma angiotensin II: Interdependence on sodium and calcium homeostasis. *Peptides* **1988**, *9*, 243–248. [CrossRef]
103. Brown, J.M.; Williams, J.S.; Luther, J.M.; Garg, R.; Garza, A.E.; Pojoga, L.H.; Ruan, D.T.; Williams, G.H.; Adler, G.K.; Vaidya, A. Human interventions to characterize novel relationships between the renin-angiotensin-aldosterone system and parathyroid hormone. *Hypertension* **2014**, *63*, 273–280. [CrossRef] [PubMed]
104. Müller, J. Aldosterone: The minority hormone of. *Steroids* **1995**, *60*, 2–9. [CrossRef]
105. Rojas, J.; Olivar, L.C.; Chavez Castillo, M.; Martinez, M.S.; Wilches-Duran, S.; Graterol, M.; Contreras-Velasquez, J.; Cerda, M.; Riaño, M.; Bermudez, V. Hormona paratiroidea, aldosterona e hipertensión arterial ¿una amenaza infravalorada? *Rev. Latinoam. Hipertens.* **2017**, *12*, 1–18.

106. Catena, C.; Colussi, G.L.; Brosolo, G.; Bertin, N.; Novello, M.; Palomba, A.; Sechi, L.A. Salt, Aldosterone, and Parathyroid Hormone: What Is the Relevance for Organ Damage? *Int. J. Endocrinol.* **2017**, *2017*, 4397028. [CrossRef] [PubMed]
107. Sabbadin, C.; Cavedon, E.; Zanon, P.; Iacobone, M.; Armanini, D. Resolution of hypertension and secondary aldosteronismafter surgical treatment of primary hyperparathyroidism. *J. Endocrinol. Investig.* **2013**, *36*, 665–666.
108. Barkan, A.; Marilus, R.; Winkelsberg, G.; Yeshurun, D.; Blum, I. Primary hyperparathyroidism: Possible cause of primary hyperaldosteronism in a 60-year-old woman. *J. Clin. Endocrinol. Metab.* **1980**, *51*, 144–147. [CrossRef]
109. Mazzocchi, G.; Aragona, F.; Malendowicz, L.K.; Nussdorfer, G.G. PTH and PTH-related peptide enhance steroid secretion from human adrenocortical cells. *Am. J. Physiol. Metab.* **2001**, *280*, E209–E213. [CrossRef] [PubMed]
110. Isales, C.M.; Barrett, P.Q.; Brines, M.; Bollag, W. Parathyroid Hormone Modulates Angiotensin II-Induced. *Endocrinology* **1991**, *129*, 489–495. [CrossRef]
111. Maniero, C.; Fassina, A.; Guzzardo, V.; Lenzini, L.; Amadori, G.; Pelizzo, M.R.; Gomez-Sanchez, C.; Rossi, G.P. Primary hyperparathyroidism with concurrent primary aldosteronism. *Hypertension* **2011**, *58*, 341–346. [CrossRef] [PubMed]
112. GBD 2017 Causes of Death Collaborators. Global, regional, and national age-sex-specific mortality for 282 causes of death in 195 countries and territories, 1980–2017: A systematic analysis for the Global Burden of Disease Study 2017. *Lancet* **2018**, *392*, 1736–1788. [CrossRef]
113. Belizán, J.M.; Villar, J.; Repke, J. The relationship between calcium intake and pregnancy-induced hypertension: Up-to-date evidence. *Am. J. Obstet. Gynecol.* **1988**, *158*, 898–902. [CrossRef]

8

Sodium Intake and Hypertension

Andrea Grillo [1], Lucia Salvi [2], Paolo Coruzzi [3], Paolo Salvi [1,*] and Gianfranco Parati [1,4]

1 IRCCS Istituto Auxologico Italiano, Cardiology Unit, 20100 Milan, Italy
2 IRCCS Policlinico San Matteo Foundation, University of Pavia, 27100 Pavia, Italy
3 Department of Medicine and Surgery, University of Parma, 43121 Parma, Italy
4 Chair of Cardiovascular Medicine, Department of Medicine and Surgery, University of Milano-Bicocca, 20100 Milan, Italy
* Correspondence: paolo.salvi@unimib.it

Abstract: The close relationship between hypertension and dietary sodium intake is widely recognized and supported by several studies. A reduction in dietary sodium not only decreases the blood pressure and the incidence of hypertension, but is also associated with a reduction in morbidity and mortality from cardiovascular diseases. Prolonged modest reduction in salt intake induces a relevant fall in blood pressure in both hypertensive and normotensive individuals, irrespective of sex and ethnic group, with larger falls in systolic blood pressure for larger reductions in dietary salt. The high sodium intake and the increase in blood pressure levels are related to water retention, increase in systemic peripheral resistance, alterations in the endothelial function, changes in the structure and function of large elastic arteries, modification in sympathetic activity, and in the autonomic neuronal modulation of the cardiovascular system. In this review, we have focused on the effects of sodium intake on vascular hemodynamics and their implication in the pathogenesis of hypertension.

Keywords: arterial stiffness; endothelial function; hypertension; salt-sensitivity; salt intake; sodium intake; sympathetic activity

---

1. Sodium Intake and Blood Pressure Values

Available evidence suggests a direct relationship between sodium intake and blood pressure (BP) values [1–4]. Excessive sodium consumption (defined by the World Health Organization as >5 g sodium per day [5]) has been shown to produce a significant increase in BP and has been linked with onset of hypertension and its cardiovascular complications [6,7]. Conversely, reduction in sodium intake not only decreases BP levels and hypertension incidence, but is also associated with a reduction in cardiovascular morbidity and mortality [8]. A large meta-analysis [9] showed that modest reduction in salt intake for four or more weeks causes a significant fall in BP in both hypertensive and normotensive individuals, irrespective of sex and ethnic group, and larger reductions in salt intake are linked to larger falls in systolic BP [9]. However, the current health policies have not reached an effective achievement for the reduction of dietary sodium in the population and the positive effects of a reduced sodium intake on BP levels tend to decrease with time, owing to poor dietary compliance.

The pathophysiological link between sodium intake and increase in BP values has been widely debated. Increased salt consumption may provoke water retention, thus leading to a condition of high flow in arterial vessels. The mechanism of pressure natriuresis has been proposed as a physiologic phenomenon where an increase in BP in the renal arteries causes increased salt and water excretion [10]. This hemodynamic load, as studies with animal models have shown [11,12], may lead to an adverse microvascular remodeling by the effects of increased BP levels. High sodium intake and increased BP levels are linked by changes in vascular resistances, but the mechanisms controlling this phenomenon may not be only viewed as a reflex pressor response aimed at increasing sodium excretion. Excessive salt intake may induce several adverse effects, causing microvascular endothelial inflammation, anatomic remodeling, and functional abnormalities, even in normotensive subjects [13]. More recent studies have shown that changes in sodium plasma levels do not only exert their effects on small resistance arteries, but may also affect the function and structure of large elastic arteries. The issue of salt-sensitivity, which refers to individual susceptibility in terms of BP variations following changes in dietary salt intake, has also been recently debated in its pathophysiological background and clinical implications [14,15].

In this paper, we have reviewed the evidence regarding the effects of sodium intake on arterial function, and their implication in the pathogenesis of hypertension. We have first addressed the debate on salt-sensitivity, in light of recent evidence, and then discussed the effects of sodium handling on arterial function and structure.

2. Low Sodium Intake and Cardiovascular Risk

Over the years, the evidence of a close relationship between high sodium intake and hypertension, and high sodium intake and increased cardiovascular risk and mortality, has become increasingly consolidated. For this reason, we are used to consider that the lower the sodium intake is, the better the patient prognosis is. However, the studies that are beginning to shake the foundations of this historic fortress are growing in number. Actually, in the analysis of this topic, several cohort studies [16–18] and meta-analyses [19,20] have shown that the relationship between sodium intake and poor patient prognosis have not a linear trend, but rather describe a J-shape curve. In these studies, an increased risk not only in high sodium intake, but also in significantly low sodium intake levels is underlined. To reach this declaration, large patient populations have been studied, including various types of healthy patients or those with different co-morbidities (i.e., diabetes, vascular disease, hypertension population), with wide numbers in all subgroups.

The relationship between cardiovascular events and sodium intake was derived from baseline urinary sodium excretion on a 24-h urine collection: urinary sodium excretion less than 3 g/day is considered to reflect a low sodium dietary intake. It was observed that a poor patient prognosis is associated with either a very high and a very low 24h urinary sodium excretion. This relationship does not depend on BP, aging, diabetes, chronic kidney disease, or cardiovascular disease. Mente et al. [19] reported that only patients with arterial hypertension have a high cardiovascular risk associated with high sodium intake, while this association was not confirmed in patients without hypertension [19].

Mechanisms linking high sodium intake and cardiovascular adverse events are well known; less defined are those that justify a relationship between low salt intake and high mortality. Sodium is an indispensable cation, essential to the action potential of all cells in the body, and its homoeostasis is under tight physiological regulation. Sodium intake is governed by neural mechanisms that regulate intake of sodium and related homoeostatic systems, and so although extreme reductions in sodium intake are possible in controlled settings for short periods, this is unlikely to be sustainable in everyday life in the long-term. Thus, as for all our body components, there may be an optimal range for its intake, below which the human body starts being damaged, at variance from what happens in case of intake of, or exposure to, potentially toxic external substances, such as tobacco smoke, drugs or environmental pollutants.

In experimental models, it is known that sodium restriction results in increased atherosclerosis [21]. In humans, the relationship between salt restriction and increased renin-angiotensin-aldosterone system activation has been described [22,23], as well as the relationship with increased sympathetic activity [24] and insulin resistance [25–27]. High renin concentrations and increased levels of catecholamines have been reported in studies in poor sodium intake population. On the other hand, several studies have shown that increases of renin, aldosterone, and catecholamines are all associated with increased cardiovascular disease events and mortality [24,28]. Regarding sympathetic activity, sodium intake restriction is associated with a persistent attenuation of the muscle sympathetic nerve activity responses to baroreceptor stimulation and deactivation [28].

Furthermore, there is a significant correlation between the reduction in baroreflex sensitivity and the increase of concomitant muscle sympathetic nerve activity. Accordingly, a reduced ability of this reflex to obtain a proper downregulation of sympathetic tone leads to the sympathostimulating effect of a very low sodium intake. As described in other studies evaluating high sodium intake, the increase in muscle sympathetic nerve traffic due to very low sodium intake is also associated with an increase in plasma norepinephrine, and a drastic reduction in sodium intake has been reported to cause, in man, an increase in renal norepinephrine removal. Moreover, sodium restriction causes insulin resistance; this may be the result of sympathetic activation but, in turn, increased insulin levels may themselves have a sympathoexcitatory influence. Lastly, low salt supply causes a reduction of central venous pressure, which may lead to an activation of the sympathetic system via unloading of cardiopulmonary receptors.

To sum up, predicting the net clinical effect of low sodium intake based on only considering the effects of sodium on BP might not provide a comprehensive view of its effects on cardiovascular disease and mortality, especially within the range of sodium intake that affects the renin system (<4 g/day). In other words, the effects of sodium intake level on clinical outcomes are only partly mediated through its effects on BP. For a full understanding of the clinical impact of sodium intake it is also necessary to consider other mechanisms that might be at play. In particular, while the potential harm of sodium excess may be BP-driven, the potential negative effects of a low sodium intake may be mediated by elevated renin-aldosterone activity and sympathetic neural activation.

Numerous methodological concerns have arisen from studies that have underlined the J-shape of the sodium intake and cardiovascular events' relationship [29,30]. It has been remarked that a single morning urine sample may offer an inaccurate measure of usual sodium intake, ignoring day-to-day variability in sodium intake, diurnal variation in sodium excretion, and the effects of medications. Another confounder could come from the fact that other prognostically negative factors might be activated in the low sodium intake interval because of dietary advice or poor appetite, or in the high sodium intake interval because of concomitant high caloric intake (typical of overweight or diabetic patients), which could have contributed to increased mortality in the low- and the high-sodium groups respectively (reverse causality). However, most studies took measures to adjust for such confounding elements.

Recent findings further support the calls for caution before applying salt restriction universally. Although more studies have confirmed the benefit of reducing sodium intake in hypertensive subjects with a high salt intake, it is unclear whether the remaining more than 90% of the population will profit from dietary sodium reduction. Therefore, until new robust data emerge from large trials, it might be prudent to recommend reduction in sodium intake only in those with high sodium intake and with hypertension. In other words, it would perhaps be more correct to start discussing about "inappropriate" rather than "excessive" salt intake.

3. Hypertension and Salt-Sensitivity

Nearly half a century ago, Guyton and Coleman proposed that whenever arterial pressure is elevated, the pressure natriuresis mechanism enhances the excretion of sodium and water until blood volume is reduced adequately in order to return BP to normal values [31]. According to this premise, hypertension may occur only when the ability of the kidney of excreting sodium is impaired. Further evidence has shown that the BP response to changes in salt intake in diet has a significant variability among individuals in the general population. This phenomenon was defined as salt-sensitivity of BP. Strains of rats whose BP was either sensitive or resistant to changes in sodium intake were developed [32], thus establishing a genetic background for the phenomenon of salt-sensitivity. However, the BP response to changing salt intake display marked inter-individual variability [33,34], and thus salt-sensitivity behaves as a continuous parameter at a population level. Although the role of salt-sensitivity is of increasing interest both in research and in a clinical setting, the existing methods to identify salt-sensitivity and resistance may be imprecise and the definitions of "salt-sensitive" and "salt-resistant" hypertension are based on relative inaccurate approaches. Generally, the definition of salt-sensitivity is based on the BP response to moderate reduction and increase of salt intake. For the clinical evaluation of BP salt-sensitivity, a commonly used protocol in clinical research is the test of Grim and Weinberger [6], which has been the reference test for the last decades. According to this protocol, patients are prescribed to follow a diet with high sodium (200 mmol NaCl per day) and with a low sodium intake (30 mmol NaCl per day) diet, each for one week, with the quantification of 24-hour urinary sodium excretion on the last day of each diet week [35,36]. A modified protocol with a more rapid execution was proposed and tested, and was able to correctly predict a significant BP response to dietary salt restriction [37]. The prescription of a long-term reduction in sodium intake is often limited because of insufficient compliance of patients to the dietary instructions, and the follow-up may be challenging for both patients and physicians. This is the reason why, more recently, Castiglioni et al. proposed a protocol based on ambulatory BP monitoring (ABPM) for a simplified clinical screening of BP salt-sensitivity [38]. These authors hypothesized that in a population following a high-sodium diet, individuals with a marked salt-sensitivity may display an altered circadian profile, with a less pronounced nocturnal dipping, as a consequence of retention of sodium and water in the daytime, accompanied by an elevated mean 24-hour heart rate. By using such an "ambulatory salt-sensitivity index", based on the combination of reduced nocturnal BP dipping and elevated 24 h heart rate, they established three classes of risk for salt-sensitivity (low, intermediate, and high) by combining the BP-dipping and heart rate levels observed during a 24h ABPM without need of changing the dietary sodium content. This index was validated through the observation that the prevalence of sodium-sensitive patients, evaluated with a traditional test, increased significantly from the class with the lowest risk for salt-sensitivity (25% of prevalence) to the intermediate risk (40%) and high risk (70%) classes, as defined by this index of ambulatory salt-sensitivity. Thus, by performing ABPM in conditions of usual daily life and with habitual diet, some useful information on the degree of salt-sensitivity of patients with hypertension may be available with an easy and direct method, without resorting to a traditional approach requiring a demanding salt-sensitivity test.

In both normotensive and hypertensive persons, current evidence suggests that salt-sensitivity is associated with an increased cardiovascular risk. The risk for developing hypertension is higher in normotensive men with a more pronounced salt-sensitivity at baseline, in a long-term follow-up [39]. Moreover, in patients with essential hypertension, the prevalence of severe hypertensive target organ damage was higher among salt-sensitive patients [40]. Cardiovascular morbidity and mortality were found to be higher both in hypertensive and even in normotensive individuals with a higher degree of salt-sensitivity [34,41]. A cluster of possible determining factors, such as high insulin levels, alterations in lipid profile, and microalbuminuria, which are known to be prevalent in salt-sensitive hypertension, may explain, at least in part, the increase in cardiovascular risk observed in salt-sensitive patients.

Recent studies have highlighted the genetic and metabolic background of salt-sensitivity, a phenomenon with remarkable variability among human subjects [33], as well as among animal models [42]. A number of genetic, hormonal, and neuro-endocrine factors are involved in the salt-sensitivity of BP [43]. The sympathetic nervous system, the renin-angiotensin-aldosterone system, natriuretic peptides, insulin, leptin, and several endothelial mediators with endocrine activity may modify BP response to salt [15]. BP salt-sensitivity may be genetically inherited, as in some rare monogenic forms of hypertension, or influenced by several genetic polymorphisms involving sodium reabsorption in the nephron or acquired by the individual subjects in their lifetime. Aging amplifies the hypertensive effects of increased sodium intake [44]. The reason of this phenomenon may be the decrease in the kidney ability of concentrating sodium in the urine with increasing age, likely due to a decline in glomerular mass with age. Similarly, chronic kidney disease leads to an impairment of volume excretion and urine sodium-concentrating ability, thus enhancing the salt-sensitivity in its more severe forms. Individuals from African descent are at an increased risk for hypertension, despite plasma volume and cardiac index similar to white population [45]. The ability of concentrating sodium in urine after salt loading seems impaired in the blacks compared to whites [46], thus supporting salt-sensitivity as a more common cause of hypertension among blacks. BP salt-sensitivity also showed a positive association with obesity, being found higher among obese rather than in lean adolescents, and is reversed after weight loss [47]. Abdominal adiposity and the metabolic syndrome [48] are associated with an increased rate of sodium reabsorption by the kidney, an effect that is at least partially mediated by insulin and leptin [49].

Although salt-sensitivity of BP is a well-established phenomenon and the correlations of this phenotype with clinical features have been established, the pathophysiologic mechanisms leading to increased BP values have been long-time debated and have not yet been completely elucidated. Until recently, according to the classic concept of Guyton [50], the prevailing theory is that high salt intake leads to an expansion in circulating volumes, an increased cardiac output, and a rise in kidney perfusion pressure. The "pressure-natriuresis" mechanism tends to increase sodium output to restore the increased circulating volume to normality. Salt-sensitivity is thus conceived and explained by a relative 'natriuretic handicap' from the kidney, which is unable to produce a sufficient excretion of sodium to preserve sodium balance and volumes without sufficiently higher pressure. Hypertension may develop only when the excretory ability of the kidney is impaired and the relation between sodium excretion and BP is shifted toward higher values. Research into the possible physiological mechanisms determining salt-sensitivity has thus been driven mostly by a conceptual framework derived from the work of Guyton, which is also highlighted in a recent scientific statement from the American Heart Association on this topic [15].

The traditional view of sodium handling has been challenged by the finding of non-osmolar storage of sodium. The traditional framework assumes that sodium and chloride are osmotically active and cause water retention in amounts which preserve an unchanged osmolarity. A high-sodium diet may expand the extracellular volume until a steady state is reached, where sodium intake and output are balanced, with a significant increase in the quantity of total body water. However, rigorous studies have demonstrated that sodium may accumulate in the body without a concomitant retention of water, both in humans [51] and in experimental models [52]. Recent clinical research has highlighted that salt-sensitive and salt-resistant patients do not show any difference in circulating volumes, cardiac output, or sodium balance after salt loading [53]. This may be explained by non-osmolar storage of sodium, without considering the effect on water retention.

An alternative to the Guyton framework of the "pressure-natriuresis" and the "natriuretic handicap" was also developed [14]. Evidence has accumulated showing that impairment in vascular function may play a relevant role in salt-sensitive hypertension. In fact, abnormal responses of vascular resistance in the renal circulation are present after salt intake in salt-sensitive individuals, without an increase in sodium retention or cardiac output [46,54]. After acute or chronic increases in salt intake, salt-sensitive patients are not subject to an increase in sodium storage and do not increase the cardiac output, when compared to normal controls [55]. Then, the increase in BP induced by salt may be mediated by abnormalities in the vascular response to salt, in particular in peripheral and renal resistances, along with changes in sodium balance and in cardiac output [56]. In normal conditions, salt-resistant individuals may show a robust decrease in systemic vascular resistances after an increase in salt intake [57]. Specifically, in salt-sensitive individuals, the effect of salt includes a failure to induce a normal decrease in vascular resistances, which may show unchanged or even increased levels. Conversely, normal salt-resistant individuals are able to induce a vasodilatory response after an increase in salt intake [58], and then BP is maintained within normal values. Thus, the preservation of normal BP levels under salt loading appears to be independent from the ability of salt resistant subjects to rapidly excrete a salt load or to better manage better the balance of sodium, of circulating volume, and of cardiac output than salt-sensitive individuals, as hypothesized in a classical view of salt-sensitivity. According to these recent theories, these alternative physiological mechanisms involved in the phenomenon of salt-sensitivity [14] could be framed in a large unifying view of the salt-sensitivity phenomenon and explain the recent observations on the effects induced by salt in the arterial vessel wall.

4. Sodium Intake and Sympathetic Activity

Diet with high salt supply can modulate the activity of the autonomic nervous system, especially sympathetic activity, in several ways. A previous study of our research group [35] showed, in salt-sensitive hypertensive patients, different changes in autonomic cardiovascular control at different levels of sodium loading. Salt-Sensitivity Index (SSI) was calculated in 34 essential hypertensive patients [35]. SSI is the ratio of the change in brachial mean arterial pressure (ΔMAP), between the high- and the low-sodium diet periods, with the corresponding change in urinary sodium excretion rate (ΔUNaV, expressed in mmol/L/day), multiplied by a factor of 1000. Autonomic cardiovascular control was evaluated by spectral analysis of beat-by-beat finger BP and pulse interval variability, and by the related assessment of spontaneous baroreflex sensitivity (sequence technique) [59–61]. The results of these studies indicate a better parasympathetic cardiac modulation (quantified by baroreflex sensitivity and indexes of heart rate variability in the high frequency band) associated with lower SSI. These results underline the presence of greater sympathetic activation in salt-sensitive patients; in fact, they exhibit the physiological reciprocal behavior that usually characterizes sympathetic and sympathetic cardiac modulation. [62]. In fact, a sodium-rich diet is reported in subjects with lower SSI who are also characterized by a preserved autonomic cardiovascular modulation. Therefore, an increased dietary salt supply can induce a reflex reduction of sympathetic efferent activity if reflex cardiovascular regulation is physiologically preserved, activating cardiopulmonary receptors through an increase in plasma volume [63]. An opposite condition occurs in the presence of low sodium intake [24]. However, this neural regulation has not been described in patients with the highest degree of salt-sensitivity. No changes in their impaired autonomic cardiovascular control are associated with changes in sodium intake. In conclusion, the increased BP associated with excessive sodium intake observed in hypertensive patients, characterized by high salt-sensitivity, may be due to the impairment of their baroreflex function or to their inability to increase baroreflex sensitivity and reduce sympathetic activity in response to the increase in plasma volume, determined by sodium loading [24,62–68]. More recently, we have also reported a blunted vagal control of heart rate in young normotensive individuals with a higher degree of sodium-sensitivity, when facing a high-salt diet [36].

5. Salt-Induced Vasodysfunction

In the pathophysiological explanation of the salt-sensitivity of BP a dysfunction in vascular modulation has also been hypothesized. An increased salt intake may clearly provoke an expansion in circulating volumes, an increase in flow and BP values, and thus an adverse remodeling of arterial wall mediated by the mechanic load through shear stress and an increase in wall tension. Beyond that, several experimental and clinical studies have recently demonstrated the adverse effects of high sodium intake in the microvascular circulation [13].

In experimental animal studies, salt intake was associated with microvascular rarefaction in normotensive and hypertensive rats, resulting from structural alterations and differing from the degenerative processes observed in experimental animals with chronic hypertension that are characterized by microvascular rarefaction [69]. Moreover, apart from microvessel rarefaction, a reduced arterial vasodilator capacity developed with high-salt diet has also been described in rats with hypertension induced by a reduced renal mass, which and was restored with low-salt diet [70]. Additional vascular effects of a high sodium intake include the potentiation of local vasoconstrictive effectors, such as alterations of endothelial Ca2+ signaling [71] or an abnormal high production of 20-hydroxyeicosatetraenoic acid [72]. The upregulation induced by a high salt intake of the cytochrome P450 ω-hydroxylase 4A)/20-hydroxyeicosatetraenoic acid system results in elevated oxidative stress and a reduced nitric oxide bioavailability, causing vascular dysfunction [73], and may thus be a key mediator linking increased salt intake to microvascular dysfunction.

A series of human studies have identified alterations in the small arteries and endothelial function in relation to salt intake. Impaired vasodilatation of the small vessels has been shown to occur in conditions of high salt intake [74]. In young, healthy normotensives, salt loading impaired vascular endothelial function along with left ventricular mechanical relaxation [75]. These results were confirmed in normotensive adults, where sodium-induced impairments in microvascular function were observed. The microvascular function was improved by the administration of the anti-oxidant ascorbic acid, suggesting a role of oxidative stress in this process [76]. An impairment in endothelial function was observed in the brachial arteries of healthy volunteers subjected to high-salt diet, with a switch in the mediator of vasodilation in the microcirculation to a non-nitric oxide-dependent mechanism, which was restored with acute exercise [77]. Moreover, in young normotensives, intravenous sodium loading had direct adverse effects on the endothelial surface layer by increasing microvascular permeability to albumin, independently from BP [78]. Furthermore, an imbalance between cardiac output and vascular resistances in salt-sensitive subjects, determined by the failure to adequately lower vascular resistances after increase of sodium intake, has been described in young normotensive subjects [36], thereby confirming data collected in normotensive black individuals [79].The restriction in dietary sodium in middle aged hypertensives largely reversed microvascular endothelial dysfunction by increasing nitric oxide and tetrahydrobiopterin bioavailability, and by the reduction of oxidative stress, supporting the role of a vascular protection induced by salt restriction beyond that attributable to its BP-lowering effects [80].

A link was hypothesized between the described vascular impairments and abnormalities in interstitial sodium storage [53]. The emerging magnetic resonance imaging–based techniques that directly detect Na^+ in tissues [81] have recently provided confirmation and further evidence about the compartmentalized sodium storage in humans, also in relation to cardiovascular morbidities [82]. Recent experiments [83–85] have shown that sodium homeostasis is regulated by negatively-charged glycosaminoglycans in the skin interstitium, where sodium is bound to glycosaminoglycans without causing an effect on extracellular volume. Negatively-charged glycosaminoglycans in the skin may be important for non-osmotic sodium accumulation and explain the observation a positive sodium balance without a concomitant volume expansion [86]. The skin is thus known to represent the main site for the storing of sodium in the body, with a buffering capacity adapting to changes in salt intake in which skin glycosaminalgycans have been shown to have the most relevant role [83]. The relationship between skin deposition of sodium and hypertension may be mediated by a molecular mechanism in which vascular-endothelial growth factor-C (VEGF-C) is the most relevant mediator. The hypertonicity of skin interstitial space, which develops during high salt intake, is accompanied by newly-developed lymphatic vessels and an increased density and hyperplasia of the lymphocapillary network, a process regulated by macrophages releasing the osmosensitive transcription factor, that in turn induces the release the VEGF-C [87,88], which enhances the production of endothelial nitric oxide synthase and of nitric oxide. Failure of this regulatory mechanism, which enhances sodium excretion via lymphatics and regulates vascular tone by increasing endothelial nitric oxide synthase protein expression, may lead to a salt-sensitive BP response [89].

Although the molecular pathway involving VEGF-C has been the most studied in animal models to explain the link between skin sodium and hypertension, other mechanisms have been proposed to play a role in this relationship. The increase in salt intake has been shown to induce the rarefaction of the skin microcapillary network in different racial groups [90], and to increase the reactivity of skin vessels in response to angiotensin-2 and noradrenaline [91]. Other works suggest that the hypoxia inducible factor (HIF) may represent a key regulator of vascular tone of the skin [83], although its role has been mainly studied in the renal medulla until now [92]. Although further works are needed to clarify the underlying mechanisms involved in this relationship, the role of skin in regulating BP, and by mediating a vasodilatory response.

6. Sodium Intake and Arterial Stiffness

The close relationship between high dietary salt content, arterial hypertension, and increased stiffness of the large arteries is not a recent discovery. In fact, Huang Ti Nei Ching Su Wein, a wise Chinese doctor who lived 3700 years ago, already argued in his studies: " ... *therefore if large amounts of salt are taken, the pulse will stiffen and harden"*. He was indeed right. In fact, in the following centuries it was confirmed that a high plasma serum sodium deeply affects the functional peculiarities of the large elastic arteries [93], and is associated with a relative increase in systemic peripheral resistance. Additionally, an effect of sodium on small resistance arteries has also been demonstrated [94]. Among the various studies that have investigated this topic, we recall the Avolio et al. research performed in the 1980s [95,96]. In their papers, urinary sodium excretion was used as a surrogate for daily dietary intake. Comparing rural and urban populations, an average excretion of 13.3 g/24 h of NaCl was found in the cities, and 7.3 g/24 h in the rural population. This difference reflects different dietary habits in the two recruited groups, which are physiologically expressed in significantly lower carotid-femoral pulse (PWV) wave velocity in the rural community [95]. Hypertension also had a higher incidence in the urban group. This topic has been further investigated in a following study on normotensive subjects [96]. Even in this case, lower aortic PWV values were detected in subjects who followed a low-salt diet compared to a reference group. As in the previous study, the difference between groups in PWV was not dependent on BP levels. In a number of studies involving hypertensive patients [97–100], aortic PWV values were significantly lower in the low-salt group than in the high-salt group; however, other studies in which no significant difference in PWV has been described in relation to dietary sodium intake can be found in the literature [101–107]. In almost all of these latter randomized controlled trials, however, the relatively small number of enrolled patients and the relatively short duration of a given level of sodium intake with the diet assigned to each group were probably the main factors affecting the failure in reaching a statistically significant difference in PWV between high- and low-salt groups. A meta-analysis recently published by D'Elia et al. tried to better clarify the relationship between sodium intake with diet and arterial stiffness [108]. The results of this study show that an average reduction in salt intake of 5 g/day is associated with a 2.8% reduction in carotid-femoral PWV. The authors also showed how this PWV reduction was independent of the reduction in BP values in hypertensive and/or pre-hypertensive middle-aged subjects. Since the relationship between arterial stiffness and sodium intake has been mostly evaluated during salt-intake manipulations, data on the effects of sodium-sensitivity condition on PWV are scarce.

The relationship between high BP values and arterial stiffness is described and confirmed in several studies [109,110]. High BP values that persist for a prolonged time interval lead to progressive structural changes in the arterial wall of the large elastic arteries, with consequent increase in arterial stiffness. In particular, the increase in the expression of collagen fibers, and the consequent reduction in the ratio between elastin and collagen fibers, can cause the progressive increase in arterial wall stiffness. In this context, the aforementioned alterations in arterial stiffness —independent of arterial pressure and due to a sodium-rich diet for prolonged periods of time—are associated with the pathophysiologically-expected interrelations between BP and PWV. It seems really difficult to discriminate between BP-dependent and BP-independent variations of the viscoelastic properties of large arteries in relation to the effects of sodium intake. An excessive sodium intake with diet induces alterations in the extracellular matrix of arterial wall, favoring a process of arterial stiffening (Figure 1). Endothelial dysfunction [111,112] and oxidative stress [113] related to high sodium intake can cause vascular damage through a pressure-independent mechanism [112]. The mechanical properties of the aorta and large elastic arteries depend on the relationship between the principal components of the extracellular matrix in arterial wall: i.e. the elastin and collagen fibers. Thus, the elastin and collagen fibers ratio characterizes the viscoelastic properties of large arteries and is regulated by matrix metalloproteinases (MMPs) [114]. A high sodium intake causes an activation of extracellular matrix metalloproteinases MMP2 and MMP9, leading to stimulation of TGFß-1 [112,114,115], inducing thinning and breakage of elastin fibers and a decrease in the elastin and collagen ratio. On the other hand, the overexpression of TGFß-1 inhibits collagenase production [116] and develops a fibrogenic effect on the extracellular matrix in the arterial wall, altering its mechanical properties [117]. An important role in the expression of the viscoelastic properties of large arteries seems to be linked to the balance between MMP2 and MMP9 (both favoring the accumulation of collagen) [114,115,118] with MMP8 and MMP13 (which instead promote collagen degradation) [119,120]. Accelerated arterial fibrosis may be responsible for increased arterial stiffness and for amplification of aging-related vascular damage.

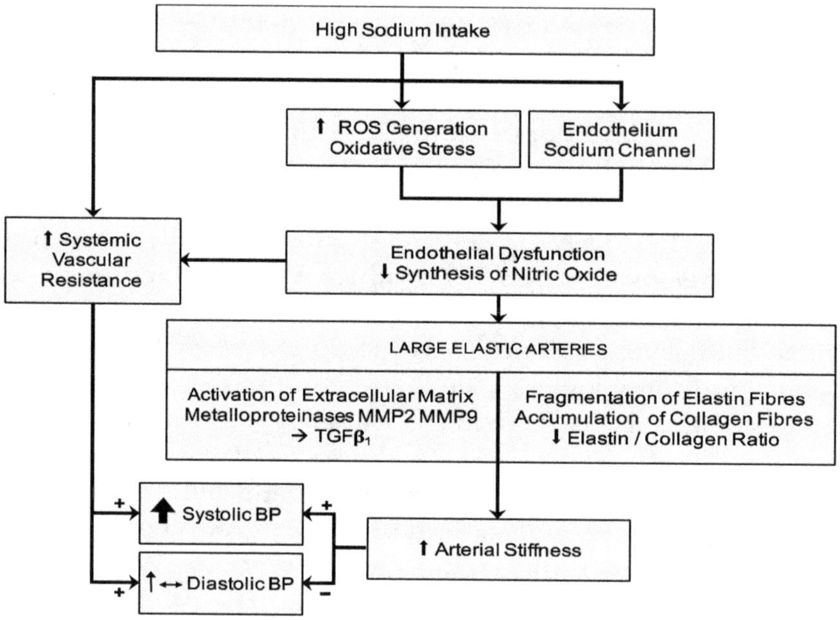

Figure 1. Relationship between high salt intake with diet, blood pressure, and arterial stiffness. Abbreviations: BP, blood pressure; MMP, matrix metalloproteinases; ROS, reactive oxygen species; TGF, transforming growth factor.

The renin-angiotensin-aldosterone system (RAAS) plays also a major role in the regulation of the mechanical properties of large elastic arteries, activating the MMPs [121] and increasing collagen I synthesis [122]. High sodium intake with diet also seems to be able to stimulate aortic Angiotensin II receptor type 1 (AT_1-receptors) [123], and the vascular damage induced by excessive sodium intake can be modulated by genetic factors, in particular by the polymorphism of AT_1-receptor genes [124] and aldosterone synthase genes [125]. These genetic polymorphisms appear to be of particular relevance in the elderly and in the hypertensive patients [117,124]. The highest mortality associated with excessive dietary sodium intake was significantly reduced in rodents when the high-sodium diet was associated with the intake of selective angiotensin II blockers [126,127].

7. Conclusions

The worldwide usual sodium intake ranges between 3.5–5.5 g per day (corresponding to 9–12 g of salt per day), with marked differences at a global level. Recommendations were made by the World Health Organization to limit sodium intake to approximately 2.0 g per day (equivalent to approximately 5.0 g salt per day) in the general population [5], and a particular effort in reducing salt intake should be made in the hypertensive population, which counts more than a billion patients globally. A reduction in salt intake can have a favorable effect on the cardiovascular system, inducing a reduction in BP values in hypertensive patients, but also with possible benefits in the vascular function and in the viscoelastic properties of the large arteries. Adequate attention should be paid to arterial structure and function when evaluating the cardiovascular outcomes of salt intake and of programs for salt reduction in the diet.

References

1. Intersalt Cooperative Research Group. An international study of electrolyte excretion and blood pressure. Results for 24 hour urinary sodium and potassium excretion. *BMJ* **1988**, *297*, 319–328. [CrossRef] [PubMed]
2. Mente, A.; O'Donnell, M.J.; Rangarajan, S.; McQueen, M.J.; Poirier, P.; Wielgosz, A.; Morrison, H.; Li, W.; Wang, X.; Di, C.; et al. Association of urinary sodium and potassium excretion with blood pressure. *N. Engl. J. Med.* **2014**, *371*, 601–611. [CrossRef] [PubMed]
3. He, F.J.; MacGregor, G.A. Effect of modest salt reduction on blood pressure: A meta-analysis of randomized trials. Implications for public health. *J. Hum. Hypertens.* **2002**, *16*, 761–770. [CrossRef] [PubMed]
4. Denton, D.; Weisinger, R.; Mundy, N.I.; Wickings, E.J.; Dixson, A.; Moisson, P.; Pingard, A.M.; Shade, R.; Carey, D.; Ardaillou, R.; et al. The effect of increased salt intake on blood pressure of chimpanzees. *Nat. Med.* **1995**, *1*, 1009–1016. [CrossRef] [PubMed]
5. World Health Organization. *Guideline: Sodium Intake for Adults and Children*; World Health Organization: Geneva, Switzerland, 2012.
6. Weinberger, M.H. Salt sensitivity of blood pressure in humans. *Hypertension* **1996**, *27*, 481–490. [CrossRef] [PubMed]
7. Strazzullo, P.; D'Elia, L.; Kandala, N.B.; Cappuccio, F.P. Salt intake, stroke, and cardiovascular disease: Meta-analysis of prospective studies. *BMJ* **2009**, *339*, b4567. [CrossRef] [PubMed]
8. Whelton, P.K.; He, J. Health effects of sodium and potassium in humans. *Curr. Opin. Lipidol.* **2014**, *25*, 75–79. [CrossRef]
9. He, F.J.; Li, J.; Macgregor, G.A. Effect of longer term modest salt reduction on blood pressure: Cochrane systematic review and meta-analysis of randomised trials. *BMJ* **2013**, *346*, f1325. [CrossRef]
10. Girardin, E.; Caverzasio, J.; Iwai, J.; Bonjour, J.P.; Muller, A.F.; Grandchamp, A. Pressure natriuresis in isolated kidneys from hypertension-prone and hypertension-resistant rats (Dahl rats). *Kidney Int.* **1980**, *18*, 10–19. [CrossRef]
11. Dajnowiec, D.; Langille, B.L. Arterial adaptations to chronic changes in haemodynamic function: Coupling vasomotor tone to structural remodelling. *Clin. Sci.* **2007**, *113*, 15–23. [CrossRef]
12. Dumont, O.; Pinaud, F.; Guihot, A.L.; Baufreton, C.; Loufrani, L.; Henrion, D. Alteration in flow (shear stress)-induced remodelling in rat resistance arteries with aging: Improvement by a treatment with hydralazine. *Cardiovasc. Res.* **2008**, *77*, 600–608. [CrossRef] [PubMed]
13. Marketou, M.E.; Maragkoudakis, S.; Anastasiou, I.; Nakou, H.; Plataki, M.; Vardas, P.E.; Parthenakis, F.I. Salt-induced effects on microvascular function: A critical factor in hypertension mediated organ damage. *J. Clin. Hypertens.* **2019**, *21*, 749–757. [CrossRef] [PubMed]
14. Kurtz, T.W.; DiCarlo, S.E.; Pravenec, M.; Morris, R.C., Jr. The American Heart association scientific statement on salt sensitivity of blood pressure: Prompting consideration of alternative conceptual frameworks for the pathogenesis of salt sensitivity? *J. Hypertens.* **2017**, *35*, 2214–2225. [CrossRef] [PubMed]
15. Elijovich, F.; Weinberger, M.H.; Anderson, C.A.; Appel, L.J.; Bursztyn, M.; Cook, N.R.; Dart, R.A.; Newton-Cheh, C.H.; Sacks, F.M.; Laffer, C.L.; et al. Salt sensitivity of blood pressure: A scientific statement from the american heart association. *Hypertension* **2016**, *68*, e7–e46. [CrossRef] [PubMed]
16. Thomas, M.C.; Moran, J.; Forsblom, C.; Harjutsalo, V.; Thorn, L.; Ahola, A.; Waden, J.; Tolonen, N.; Saraheimo, M.; Gordin, D.; et al. The association between dietary sodium intake, ESRD, and all-cause mortality in patients with type 1 diabetes. *Diabetes Care* **2011**, *34*, 861–866. [CrossRef] [PubMed]
17. Saulnier, P.J.; Gand, E.; Hadjadj, S.; Group, S.S. Sodium and cardiovascular disease. *N. Engl. J. Med.* **2014**, *371*, 2135–2136. [CrossRef] [PubMed]
18. O'Donnell, M.; Mente, A.; Rangarajan, S.; McQueen, M.J.; Wang, X.; Liu, L.; Yan, H.; Lee, S.F.; Mony, P.; Devanath, A.; et al. Urinary sodium and potassium excretion, mortality, and cardiovascular events. *N. Engl. J. Med.* **2014**, *371*, 612–623. [CrossRef]
19. Mente, A.; O'Donnell, M.; Rangarajan, S.; Dagenais, G.; Lear, S.; McQueen, M.; Diaz, R.; Avezum, A.; Lopez-Jaramillo, P.; Lanas, F.; et al. Associations of urinary sodium excretion with cardiovascular events in individuals with and without hypertension: A pooled analysis of data from four studies. *Lancet* **2016**, *388*, 465–475. [CrossRef]

20. Graudal, N.; Jurgens, G.; Baslund, B.; Alderman, M.H. Compared with usual sodium intake, low- and excessive-sodium diets are associated with increased mortality: A meta-analysis. *Am. J. Hypertens.* **2014**, *27*, 1129–1137. [CrossRef]
21. Catanozi, S.; Rocha, J.C.; Passarelli, M.; Guzzo, M.L.; Alves, C.; Furukawa, L.N.; Nunes, V.S.; Nakandakare, E.R.; Heimann, J.C.; Quintao, E.C. Dietary sodium chloride restriction enhances aortic wall lipid storage and raises plasma lipid concentration in LDL receptor knockout mice. *J. Lipid Res.* **2003**, *44*, 727–732. [CrossRef]
22. Graudal, N.A.; Galloe, A.M.; Garred, P. Effects of sodium restriction on blood pressure, renin, aldosterone, catecholamines, cholesterols, and triglyceride: A meta-analysis. *JAMA* **1998**, *279*, 1383–1391. [CrossRef] [PubMed]
23. Brunner, H.R.; Laragh, J.H.; Baer, L.; Newton, M.A.; Goodwin, F.T.; Krakoff, L.R.; Bard, R.H.; Buhler, F.R. Essential hypertension: Renin and aldosterone, heart attack and stroke. *N. Engl. J. Med.* **1972**, *286*, 441–449. [CrossRef] [PubMed]
24. Grassi, G.; Dell'Oro, R.; Seravalle, G.; Foglia, G.; Trevano, F.Q.; Mancia, G. Short- and long-term neuroadrenergic effects of moderate dietary sodium restriction in essential hypertension. *Circulation* **2002**, *106*, 1957–1961. [CrossRef] [PubMed]
25. Petrie, J.R.; Morris, A.D.; Minamisawa, K.; Hilditch, T.E.; Elliott, H.L.; Small, M.; McConnell, J. Dietary sodium restriction impairs insulin sensitivity in noninsulin-dependent diabetes mellitus. *J. Clin. Endocrinol. Metab.* **1998**, *83*, 1552–1557. [CrossRef] [PubMed]
26. Garg, R.; Williams, G.H.; Hurwitz, S.; Brown, N.J.; Hopkins, P.N.; Adler, G.K. Low-salt diet increases insulin resistance in healthy subjects. *Metabolism* **2011**, *60*, 965–968. [CrossRef]
27. Nakandakare, E.R.; Charf, A.M.; Santos, F.C.; Nunes, V.S.; Ortega, K.; Lottenberg, A.M.; Mion, D., Jr.; Nakano, T.; Nakajima, K.; D'Amico, E.A.; et al. Dietary salt restriction increases plasma lipoprotein and inflammatory marker concentrations in hypertensive patients. *Atherosclerosis* **2008**, *200*, 410–416. [CrossRef]
28. Grassi, G.; Cattaneo, B.M.; Seravalle, G.; Lanfranchi, A.; Bolla, G.; Mancia, G. Baroreflex impairment by low sodium diet in mild or moderate essential hypertension. *Hypertension* **1997**, *29*, 802–807. [CrossRef]
29. Cook, N.R. Sodium and cardiovascular disease. *N. Engl. J. Med.* **2014**, *371*, 2134. [CrossRef]
30. Batuman, V. Sodium and cardiovascular disease. *N. Engl. J. Med.* **2014**, *371*, 2134–2135. [CrossRef]
31. Hall, J.E.; Guyton, A.C.; Coleman, T.G.; Mizelle, H.L.; Woods, L.L. Regulation of arterial pressure: Role of pressure natriuresis and diuresis. *Fed. Proc.* **1986**, *45*, 2897–2903.
32. Rapp, J.P.; Dene, H. Development and characteristics of inbred strains of Dahl salt-sensitive and salt-resistant rats. *Hypertension* **1985**, *7*, 340–349. [CrossRef] [PubMed]
33. Kawasaki, T.; Delea, C.S.; Bartter, F.C.; Smith, H. The effect of high-sodium and low-sodium intakes on blood pressure and other related variables in human subjects with idiopathic hypertension. *Am. J. Med.* **1978**, *64*, 193–198. [CrossRef]
34. Weinberger, M.H.; Miller, J.Z.; Luft, F.C.; Grim, C.E.; Fineberg, N.S. Definitions and characteristics of sodium sensitivity and blood pressure resistance. *Hypertension* **1986**, *8*, II127–II134. [CrossRef] [PubMed]
35. Coruzzi, P.; Parati, G.; Brambilla, L.; Brambilla, V.; Gualerzi, M.; Novarini, A.; Castiglioni, P.; Di Rienzo, M. Effects of salt sensitivity on neural cardiovascular regulation in essential hypertension. *Hypertension* **2005**, *46*, 1321–1326. [CrossRef] [PubMed]
36. Castiglioni, P.; Parati, G.; Lazzeroni, D.; Bini, M.; Faini, A.; Brambilla, L.; Brambilla, V.; Coruzzi, P. Hemodynamic and autonomic response to different salt intakes in normotensive individuals. *J. Am. Heart Assoc.* **2016**, *5*, e003736. [CrossRef] [PubMed]
37. Galletti, F.; Ferrara, I.; Stinga, F.; Iacone, R.; Noviello, F.; Strazzullo, P. Evaluation of a rapid protocol for the assessment of salt sensitivity against the blood pressure response to dietary sodium chloride restriction. *Am. J. Hypertens.* **1997**, *10*, 462–466. [CrossRef]
38. Castiglioni, P.; Parati, G.; Brambilla, L.; Brambilla, V.; Gualerzi, M.; Di Rienzo, M.; Coruzzi, P. Detecting sodium-sensitivity in hypertensive patients: Information from 24-hour ambulatory blood pressure monitoring. *Hypertension* **2011**, *57*, 180–185. [CrossRef]
39. Barba, G.; Galletti, F.; Cappuccio, F.P.; Siani, A.; Venezia, A.; Versiero, M.; Della Valle, E.; Sorrentino, P.; Tarantino, G.; Farinaro, E.; et al. Incidence of hypertension in individuals with different blood pressure salt-sensitivity: Results of a 15-year follow-up study. *J. Hypertens.* **2007**, *25*, 1465–1471. [CrossRef]

40. Bihorac, A.; Tezcan, H.; Ozener, C.; Oktay, A.; Akoglu, E. Association between salt sensitivity and target organ damage in essential hypertension. *Am. J. Hypertens.* **2000**, *13*, 864–872. [CrossRef]
41. Morimoto, A.; Uzu, T.; Fujii, T.; Nishimura, M.; Kuroda, S.; Nakamura, S.; Inenaga, T.; Kimura, G. Sodium sensitivity and cardiovascular events in patients with essential hypertension. *Lancet* **1997**, *350*, 1734–1737. [CrossRef]
42. Elliott, P.; Walker, L.L.; Little, M.P.; Blair-West, J.R.; Shade, R.E.; Lee, D.R.; Rouquet, P.; Leroy, E.; Jeunemaitre, X.; Ardaillou, R.; et al. Change in salt intake affects blood pressure of chimpanzees: Implications for human populations. *Circulation* **2007**, *116*, 1563–1568. [CrossRef]
43. Galletti, F.; Strazzullo, P. The blood pressure-salt sensitivity paradigm: Pathophysiologically sound yet of no practical value. *Nephrol. Dial. Transplant.* **2016**, *31*, 1386–1391. [CrossRef]
44. Aburto, N.J.; Ziolkovska, A.; Hooper, L.; Elliott, P.; Cappuccio, F.P.; Meerpohl, J.J. Effect of lower sodium intake on health: Systematic review and meta-analyses. *BMJ* **2013**, *346*, f1326. [CrossRef]
45. Frohlich, E.D. Hemodynamic differences between black patients and white patients with essential hypertension. State of the art lecture. *Hypertension* **1990**, *15*, 675–680. [CrossRef]
46. Wedler, B.; Brier, M.E.; Wiersbitzky, M.; Gruska, S.; Wolf, E.; Kallwellis, R.; Aronoff, G.R.; Luft, F.C. Sodium kinetics in salt-sensitive and salt-resistant normotensive and hypertensive subjects. *J. Hypertens.* **1992**, *10*, 663–669. [CrossRef]
47. Rocchini, A.P.; Key, J.; Bondie, D.; Chico, R.; Moorehead, C.; Katch, V.; Martin, M. The effect of weight loss on the sensitivity of blood pressure to sodium in obese adolescents. *N. Engl. J. Med.* **1989**, *321*, 580–585. [CrossRef]
48. Strazzullo, P.; Barbato, A.; Galletti, F.; Barba, G.; Siani, A.; Iacone, R.; D'Elia, L.; Russo, O.; Versiero, M.; Farinaro, E.; et al. Abnormalities of renal sodium handling in the metabolic syndrome. Results of the Olivetti heart study. *J. Hypertens.* **2006**, *24*, 1633–1639. [CrossRef]
49. Barba, G.; Russo, O.; Siani, A.; Iacone, R.; Farinaro, E.; Gerardi, M.C.; Russo, P.; Della Valle, E.; Strazzullo, P. Plasma leptin and blood pressure in men: Graded association independent of body mass and fat pattern. *Obes. Res.* **2003**, *11*, 160–166. [CrossRef]
50. Guyton, A.C. Blood pressure control—Special role of the kidneys and body fluids. *Science* **1991**, *252*, 1813–1816. [CrossRef]
51. Heer, M.; Baisch, F.; Kropp, J.; Gerzer, R.; Drummer, C. High dietary sodium chloride consumption may not induce body fluid retention in humans. *Am. J. Physiol. Physiol.* **2000**, *278*, F585–F595. [CrossRef]
52. Titze, J.; Bauer, K.; Schafflhuber, M.; Dietsch, P.; Lang, R.; Schwind, K.H.; Luft, F.C.; Eckardt, K.U.; Hilgers, K.F. Internal sodium balance in DOCA-salt rats: A body composition study. *Am. J. Physiol. Physiol.* **2005**, *289*, F793–F802. [CrossRef]
53. Laffer, C.L.; Scott, R.C., 3rd; Titze, J.M.; Luft, F.C.; Elijovich, F. Hemodynamics and salt-and-water balance link sodium storage and vascular dysfunction in salt-sensitive subjects. *Hypertension* **2016**, *68*, 195–203. [CrossRef]
54. Schmidlin, O.; Forman, A.; Leone, A.; Sebastian, A.; Morris, R.C., Jr. Salt sensitivity in blacks: Evidence that the initial pressor effect of NaCl involves inhibition of vasodilatation by asymmetrical dimethylarginine. *Hypertension* **2011**, *58*, 380–385. [CrossRef]
55. Morris, R.C., Jr.; Schmidlin, O.; Sebastian, A.; Tanaka, M.; Kurtz, T.W. Vasodysfunction that involves renal vasodysfunction, not abnormally increased renal retention of sodium, accounts for the initiation of salt-induced hypertension. *Circulation* **2016**, *133*, 881–893. [CrossRef]
56. Kurtz, T.W.; DiCarlo, S.E.; Pravenec, M.; Schmidlin, O.; Tanaka, M.; Morris, R.C., Jr. An alternative hypothesis to the widely held view that renal excretion of sodium accounts for resistance to salt-induced hypertension. *Kidney Int.* **2016**, *90*, 965–973. [CrossRef]
57. Bech, J.N.; Nielsen, C.B.; Ivarsen, P.; Jensen, K.T.; Pedersen, E.B. Dietary sodium affects systemic and renal hemodynamic response to NO inhibition in healthy humans. *Am. J. Physiol.* **1998**, *274*, F914–F923. [CrossRef]
58. Van Paassen, P.; de Zeeuw, D.; Navis, G.; de Jong, P.E. Does the renin-angiotensin system determine the renal and systemic hemodynamic response to sodium in patients with essential hypertension? *Hypertension* **1996**, *27*, 202–208. [CrossRef]
59. Parati, G.; Di Rienzo, M.; Bertinieri, G.; Pomidossi, G.; Casadei, R.; Groppelli, A.; Pedotti, A.; Zanchetti, A.; Mancia, G. Evaluation of the baroreceptor-heart rate reflex by 24-hour intra-arterial blood pressure monitoring in humans. *Hypertension* **1988**, *12*, 214–222. [CrossRef]

60. Di Rienzo, M.; Parati, G.; Castiglioni, P.; Tordi, R.; Mancia, G.; Pedotti, A. Baroreflex effectiveness index: An additional measure of baroreflex control of heart rate in daily life. *Am. J. Physiol. Integr. Comp. Physiol.* **2001**, *280*, R744–R751. [CrossRef]
61. Parati, G.; Saul, J.P.; Di Rienzo, M.; Mancia, G. Spectral analysis of blood pressure and heart rate variability in evaluating cardiovascular regulation. A critical appraisal. *Hypertension* **1995**, *25*, 1276–1286. [CrossRef]
62. Campese, V.M.; Romoff, M.S.; Levitan, D.; Saglikes, Y.; Friedler, R.M.; Massry, S.G. Abnormal relationship between sodium intake and sympathetic nervous system activity in salt-sensitive patients with essential hypertension. *Kidney Int.* **1982**, *21*, 371–378. [CrossRef]
63. Mark, A.; Mancia, G. Cardiopulmonary baroreflexes in humans. In *Handbook of Physiology. The Cardiovascular System*; Shepherd, J.T., Abboud, F.M., Eds.; American Physiological Society: Bethesda, MD, USA, 1983; pp. 795–813.
64. Mancia, G.; Parati, G.; Pomidossi, G.; Casadei, R.; Di Rienzo, M.; Zanchetti, A. Arterial baroreflexes and blood pressure and heart rate variabilities in humans. *Hypertension* **1986**, *8*, 147–153. [CrossRef]
65. Parlow, J.; Viale, J.P.; Annat, G.; Hughson, R.; Quintin, L. Spontaneous cardiac baroreflex in humans. Comparison with drug-induced responses. *Hypertension* **1995**, *25*, 1058–1068. [CrossRef]
66. Eckberg, D.L.; Drabinsky, M.; Braunwald, E. Defective cardiac parasympathetic control in patients with heart disease. *N. Engl. J. Med.* **1971**, *285*, 877–883. [CrossRef]
67. Pagani, M.; Somers, V.; Furlan, R.; Dell'Orto, S.; Conway, J.; Baselli, G.; Cerutti, S.; Sleight, P.; Malliani, A. Changes in autonomic regulation induced by physical training in mild hypertension. *Hypertension* **1988**, *12*, 600–610. [CrossRef]
68. Berntson, G.G.; Bigger, J.T., Jr.; Eckberg, D.L.; Grossman, P.; Kaufmann, P.G.; Malik, M.; Nagaraja, H.N.; Porges, S.W.; Saul, J.P.; Stone, P.H.; et al. Heart rate variability: Origins, methods, and interpretive caveats. *Psychophysiology* **1997**, *34*, 623–648. [CrossRef]
69. Hansen-Smith, F.M.; Morris, L.W.; Greene, A.S.; Lombard, J.H. Rapid microvessel rarefaction with elevated salt intake and reduced renal mass hypertension in rats. *Circ. Res.* **1996**, *79*, 324–330. [CrossRef]
70. Frisbee, J.C.; Lombard, J.H. Development and reversibility of altered skeletal muscle arteriolar structure and reactivity with high salt diet and reduced renal mass hypertension. *Microcirculation* **1999**, *6*, 215–225. [CrossRef]
71. Zhu, J.; Drenjancevic-Peric, I.; McEwen, S.; Friesema, J.; Schulta, D.; Yu, M.; Roman, R.J.; Lombard, J.H. Role of superoxide and angiotensin II suppression in salt-induced changes in endothelial Ca2+ signaling and NO production in rat aorta. *Am. J. Physiol. Heart Circ. Physiol.* **2006**, *291*, H929–H938. [CrossRef]
72. Wang, J.; Roman, R.J.; Falck, J.R.; de la Cruz, L.; Lombard, J.H. Effects of high-salt diet on CYP450-4A omega-hydroxylase expression and active tone in mesenteric resistance arteries. *Am. J. Physiol. Heart Circ. Physiol.* **2005**, *288*, H1557–H1565. [CrossRef]
73. Lukaszewicz, K.M.; Falck, J.R.; Manthati, V.L.; Lombard, J.H. Introgression of Brown Norway CYP4A genes on to the Dahl salt-sensitive background restores vascular function in SS-5(BN) consomic rats. *Clin. Sci.* **2013**, *124*, 333–342. [CrossRef]
74. Abularrage, C.J.; Sidawy, A.N.; Aidinian, G.; Singh, N.; Weiswasser, J.M.; Arora, S. Evaluation of the microcirculation in vascular disease. *J. Vasc. Surg.* **2005**, *42*, 574–581. [CrossRef]
75. Tzemos, N.; Lim, P.O.; Wong, S.; Struthers, A.D.; MacDonald, T.M. Adverse cardiovascular effects of acute salt loading in young normotensive individuals. *Hypertension* **2008**, *51*, 1525–1530. [CrossRef]
76. Greaney, J.L.; DuPont, J.J.; Lennon-Edwards, S.L.; Sanders, P.W.; Edwards, D.G.; Farquhar, W.B. Dietary sodium loading impairs microvascular function independent of blood pressure in humans: Role of oxidative stress. *J. Physiol.* **2012**, *590*, 5519–5528. [CrossRef]
77. Cavka, A.; Jukic, I.; Ali, M.; Goslawski, M.; Bian, J.T.; Wang, E.; Drenjancevic, I.; Phillips, S.A. Short-term high salt intake reduces brachial artery and microvascular function in the absence of changes in blood pressure. *J. Hypertens.* **2016**, *34*, 676–684. [CrossRef]
78. Rorije, N.M.G.; Olde Engberink, R.H.G.; Chahid, Y.; van Vlies, N.; van Straalen, J.P.; van den Born, B.H.; Verberne, H.J.; Vogt, L. Microvascular permeability after an acute and chronic salt load in healthy subjects: A randomized open-label crossover intervention study. *Anesthesiology* **2018**, *128*, 352–360. [CrossRef]
79. Schmidlin, O.; Sebastian, A.F.; Morris, R.C., Jr. What initiates the pressor effect of salt in salt-sensitive humans? Observations in normotensive blacks. *Hypertension* **2007**, *49*, 1032–1039. [CrossRef]

80. Jablonski, K.L.; Racine, M.L.; Geolfos, C.J.; Gates, P.E.; Chonchol, M.; McQueen, M.B.; Seals, D.R. Dietary sodium restriction reverses vascular endothelial dysfunction in middle-aged/older adults with moderately elevated systolic blood pressure. *J. Am. Coll. Cardiol.* **2013**, *61*, 335–343. [CrossRef]
81. Kopp, C.; Linz, P.; Dahlmann, A.; Hammon, M.; Jantsch, J.; Muller, D.N.; Schmieder, R.E.; Cavallaro, A.; Eckardt, K.U.; Uder, M.; et al. 23Na magnetic resonance imaging-determined tissue sodium in healthy subjects and hypertensive patients. *Hypertension* **2013**, *61*, 635–640. [CrossRef]
82. Nijst, P.; Verbrugge, F.H.; Grieten, L.; Dupont, M.; Steels, P.; Tang, W.H.W.; Mullens, W. The pathophysiological role of interstitial sodium in heart failure. *J. Am. Coll. Cardiol.* **2015**, *65*, 378–388. [CrossRef]
83. Selvarajah, V.; Connolly, K.; McEniery, C.; Wilkinson, I. Skin sodium and hypertension: A paradigm shift? *Curr. Hypertens. Rep.* **2018**, *20*, 94. [CrossRef]
84. Titze, J.; Krause, H.; Hecht, H.; Dietsch, P.; Rittweger, J.; Lang, R.; Kirsch, K.A.; Hilgers, K.F. Reduced osmotically inactive Na storage capacity and hypertension in the Dahl model. *Am. J. Physiol. Physiol.* **2002**, *283*, F134–F141. [CrossRef]
85. Titze, J.; Lang, R.; Ilies, C.; Schwind, K.H.; Kirsch, K.A.; Dietsch, P.; Luft, F.C.; Hilgers, K.F. Osmotically inactive skin Na+ storage in rats. *Am. J. Physiol. Physiol.* **2003**, *285*, F1108–F1117. [CrossRef]
86. Titze, J.; Shakibaei, M.; Schafflhuber, M.; Schulze-Tanzil, G.; Porst, M.; Schwind, K.H.; Dietsch, P.; Hilgers, K.F. Glycosaminoglycan polymerization may enable osmotically inactive Na+ storage in the skin. *Am. J. Physiol. Heart Circ. Physiol.* **2004**, *287*, H203–H208. [CrossRef]
87. Machnik, A.; Neuhofer, W.; Jantsch, J.; Dahlmann, A.; Tammela, T.; Machura, K.; Park, J.K.; Beck, F.X.; Muller, D.N.; Derer, W.; et al. Macrophages regulate salt-dependent volume and blood pressure by a vascular endothelial growth factor-C-dependent buffering mechanism. *Nat. Med.* **2009**, *15*, 545–552. [CrossRef]
88. Wiig, H.; Schroder, A.; Neuhofer, W.; Jantsch, J.; Kopp, C.; Karlsen, T.V.; Boschmann, M.; Goss, J.; Bry, M.; Rakova, N.; et al. Immune cells control skin lymphatic electrolyte homeostasis and blood pressure. *J. Clin. Investig.* **2013**, *123*, 2803–2815. [CrossRef]
89. Machnik, A.; Dahlmann, A.; Kopp, C.; Goss, J.; Wagner, H.; van Rooijen, N.; Eckardt, K.U.; Muller, D.N.; Park, J.K.; Luft, F.C.; et al. Mononuclear phagocyte system depletion blocks interstitial tonicity-responsive enhancer binding protein/vascular endothelial growth factor C expression and induces salt-sensitive hypertension in rats. *Hypertension* **2010**, *55*, 755–761. [CrossRef]
90. He, F.J.; Marciniak, M.; Markandu, N.D.; Antonios, T.F.; MacGregor, G.A. Effect of modest salt reduction on skin capillary rarefaction in white, black, and Asian individuals with mild hypertension. *Hypertension* **2010**, *56*, 253–259. [CrossRef]
91. Helle, F.; Karlsen, T.V.; Tenstad, O.; Titze, J.; Wiig, H. High-salt diet increases hormonal sensitivity in skin pre-capillary resistance vessels. *Acta Physiol.* **2013**, *207*, 577–581. [CrossRef]
92. Zhu, Q.; Hu, J.; Han, W.Q.; Zhang, F.; Li, P.L.; Wang, Z.; Li, N. Silencing of HIF prolyl-hydroxylase 2 gene in the renal medulla attenuates salt-sensitive hypertension in Dahl S rats. *Am. J. Hypertens.* **2014**, *27*, 107–113. [CrossRef]
93. Safar, M.; Laurent, S.; Safavian, A.; Pannier, B.; Asmar, R. Sodium and large arteries in hypertension. Effects of indapamide. *Am. J. Med.* **1988**, *84*, 15–19. [CrossRef]
94. Blaustein, M.P. Sodium ions, calcium ions, blood pressure regulation, and hypertension: A reassessment and a hypothesis. *Am. J. Physiol.* **1977**, *232*, C165–C173. [CrossRef]
95. Avolio, A.P.; Deng, F.Q.; Li, W.Q.; Luo, Y.F.; Huang, Z.D.; Xing, L.F.; O'Rourke, M.F. Effects of aging on arterial distensibility in populations with high and low prevalence of hypertension: Comparison between urban and rural communities in China. *Circulation* **1985**, *71*, 202–210. [CrossRef]
96. Avolio, A.P.; Clyde, K.M.; Beard, T.C.; Cooke, H.M.; Ho, K.K.; O'Rourke, M.F. Improved arterial distensibility in normotensive subjects on a low salt diet. *Arteriosclerosis* **1986**, *6*, 166–169. [CrossRef]
97. Todd, A.S.; Macginley, R.J.; Schollum, J.B.; Johnson, R.J.; Williams, S.M.; Sutherland, W.H.; Mann, J.I.; Walker, R.J. Dietary salt loading impairs arterial vascular reactivity. *Am. J. Clin. Nutr.* **2010**, *91*, 557–564. [CrossRef]
98. McMahon, E.J.; Bauer, J.D.; Hawley, C.M.; Isbel, N.M.; Stowasser, M.; Johnson, D.W.; Campbell, K.L. A randomized trial of dietary sodium restriction in CKD. *J. Am. Soc. Nephrol.* **2013**, *24*, 2096–2103. [CrossRef]

99. Jablonski, K.L.; Fedorova, O.V.; Racine, M.L.; Geolfos, C.J.; Gates, P.E.; Chonchol, M.; Fleenor, B.S.; Lakatta, E.G.; Bagrov, A.Y.; Seals, D.R. Dietary sodium restriction and association with urinary marinobufagenin, blood pressure, and aortic stiffness. *Clin. J. Am. Soc. Nephrol.* **2013**, *8*, 1952–1959. [CrossRef]
100. He, F.J.; Marciniak, M.; Visagie, E.; Markandu, N.D.; Anand, V.; Dalton, R.N.; MacGregor, G.A. Effect of modest salt reduction on blood pressure, urinary albumin, and pulse wave velocity in white, black, and Asian mild hypertensives. *Hypertension* **2009**, *54*, 482–488. [CrossRef]
101. Todd, A.S.; Macginley, R.J.; Schollum, J.B.; Williams, S.M.; Sutherland, W.H.; Mann, J.I.; Walker, R.J. Dietary sodium loading in normotensive healthy volunteers does not increase arterial vascular reactivity or blood pressure. *Nephrology* **2012**, *17*, 249–256. [CrossRef]
102. Dickinson, K.M.; Keogh, J.B.; Clifton, P.M. Effects of a low-salt diet on flow-mediated dilatation in humans. *Am. J. Clin. Nutr.* **2009**, *89*, 485–490. [CrossRef]
103. Dickinson, K.M.; Clifton, P.M.; Keogh, J.B. A reduction of 3 g/day from a usual 9 g/day salt diet improves endothelial function and decreases endothelin-1 in a randomised cross_over study in normotensive overweight and obese subjects. *Atherosclerosis* **2014**, *233*, 32–38. [CrossRef]
104. Van der Graaf, A.M.; Paauw, N.D.; Toering, T.J.; Feelisch, M.; Faas, M.M.; Sutton, T.R.; Minnion, M.; Lefrandt, J.D.; Scherjon, S.A.; Franx, A.; et al. Impaired sodium-dependent adaptation of arterial stiffness in formerly preeclamptic women: The RETAP-vascular study. *Am. J. Physiol. Heart Circ. Physiol.* **2016**, *310*, H1827–H1833. [CrossRef]
105. Suckling, R.J.; He, F.J.; Markandu, N.D.; MacGregor, G.A. Modest salt reduction lowers blood pressure and albumin excretion in impaired glucose tolerance and type 2 diabetes mellitus: A randomized double-blind trial. *Hypertension* **2016**, *67*, 1189–1195. [CrossRef]
106. Gijsbers, L.; Dower, J.I.; Mensink, M.; Siebelink, E.; Bakker, S.J.; Geleijnse, J.M. Effects of sodium and potassium supplementation on blood pressure and arterial stiffness: A fully controlled dietary intervention study. *J. Hum. Hypertens.* **2015**, *29*, 592–598. [CrossRef]
107. Pimenta, E.; Gaddam, K.K.; Oparil, S.; Aban, I.; Husain, S.; Dell'Italia, L.J.; Calhoun, D.A. Effects of dietary sodium reduction on blood pressure in subjects with resistant hypertension: Results from a randomized trial. *Hypertension* **2009**, *54*, 475–481. [CrossRef]
108. D'Elia, L.; Galletti, F.; La Fata, E.; Sabino, P.; Strazzullo, P. Effect of dietary sodium restriction on arterial stiffness: Systematic review and meta-analysis of the randomized controlled trials. *J. Hypertens.* **2018**, *36*, 734–743. [CrossRef]
109. Salvi, P.; Palombo, C.; Salvi, G.M.; Labat, C.; Parati, G.; Benetos, A. Left ventricular ejection time, not heart rate, is an independent correlate of aortic pulse wave velocity. *J. Appl. Physiol.* **2013**, *115*, 1610–1617. [CrossRef]
110. Salvi, P. *Pulse Waves. How Vascular Hemodynamics Affects Blood Pressure*, 2nd ed.; Springer Nature: Heidelberg, Germany, 2017.
111. Matrougui, K.; Schiavi, P.; Guez, D.; Henrion, D. High sodium intake decreases pressure-induced (myogenic) tone and flow-induced dilation in resistance arteries from hypertensive rats. *Hypertension* **1998**, *32*, 176–179. [CrossRef]
112. Ying, W.Z.; Sanders, P.W. Dietary salt increases endothelial nitric oxide synthase and TGF-beta1 in rat aortic endothelium. *Am. J. Physiol.* **1999**, *277*, H1293–H1298.
113. Edwards, D.G.; Farquhar, W.B. Vascular effects of dietary salt. *Curr. Opin. Nephrol. Hypertens.* **2015**, *24*, 8–13. [CrossRef]
114. Harvey, A.; Montezano, A.C.; Lopes, R.A.; Rios, F.; Touyz, R.M. Vascular fibrosis in aging and hypertension: Molecular mechanisms and clinical implications. *Can. J. Cardiol.* **2016**, *32*, 659–668. [CrossRef]
115. Wang, M.; Zhao, D.; Spinetti, G.; Zhang, J.; Jiang, L.Q.; Pintus, G.; Monticone, R.; Lakatta, E.G. Matrix metalloproteinase 2 activation of transforming growth factor-beta1 (TGF-beta1) and TGF-beta1-type II receptor signaling within the aged arterial wall. *Arter. Thromb. Vasc. Biol.* **2006**, *26*, 1503–1509. [CrossRef]
116. Duncan, M.R.; Frazier, K.S.; Abramson, S.; Williams, S.; Klapper, H.; Huang, X.; Grotendorst, G.R. Connective tissue growth factor mediates transforming growth factor beta-induced collagen synthesis: Down-regulation by cAMP. *FASEB J.* **1999**, *13*, 1774–1786. [CrossRef]
117. Safar, M.E.; Thuilliez, C.; Richard, V.; Benetos, A. Pressure-independent contribution of sodium to large artery structure and function in hypertension. *Cardiovasc. Res.* **2000**, *46*, 269–276. [CrossRef]

118. Prakobwong, S.; Yongvanit, P.; Hiraku, Y.; Pairojkul, C.; Sithithaworn, P.; Pinlaor, P.; Pinlaor, S. Involvement of MMP-9 in peribiliary fibrosis and cholangiocarcinogenesis via Rac1-dependent DNA damage in a hamster model. *Int. J. Cancer* **2010**, *127*, 2576–2587. [CrossRef]
119. Newby, A.C. Dual role of matrix metalloproteinases (matrixins) in intimal thickening and atherosclerotic plaque rupture. *Physiol. Rev.* **2005**, *85*, 1–31. [CrossRef]
120. Wang, M.; Kim, S.H.; Monticone, R.E.; Lakatta, E.G. Matrix metalloproteinases promote arterial remodeling in aging, hypertension, and atherosclerosis. *Hypertension* **2015**, *65*, 698–703. [CrossRef]
121. Pons, M.; Cousins, S.W.; Alcazar, O.; Striker, G.E.; Marin-Castano, M.E. Angiotensin II-induced MMP-2 activity and MMP-14 and basigin protein expression are mediated via the angiotensin II receptor type 1-mitogen-activated protein kinase 1 pathway in retinal pigment epithelium: Implications for age-related macular degeneration. *Am. J. Pathol.* **2011**, *178*, 2665–2681. [CrossRef]
122. Savoia, C.; Touyz, R.M.; Amiri, F.; Schiffrin, E.L. Selective mineralocorticoid receptor blocker eplerenone reduces resistance artery stiffness in hypertensive patients. *Hypertension* **2008**, *51*, 432–439. [CrossRef]
123. Wang, D.H.; Du, Y. Regulation of vascular type 1 angiotensin II receptor in hypertension and sodium loading: Role of angiotensin II. *J. Hypertens.* **1998**, *16*, 467–475. [CrossRef]
124. Benetos, A.; Gautier, S.; Ricard, S.; Topouchian, J.; Asmar, R.; Poirier, O.; Larosa, E.; Guize, L.; Safar, M.; Soubrier, F.; et al. Influence of angiotensin-converting enzyme and angiotensin II type 1 receptor gene polymorphisms on aortic stiffness in normotensive and hypertensive patients. *Circulation* **1996**, *94*, 698–703. [CrossRef]
125. Pojoga, L.; Gautier, S.; Blanc, H.; Guyene, T.T.; Poirier, O.; Cambien, F.; Benetos, A. Genetic determination of plasma aldosterone levels in essential hypertension. *Am. J. Hypertens.* **1998**, *11*, 856–860. [CrossRef]
126. Mercier, N.; Labat, C.; Louis, H.; Cattan, V.; Benetos, A.; Safar, M.E.; Lacolley, P. Sodium, arterial stiffness, and cardiovascular mortality in hypertensive rats. *Am. J. Hypertens.* **2007**, *20*, 319–325. [CrossRef]
127. Safar, M.E.; Temmar, M.; Kakou, A.; Lacolley, P.; Thornton, S.N. Sodium intake and vascular stiffness in hypertension. *Hypertension* **2009**, *54*, 203–209. [CrossRef]

9

Relation between Dietary Habits, Physical Activity and Anthropometric and Vascular Parameters in Children Attending the Primary School in the Verona South District

Alice Giontella [1], Sara Bonafini [1,*], Angela Tagetti [1], Irene Bresadola [2], Pietro Minuz [1], Rossella Gaudino [2], Paolo Cavarzere [2], Diego Alberto Ramaroli [2], Denise Marcon [1], Lorella Branz [1], Lara Nicolussi Principe [1], Franco Antoniazzi [2], Claudio Maffeis [2] and Cristiano Fava [1]

[1] Department of Medicine, University of Verona, 37129 Verona, Italy; alice.giontella@gmail.com (A.G.); angela.tagetti@libero.it (A.T.); pietro.minuz@univr.it (P.M.); denise.m@hotmail.it (D.M.); lorellabranz@yahoo.com (L.B.); lara.nicolussiprincipe@studenti.univr.it (L.N.P.); cristiano.fava@univr.it (C.F.)

[2] Department of Surgery, Dentistry, Paediatrics and Gynaecology, University of Verona, 37129 Verona, Italy; ire.bre@hotmail.it (I.B.); rossella.gaudino@univr.it (R.G.); paolo.cavarzere@ospedaleuniverona.it (P.C.); diegoalberto.ramaroli@univr.it (D.A.R.); franco.antoniazzi@univr.it (F.A.); claudio.maffeis@univr.it (C.M.)

* Correspondence: bonafinisara@gmail.com

Abstract: The aim of this school-based study was to identify the possible association between diet and physical activity, as well as the anthropometric, vascular, and gluco-lipid parameters. We administered two validated questionnaires for diet and physical activity (Food Frequency questionnaire (FFQ), Children-Physical Activity Questionnaire (PAQ-C)) to children at four primary schools in Verona South (Verona, Italy). Specific food intake, dietary pattern, and physical activity level expressed in Metabolic Equivalent of Task (MET) and PAQ-C score were inserted in multivariate linear regression models to assess the association with anthropometric, hemodynamic, and gluco-lipid measures. Out of 309 children included in the study, 300 (age: 8.6 ± 0.7 years, male: 50%; Obese (OB): 13.6%; High blood pressure (HBP): 21.6%) compiled to the FFQ. From this, two dietary patterns were identified: "healthy" and "unhealthy". Direct associations were found between (i) "fast food" intake, Pulse Wave Velocity (PWV), and (ii) animal-derived fat and capillary cholesterol, while inverse associations were found between vegetable, fruit, and nut intake and capillary glucose. The high prevalence of OB and HBP and the significant correlations between some categories of food and metabolic and vascular parameters suggest the importance of life-style modification politics at an early age to prevent the onset of overt cardiovascular risk factors in childhood.

Keywords: children; diet; physical activity; cardiovascular risk factors; obesity; hypertension; blood pressure; pulse wave velocity

---

1. Introduction

Since childhood, the presence of cardiometabolic risk factors such as obesity, hypertension, high levels of cholesterol, and triglycerides [1] may lead to the development of an atherosclerotic fatty streak in the intima of arteries [2,3]. Childhood obesity—considered by the "World Health Organization" (WHO) to be one of the most serious problem of 21st century—is a well-known cause of noncommunicable disease in adults [4]. High blood pressure (HBP) in children is responsible for haemodynamic changes, including altered artery elasticity [5]. At a young age, the process is considered reversible [2] and can be prevented or minimized by implementing a healthy lifestyle [3]. Dietary habits and physical activity represent key points in the prevention of cardiovascular risk factors [6]. Diet is considered one of the major modifiable determinants of chronic diseases, with more and more scientific evidences supporting the fact that a "healthy" diet pattern could protect [5] a diet consisting of a daily intake of fruits and vegetables combined with a low consumption of salt, sugar, and saturated fat, in addition to industrially-produced-trans-fatty acids; this is still considered as a "high-quality" diet [5]. It is associated with a better cardiometabolic profile both in adults and in children [1,5]. Many studies have investigated the association between food intake and cardiovascular risk factors. With globalization and urbanization, children are exposed to ultra-processed, energy-dense, and nutrient-poor foods, which are cheap and readily available [7]. The intake of this kind of food increases the risk for young people to develop obesity in childhood and in adulthood [8]. To the contrary, "healthy diets" such as a Mediterranean-like dietary pattern rich in vegetables, fruit, fish, nuts, and olive oil, have been associated with not only to a reduction of blood pressure, improvement in lipid profile, endothelial function, and vascular inflammation in adults [9] but also to a reduction of inflammation already present in the younger population [10].

Physical activity influences body composition in terms of the amount of fat and muscle [7]. Because sedentary lifestyles are a rapidly increasing problem in both developed and developing countries [7], an appropriate level of physical activity provides health beneficial for musculoskeletal tissue, cardiovascular system, neuromuscular awareness, body weight control, and psychological benefits [11]. WHO reports that more than 80% of adolescents do not acheive the recommended level of daily physical activity [7]. WHO guidelines recommend that for at least one hour a day children engage in moderate-to vigorous physical activity, including games, sports, transportation, chores, recreation, physical education, or planned exercise, in the context of family, school, and community activities [12].

This study is a part of an observational school-based study set up with the aim to assess the relationship between food, physical activity, and the main cardiovascular risk factors in children attending their third and fourth class of primary school in the Verona South district. In particular, we aimed at assessing the prevalence of obesity (OB) and HBP in a defined age group and the possible associations between (i) dietary pattern and physical activity level, as well as (ii) anthropometric, gluco-lipid, and hemodynamic measures. This study could be useful to clarify how many children carry either overt or potential CV risk factors and additionally clarify how strong the association is between these factors and lifestyle.

2. Materials and Methods

2.1. Study Design

Children were recruited from the third and fourth classes of four primary schools in the Verona south district. The choice of the sample was determined by the age range (7–10), which was considered well suited for the aims of the study, as mostly prepuberal children were willing to participate.

The Verona South district was chosen because of the headmasters' willingness to allow us to perform the investigation. Subjects who refused to participate in the study or did not have their parents' consensus were excluded. The study was conducted according to a cross-sectional observational design and was approved by the Ethical Committee of Verona and Rovigo (CESC) (n = 375). Written inform consent was signed by all children's parents.

In their school gym, children were evaluated in the morning starting at 8:30 a.m. Anthropometric measurements were collected with children wearing light clothes without shoes. Weight and height were measured with a calibrated balance and stadiometer; body mass index (BMI, kg/m2) was calculated. Children were classified as overweight (the percentile BMI for their age was above the 85th) or obese (the percentile BMI for their age was above the 95th) using the WHO child growth standard [13,14]. Waist-height ratio was measured and values were transformed in z-score and percentile [15,16]. Brachial blood pressure (BP) was the average of the three measurements in the supine positions, using a children-validated semiautomatic oscillometric device (Omron 750 IT) [17]; the measurments were expressed as a Z-Score and percentiles were indicated by the guidelines [18,19]. Subjects whose BP was between the 90th and 95th percentile were considered to have normal-high BP, while those with a BP equal or above the 95th percentile were defined as having a high BP.

Besides brachial BP, even central aortic pressure waveform (cSBP, mmHg) and carotid-femoral pulse wave velocity (PWV, m/s) were derived using the SphygmoCor XCEL device. The cuff pulsations were recorded at the brachial artery, then a general transfer function was applied to calculate aortic waveform [20] using a cuff around the femoral artery that captures the femoral waveform and a tonometer that captures the carotid waveform. The velocity is computed by dividing the distance between the carotid and femoral arteries, using the pulse transit time. Z-score and percentiles were computed for cSBP and PWV [21,22]. Capillary cholesterol, triglycerides, and glucose were measured from fingerpick blood drops with two point-of-care testing (POCT) instruments (for cholesterol and triglycerides: HPS Multicare-in, Biochemical System International, Arezzo, Italy; for glucose: and Nova Biomedical, Waltham, MA, USA) [23,24], while children were fasting for at least four hours. Two questionnaires, both previously validated for children, were administered: "Food Frequency Questionnaire" (FFQ) [25] and a Physical Activity Questionnaire for Older Children (PAQ-C) [26,27]. Questionnaires were explained to the children and their parents on a previous informative day, then compiled at home along with parents and revised at the evaluation day with each child by a dedicated dietician.

2.2. *Food Frequency Questionnaire (FFQ)*

Children indicated their usual consumption of 61 items on the FFQ, using a 5-point scale (never; 1–2 times a month; 1–3 times weekly; 4–5 times weekly; one a day; more than once daily). Association of diet to diseases needed to be determined through different approaches because diet is a complex exposure variable [28]. Thus, we investigated a single FFQ intake (eggs, oil, seed oil, and nuts), main food groups intake (cereals and tubers, dairy products, legumes, fish, vegetables, fresh and dried fruit, meat, FFQ category of fast food, sweets, animal fat-derived condiments, junk food) and dietary patterns in relation to other collected variables. The patterns were extrapolated using the exploratory Principal Components Analysis (PCA), which represents one of the most used tools to derive behavioral patterns [29]. Dietary patterns could be representative of the intake of the usual combinations of individual food or groups of foods [29,30] and could provide more information regarding the association diet-disease since it reflects individual dietary behaviors [31].

2.3. *Physical Activity*

PAQ-C is a seven-day recall composed of nine statements about the frequency of physical activities at school, at home, and during leisure time. A score from 1 to 5 is assigned to each item and a mean total score of physical activity, the PAQ-C score, is then computed [32]. PAQ-C represents a valid and reliable method to assess general levels of physical activities but does not provide specific information about frequency, time, and intensity. For this reason, the first item of PAQ-C has been integrated with a semiquantitative question asked to define one's physical activity level in terms of Metabolic Equivalent of Task (MET), which is defined as the energetic cost of sitting quietly [33]. A total MET-minutes/week has been obtained, as described in Supplementary methods 1.1. The threshold indicated in the "Guidelines for data processing and analysis of the IPAQ" of 600 and 3000 MET-minutes/week has been used, respectively, to categorize subjects in "low", "medium", or "high" adherence to moderate-vigorous physical activity [32].

2.4. *Statistics*

Data are expressed as mean ± standard deviation (SD) for continuous variables or percentages for categorical ones. The level of the p-value was set at 0.05. The Spearman correlation coefficient was used to quantify linear relationship between variables. The Student's T-test was used to compare variables among two groups, while the ANOVA with Tukey post-hoc test was used for several groups. The relationship between categorical data was tested using the chi-square test. A power calculation based on an estimated prevalence of 9% obesity, as previously reported in Italian children [34], indicates that with our actual sample size of 300 children, we have 80% power to detect the true prevalence of obesity with a precision of 3.24% (that is a 95% CI of the estimate, between 5.76% and 12.24%). PCA was set as described in Supplementary methods 1.1. Adequacy of the sample to perform PCA were tested with Kaiser-Meyer-Olkin (KMO) test. Multivariate linear regression models were performed in order to test if diet pattern and/or physical activity remained associated with hemodynamic and metabolic variables, with results that were correlated by univariate analysis after adjustment. Age, sex, ethnicity, BMI, quartiles of kilocalorie intake, and quartiles of PAQ-C scores were used as covariates in the models. Statistics were performed with SPSS (IBM Corp. Released 2015. IBM SPSS Statistics for Windows, Version 23.0. Armonk, NY: IBM Corp, USA) and R (R Core Team (2014). R: A language and environment for statistical computing. R Foundation for Statistical Computing, Vienna, Austria). Graphs have been created with GraphPad Prism version 7.00 for Windows (GraphPad Software, La Jolla, San Diego, CA, USA).

3. Results

3.1. Characteristics of the Population

A total of 309 out of 413 children chose to participate in the study (participation rate 74.8%). Out of the 309 children recruited in the study (97.1% of population), 300 children (Age: 8.6 ± 0.7 years, male: 50%) filled out the questionnaires correctly. Baseline characteristics are shown in Table 1.

Table 1. General characteristics of the population.

Characteristics	Male (n = 150)	Female (n = 150)	p-Value
	mean ± SD	mean ± SD	
Age; ys	8.7 ± 0.8	8.6 ± 0.7	n.s.
Caucasian ethnicity; n (%)	102 (68.0)	94 (62.7)	n.s.
Other ethnicities; n (%)	48 (32.0)	56 (37.3)	
BMI; kg/m2	18.1 ± 3.2	18.2 ± 3.6	n.s
BMI; percentile for age	63.9 ± 30.1	61.6 ± 31.6	n.s.
Normal weight; n (%)	95.0 (63.3)	102.0 (68.0)	
Overweight; n (%)	35.0 (20.3)	29.0 (19.3)	n.s.
Obese; n (%)	20.0 (13.4)	19.0 (12.7)	
Waist-height ratio	0.46 ± 0.8	0.46 ± 0.8	n.s.
Waist-height ratio; percentile	44.4 ± 31.7	48.0 ± 31.3	n.s.
Brachial SBP; mmHg	110.5 ± 9.5	110.2 ± 10.3	n.s.
Brachial DBP; mmHg	66.3 ± 7.4	67.2 ± 8.1	n.s.
Brachial SBP; percentile	75.9 ± 20.5	75.9 ± 20.5	n.s.
Brachial DBP; percentile	70.2 ± 19.2	71.6 ± 20.5	n.s.
Normal BP; n (%)	95 (63.3)	87 (58)	n.s.
High BP; n (%)	55 (36.7)	63 (42)	
Pulse Wave Velocity; m/s	4.6 ± 1.0	4.6 ± 0.8	n.s.
Pulse Wave Velocity; percentile for height	61.6 ± 40.2	58.4 ± 38.5	n.s.
cSBP; mmHg	100.2 ± 9.3	101.5 ± 10.7	n.s.
cSBP <90° percentile for height; n (%)	76.4 ± 27.2	78.1 ± 28.5	n.s.
cSBP >90° percentile for height; n (%)	68 (46.3)	78 (53.4)	n.s.
Capillary Triglycerides; mg/dl	178.4 ± 84.0	165.7 ± 62.4	$p < 0.001$
Capillary Cholesterol; mg/dl	241.5 ± 36.4	221.2 ± 38.5	n.s.
Capillary Glucose; mg/dl	92.3 ± 8.8	86.0 ± 10.4	$p < 0.001$
Energy intake kcal/die	2933.2 ± 932.0	3031.6 ± 1138.0	n.s.
PAQ-C Score	1.9 ± 0.4	1.8 ± 0.5	$p < 0.05$
Moderate-vigorous activity (MET-min/wk)	3825.2 ± 4230.7	2721.1 ± 3578.2	$p < 0.05$

BMI, Body Mass Index.

The prevalence of overweight and obesity were 21.3% and 13%, respectively, while the prevalence of normal-high BP and HBP were 17.6% and 21.7% (Figure 1), respectively. Among obese children, the prevalence of HBP was 30.8%, whereas among overweight children, the prevalence of HBP was 20.3%. Moreover, 150 (50%) and 121 children (41.3%) were found to have cSBP higher than either the 90th or 95th percentile for height, respectively. Among the 55 (18.3%) children classified as HBP by brachial SBP, 45 (81.8%) and 41 (78.8%) present cSBP over either the 90th or 95th percentile for height, respectively. We found higher consumption of vegetables in children categorized as normal weight group, compared to the overweight and obese group (Supplementary Table S1), as well as in normotensive children compared to children with normal-high or HBP (Supplementary Table S2).

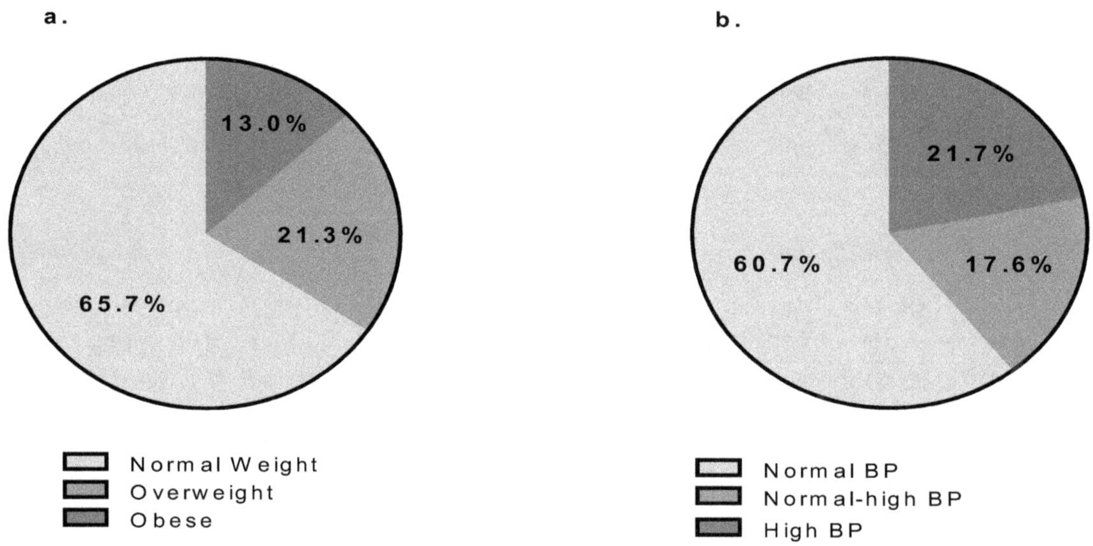

Figure 1. Prevalence of overweight/obese (**a**) and normal high/high blood pressure (BP) (**b**). Legend: "Normal weight": percentile body mass index (BMI)—age < 85th; "Overweight": 85th < P percentile BMI—age < 95th; "Obese": percentile BMI—age > 95th; "Normal blood pressure (BP)": percentile SBP and DBP < 90th; "Normal-high blood pressure (BP)": 90th < percentile SBP or DBP < 95th; "High blood pressure (BP)": percentile SBP or DBP > 95th.

3.2. FFQ

3.2.1. Single FFQ Category

In univariate analysis, some significant correlations between the FFQ categories and anthropometric, haemodynamic, and gluco-lipid parameters were found (Table 2). In particular, we underlined the direct association between "fast food" and BMI, PWV, brachial, and central BP, capillary triglycerides. Meat intake was associated with a higher PWV and brachial DBP, whereas vegetables and fruit (fresh and nuts) intake were associated with a lower level of capillary glucose. Nut intake confirms the inverse correlation with capillary glucose that was already evident in the fruit group (r_s = -0.162, $p < 0.05$). Among condiments, those derived from animal fat (butter and lard) correlated positively with the level of capillary cholesterol, while among vegetable fats, seed oil intake is associated to a higher value of central systolic blood pressure ($r_s = 0.117$, $p < 0.05$).

Table 2. Correlations between food intake and anthropometric, hemodynamic, and gluco-lipidic parameters.

Characteristics	Fast Food	Cereals and Tubers	Vegetables	Fruit	Eggs	Meat	Dairy Product	Sweets	Legumes	Fish	Nuts	EVO Oil	Animal-Derived Fat	Seed Oil
BMI, kg/m^2	**0.129***	−0.080	−0.093	0.067	−0.028	0.042	0.102	−0.052	−0.020	−0.040	−0.049	0.076	0.057	0.07
Z-score BMI	**0.141***	−0.081	−0.090	0.044	−0.040	0.044	0.091	−0.039	−0.021	−0.030	−0.064	0.092	0.064	0.093
Waist-height ratio	0.062	−0.048	−0.105	0.025	−0.093	0.051	0.37	−0.045	−0.062	−0.085	−0.027	0.060	0.006	0.046
Z-score waist-height ratio	0.074	−0.036	−0.095	0.018	−0.106	0.044	0.031	−0.039	−0.083	−0.088	−0.041	0.057	0.007	0.034
Brachial SBP, mmHg	0.013	0.043	−0.052	0.106	−0.003	0.042	0.091	0.026	0.010	0.084	0.066	−0.091	0.064	**0.117***
Z-score Brachial SBP	−0.005	0.069	−0.051	0.087	−0.042	0.034	0.063	0.020	0.000	0.078	0.069	−0.260	0.025	0.076
Brachial DBP, mmHg	**0.124***	0.025	−0.101	0.006	0.019	**0.128***	0.027	0.048	−0.020	0.017	−0.057	−0.006	0.008	0.09
Z-score Brachial DBP	**0.118***	0.023	−0.107	−0.029	−0.010	**0.121***	0.009	0.061	−0.033	0.006	−0.057	−0.064	0.008	0.079
PWV, m/s	**0.178****	0.017	−0.021	**0.154****	0.035	0.110	−0.030	−0.022	0.037	0.013	0.040	−.056	0.048	0.111
Z-score PWV	**0.158****	0.002	−0.003	**0.130***	0.009	**0.126***	−0.052	−0.020	0.023	0.022	0.036	−0.075	0.011	0.090
cSBP, mmHg	**0.140***	0.021	0.011	0.102	−0.013	0.073	0.004	0.047	0.039	0.076	0.043	−0.075	−0.038	0.07
Z-score cSBP	**0.123***	0.026	0.009	0.082	−0.056	0.051	−0.021	0.032	0.026	0.053	0.050	−0.070	−0.028	0.07
C-Triglycerides mg/dl	**0.145***	−0.013	−0.062	−0.029	−0.072	−0.038	−0.024	−0.083	−0.077	−0.120	0.019	−0.039	0.023	−0.390
C-Cholesterol mg/dl	0.087	−0.062	0.029	−0.092	−0.029	−0.077	−0.129	−0.066	−0.011	0.074	0.096	−0.036	**0.164***	−0.015
C-Glucose mg/dl	−0.018	−0.088	**−0.142***	**−0.250****	−0.035	−0.066	−0.080	−0.088	−0.100	−0.110	**−0.16***	−0.024	0.071	−0.056

BMI: Body Mass Index; EVO oil: Extra Virgin Olive oil; SBP: systolic Blood Pressure; DBP: Diastolic Blood pressure; PWV: pulse wave velocity; c-: capillary. Significant Spearman correlations are expressed in bold (*= p-value<0.05; **= p-value<0.01)

3.2.2. Dietary Pattern

A KMO of 0.802 attested to the adequacy of data to perform factor analysis. PCA identifies two main patterns. The first principal component was represented by high factor loadings for fish, legumes, vegetables, fresh and dried fruit, and dairy products intake. This pattern was considered a "healthy" diet. Moreover, the second principal component, characterized by high factor loadings for cereals and tubers, sweets, fast food, meat, and eggs intake was considered a "unhealthy" pattern (Supplementary Table S3). Individual scores were used to correlate with specific parameters. (Supplementary Table S4). The "healthy" pattern correlated with lower level of capillary glucose ($r_s = -0.191$, $p < 0.01$), while the "unhealthy" pattern directly correlates with brachial DBP ($r_s = 0.130$, $p < 0.05$) (Supplementary Table S4).

3.3. *Physical Activity*

PAQ-C data were available for 286 (95.3%) children that completed the questionnaire correctly. Then, the PAQ-C score (1.8 ± 0.5) and total MET-min/week (3278.9 ± 3953.4) were computed (Table 1). The results found that 42 (14.0%) children spent less than 600 MET-min/week in moderate-vigorous activities. Further, 136 (50%) and 96 (35.3%), respectively, spent from 600 to 3000 and more than 3000 MET-min/week. MET min-week spent in moderate-vigorous activity was inversely correlated with central SBP, brachial DBP, and triglycerides. No significant correlation was found with the PAQ-C score (Supplementary Table S5). With regard to categories that asked about physical activity measured as MET, central SBP was significantly higher in the "low" category versus "medium" and versus "high" category (Supplementary Table S6) (Figure 2).

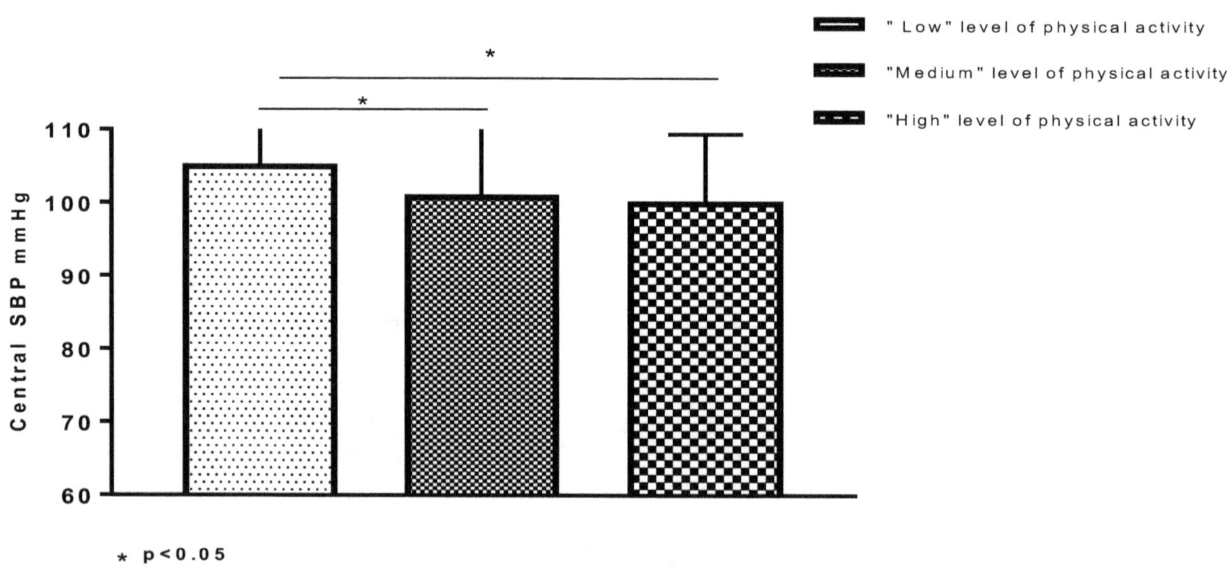

Figure 2. Difference of central blood pressure (cSBP, mmHg) among levels of moderate-vigorous physical activity. Legend: "Low": <600 MET-minutes/week; "Medium": 600–3000 MET-minutes/week; "High": >3000 MET-minutes/week. SBP: systolic blood pressure.

3.4. *Multivariate Models*

Linear regression models confirmed that even after adjustment for age, sex, ethnicity, and BMI, quartile of kcal intake and quartile of PAQ-C score had significant associations between fast food intake and PWV ($\beta = 0.337$; 95% CI: 0.140/0.534; $p < 0.01$). In addition, vegetable and fruit intake remained significantly associated to a decreased capillary glucose level [($\beta = -0.173$; 95% CI: −3.251/−0.207; $p < 0.05$); ($\beta = -2.530$; 95% CI: −4.274/−0.785; $p < 0.01$)]. Nut intake was inversely associated to capillary glucose ($\beta = -2.500$; 95% CI: −0.011/−1.255; $p < 0.05$). Higher animal fat-derived condiment intake remained independently associated to a higher level of capillary cholesterol ($\beta = 11.009$;

95% CI: 1.349/20.669; $p < 0.05$) (Figure 3a–e) (Supplementary Table S7a–e). The "healthy" pattern remained independently associated with capillary glucose levels after adjusting for cofounder variables ($\beta = -0.016$; 95% CI: $-0.027/-0.005$; $p < 0.01$), which is contrary to the association between the "unhealthy" pattern and brachial DBP ($\beta = 0.911$; 95% CI: $-0.150/1.972$; p = n.s.) (Supplementary Table S7g–f)) (Figure 4a–b).

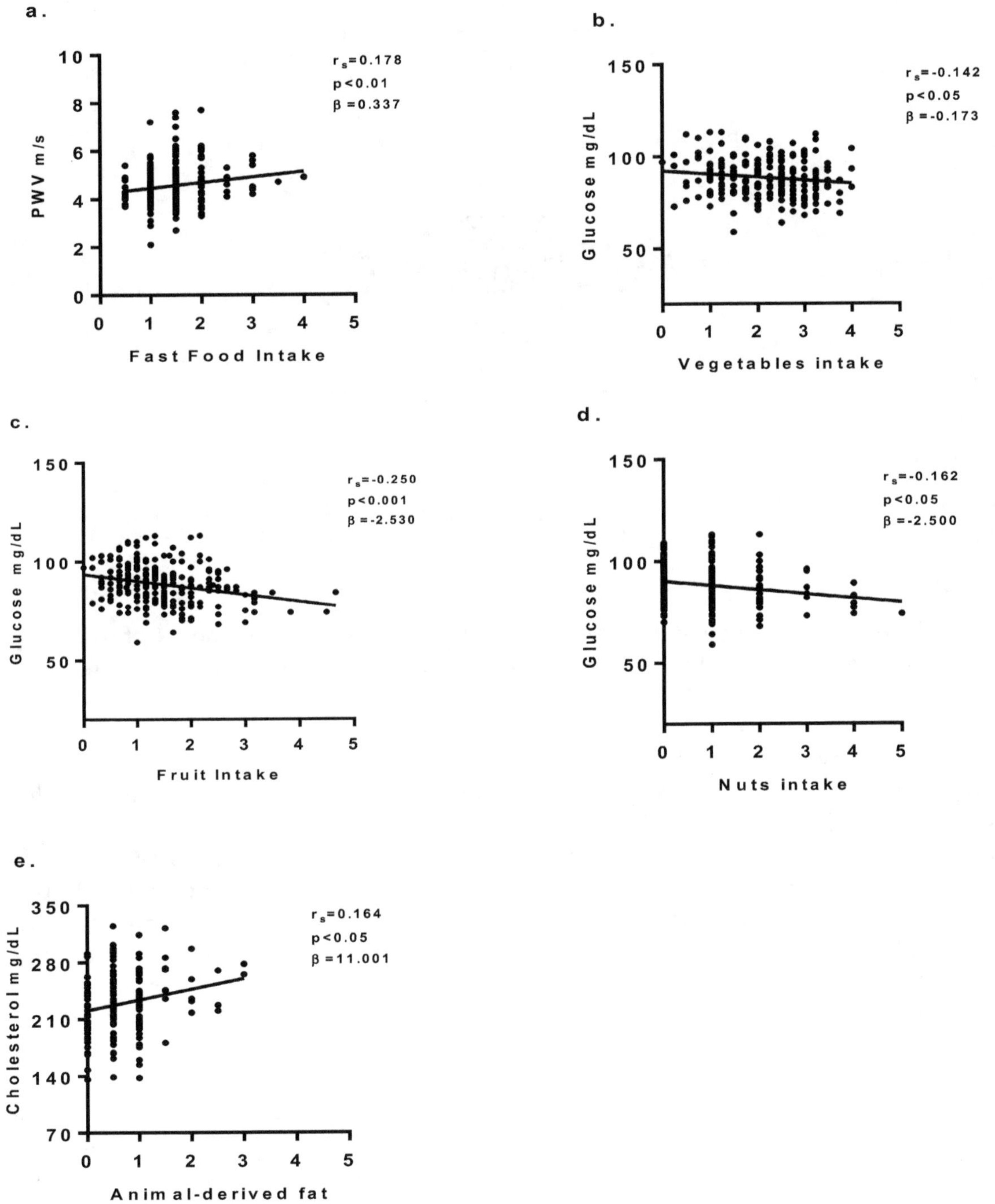

Figure 3. (**a–e**) Correlations between food intake and hemodynamic and gluco-lipid parameters. Correlation between: fast food intake and PWV (**a**); vegetables intake and glucose (**b**); fruit intake and glucose (**c**); nuts intake and glucose (**d**); animal-derived fat and cholesterol (**e**). PWV: Pulse Wave Velocity.

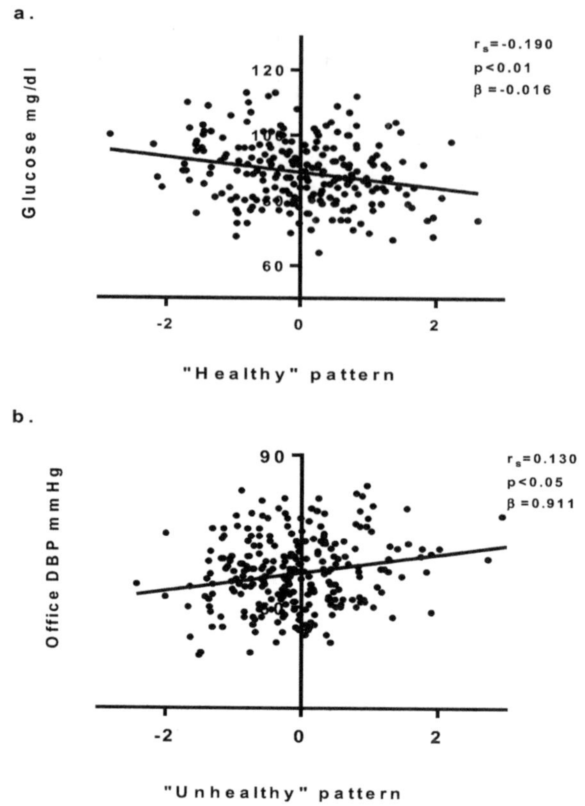

Figure 4. (**a–b**) Associations between "healthy pattern" and capillary glucose level (**a**) and between "unhealthy pattern" brachial diastolic blood pressure (**b**) DBP: diastolic blood pressure.

4. Discussion

Perhaps the most alarming result of the present study is the high prevalence of overweight-obesity and high blood pressure in children attending their third and fourth years of primary school in the Verona South district. More than 30% of children are overweight (21.3%) or obese (13.0%), which is in line with data reported in 2016 by the Italian National Surveillance System "Okkio alla salute" related to the prevalence of overweight and obese children (8–9 years) of 21.3% and 9.3%, respectively [34]. Further, in 2016 WHO estimated that 17% of children and adolescents (5–19 years) worldwide were overweight [7].

Our sample results show a high prevalence of normal high-BP and HBP (respectively 17.6% and 21.7%), with a further increased frequency in obese children. However, data about BP should be considered cautiously because despite having the average of three measurements, using a device validated in children, the measures were recorded in a single occasion, with children not in seated position, and thus cannot be considered diagnostic for hypertension. Moreover, in a subgroup of 25 children with BP ≥ 95th percentile, BP was measured in a follow-up visit in standard conditions, as requested in clinical guidelines, to confirm the presence of hypertension [19]. Only one child resulted to maintain a brachial BP higher than the 95th percentile for SBP or DBP, whereas two children were reclassified as normal-high BP (<90th percentile of brachial SBP or DBP <95th) and seventeen children had normal BP. It is important to note that of the children with brachial SBP higher than the 95th percentile, they also had a cSBP higher the 95th percentile for height, at least suggesting that these values were not driven by an abnormal amplification of the pressure wave, which is common in young subjects [35].

The prevalence of hypertension in the adult population of the United States and Europe has been estimated at nearly 15–30%, while the prevalence in children is 2–4%. However, it is common opinion that hypertension is under-diagnosed in clinical practice [36]. Moreover, the estimated percentage of school-children in Italy with high BP is reported to be 2–4% [37,38]. Many children today grow up in an obesogenic environment that encourages weight gain and obesity, caused by the changes in dietary habits and food availability and from the decline of physical activity [7]. Promoting the intake of healthy food and reducing the exposure of children to unhealthy dietary patterns is one of the programs declared by World Health Organization (WHO) to deal with childhood obesity [7]. From our data, it emerged that both "at risk" groups of overweight/obese children and those with normal-high/high BP values (percentile brachial SBP or brachial DBP >90°) eat less quantity of vegetables with respect to the normal weight or normotensive group at their same age. Many global health programs endorse an increased consumption of plant-based foods because of their inverse association with several chronic disease [39].

Data from the multi-center International Study of Asthma and Allergies in Childhood (ISAAC), which included 77243 children, demonstrated an inverse association between BMI and the consumption of vegetables [40]. Apart from the above-mentioned difference in vegetables intake, from our results, no clear association emerged between any type of food intake or grade of physical activity and markers of obesity (BMI and waist/height ratio). The relationship between BMI and fast food consumption has been widely reported. In a previous analysis, Braithwaith et al., within the aforementioned ISSAC, reported that more frequent fast food consumption was associated to a BMI of 0.14 kg/m2, which is higher than the infrequent consumption in a sample of 72900 children aged 6–7 [41]. Other studies reported the beneficial effect that physical activity has on weight [42–44], when physical activities was assessed using objective method like accelerometers. In a systematic review by Janssen et al., they included most of the studies with self- or parental-assessed physical activity, wherein the association between physical activity and weight was weak and associated to a not-significant risk [45] further underlining that data from questionnaire.

Conversely, we found associations between the intake of some food groups and haemodynamic and gluco-lipid variables. In particular, fast food intake resulted to be associated to an increased PWV. This correlation, although weak, remained significant after adjusting for age, sex, ethnicity, BMI, quartiles of daily kilocalories intake, and quartile of PAQ-C score. Even if to our knowledge there is no study that directly correlates fast-food intake and PWV, it has already been reported that PWV is inversely associated to healthy lifestyle and Mediterranean Diet [46,47]. "The Cardiovascular Risk in Young Finns Study" collected lifestyle data from childhood and had a 27-year follow-up. They reported that vegetable intake in childhood is an independent predictor of PWV in adulthood [46].

In the EVIDENT cohort study, a higher adherence to the Mediterranean diet—expressed as EVIDENT, a diet index derived from the FFQ—was associated to lower values of PWV [47]. In another sample including 77 12-year-old children, adherence to the Mediterranean diet was estimated by the KIDMED index and had negative results that correlated with the Augmentation Index, independent of obesity [48].

As for gluco-lipid measurements, we found that a higher intake of animal-derived fat that are rich in cholesterol was associated with a higher level of capillary cholesterol consistent with the fact that cholesterol intake reflects cholesterol blood concentration [49]. We found also that glucose level was lower in children consuming most frequently vegetables and fruit (fresh and nuts). In a meta-analysis, Wang PY et al. investigated the influence of vegetable and fruit intake on the risk of type-2 diabetes. It emerged that several studies reported the beneficial role of these food groups [50]. Fruit and vegetables are rich sources of fiber, flavonoids, and anti-oxidant compounds (carotenoids, vitamin C and E), folate, and potassium, which could explain the protective effects of fruit and vegetables on type 2 diabetes [50].

Among fruit we found that especially nuts are associated to lower glucose level. Nuts have an increased interest in research for its association to healthy outcomes [51]. Nuts are mainly composed of polyunsaturated fatty acids (PUFA) in addition to complex carbohydrate and fiber, tocopherols, minerals, phytosterols, and polyphenols [52]. Its consumption, in moderate quantity, is considered a part of the Mediterranean Diet pattern and recommended to an all-world population [51]. In a previous study conducted in a sample of obese children, we found an inverse correlation between omega-6 fatty acids (FA), whose nuts are particularly rich, and several parameters of the metabolic syndrome including glucose, suggesting that this kind of fruit can be particularly healthful in children [53]. When nut intake is high, randomized control trials (RCT), a large prospective study and meta-analysis, showed improved cardiovascular disease (CVD) outcomes in adults [49]. Further, the PREDIMED trial study showed the beneficial effects of nut intake, as well as olive oil, on the occurrence of chronic diseases including cardiovascular disease and type 2 diabetes [54]. In other trials including patients affected by type-2 diabetes, a higher nut intake was associated with an improved blood glucose control [52]. Even if there is coherence with literature, a limitation of these evidences is collected from capillary levels of cholesterol, triglycerides, and glucose and children not properly fasting.

Previous studies have shown that dietary patterns could be more strongly associated to executive functions than a single food intake [55]. This is due to the fact that FFQ has some intrinsic bias, such as the missing information about portion size that does not allow for a nutrient quantification. Through principal component analysis, we identified two patterns, defined as "healthy" and "unhealthy". These patterns are slightly similar to the patterns identified in literature as the "Mediterranean" and the "Western" pattern [56]. The "healthy" pattern, composed of vegetables, fruits, legumes, and dairy products, reflects the combination of food characteristics of the Mediterranean Diet that is rich in minerals, vitamins, polyphenols, fibers, polyunsaturated fatty acids (PUFAs), and monounsaturated fatty acids (MUFAs) [57]. These nutrients are mainly considered protective against CVD through the modulation of blood pressure, lipid profile, body weight, and fasting blood glucose [53,58,59]. There is strong evidence that the promotion of the Mediterranean Diet along with physical activity results in healthier effects [60]. In our sample, the higher adherence to the "healthy" pattern was associated with lower glucose levels, whereas children classified as "more active" had lower values of central systolic BP and brachial diastolic BP. This association did not remain significant after adjustment for cofounder variables, in which only BMI remained significant, suggesting that BMI could mediate this deleterious hemodynamic effect.

Physical activity contributes to a healthy lifestyle and it is a well-known fact that regular exercise is associated with minor incidence of future cardiovascular disease and mortality [61], which also contributes to epigenetic modifications in the regulation of CVD-associated genes [62]. Gerage et al. found a beneficial association of physical activity on central BP in a population of hypertensive adults [63], whereas in another study central, SBP was determined by body weight rather than exercise capacity in a population of children and adolescents [64]. We also found an inverse correlation between the total amount of MET min/wk spent in moderate physical activity and level of capillary triglycerides. Within the longitudinal "The Cardiovascular Risk in Young Finns Study", Raitakari et al. found a lower triglyceride level among children and adolescents who spent more time in physical activity. However, like in our case, the association did not persist after adjusting for cofounders [65].

We did not find any significant association using the PAQ-C score. Obtaining accurate measures of physical activity is challenging, particularly in children [66]. The PAQ-C questionnaire is a convenient and cost-effective method [66] but has some limitations in terms of accuracy because children tend to overreport [66]. Moreover, there is an ongoing debate on the quantification of physical activity across different populations. The standardization of operating procedures aimed at assessing more objective physical activity like the ALPHA-fitness test battery, already adopted in adolescents, could allow a more direct comparison between children and adolescents in different countries [67,68]. The combined association of diet and physical activity was associated as expected to better cardiometabolic values.

5. Conclusions

A strength of this work is that we investigated the lifestyle behavior in relation to cardiovascular risk factors in school-age children, highlighting the prevalence of obesity and high-blood pressure in this age group. This could be useful to detect children that could be considered at a higher risk of these things at earlier ages. Another strength is the measure of both central and brachial blood pressure the former being considered a better predictor of cardiovascular events than brachial blood pressure [64]. With regard to limitations, the cross-sectional design of our study represents a limitation for the emerged associations that cannot be considered causal, even if the biological plausibility of their link is high. Even the sample size is relatively limited and along with the choice of the sample, considerable "of convenience", can imply a problem of generalizability of our results. Anyhow, as stated before, our data of prevalence especially for overweight and obesity are in line with other Italian surveys, and the sample size was sufficient to detect statistically significant correlations with a correlation coefficient as low as 0.13. There are also intrinsic limitations of the method of assessment of dietary and physical activity data using questionnaires, such as misreporting, usual food, and/or activities that are not reported in the list of questions. In conclusion, our results launch an alarm for the high prevalence of obesity in pre-adolescent children in Verona and also strengthen the importance that diet and physical activity have on vascular and metabolic function starting in childhood. Our data also supports the need to improve diet and physical activity programs as claimed from the World Health Organization (WHO).

Supplementary Materials
Supplementary methods; Supplementary tables: Supplementary Table S1: Difference in food intake and physical activity between overweight (BMI > 85° percentile for age) or obese (BMI > 95° percentile for age) and normal weight, Supplementary Table S2: Difference in food intake and physical activity between normal-high BP (Brachial SBP or Brachial DBP > 90° percentile) or high BP (Brachial SBP or Brachial DBP > 95°) and normal BP group, Supplementary Table S3: Factor loadings > |200| associated to the dietary pattern, Supplementary Table S4: Correlation between dietary pattern and anthropometric, hemodynamic, and gluco-lipid parameters, Supplementary Table S5: Correlation between physical activity, expressed in PAQC score and MET-min/week, and anthropometric, hemodynamic and gluco-lipid parameters, Supplementary Table S6: Difference of anthropometric, hemodynamic, and gluco-lipidic parameters among categories of "low", "medium", and "high" adherence to moderate-vigorous physical activity, Supplementary Table S7 (a–f): Multivariate models including dietary intake and physical activity in relation to anthropometric, hemodynamic and gluco-lipidic parameters.

Author Contributions: Conceptualization, C.F., S.B., A.T., and F.A., C.M. methodology, C.F., S.B., A.T., I.B., R.G., P.C., D.A.R., F.A., and C.M.; software, A.G.; formal analysis, A.G., S.B., and L.N.P.; investigation, A.G., A.T., S.B., I.B., L.N.P., R.G., P.C., D.A.R., D.M., and L.B.; data curation, A.G., A.T., and S.B.; writing—original draft preparation, A.G.; writing—review and editing, C.F., S.B., A.T., F.A., and C.M.; supervision C.F, S.B., and P.M.; funding acquisition, C.F.

References

1. Funtikova, A.N.; Navarro, E.; Bawaked, R.A.; Fíto, M.; Schröder, H. Impact of diet on cardiometabolic health in children and adolescents. *Nutr. J.* **2015**, *14*, 118. [CrossRef]
2. Rodrigues, A.N.; Abreu, G.R.; Resende, R.S.; Goncalves, W.L.; Gouvea, S.A. Cardiovascular risk factor investigation: A pediatric issue. *Int. J. Gen. Med.* **2013**, *6*, 57–66. [CrossRef] [PubMed]
3. Hong, Y.M. Atherosclerotic cardiovascular disease beginning in childhood. *Korean Circ. J.* **2010**, *40*, 1–9. [CrossRef]
4. Childhood overweight and obesity. Available online: http://www.who.int/dietphysicalactivity/childhood/en/ (accessed on 8 October 2018).
5. WHO. *Diet, Nutrition and the Prevention of Chronic Diseases*; WHO: Geneva, Switzerland, 2003; Volume 916.
6. Cardiovascular risk factors. Available online: https://www.world-heart-federation.org/resources/risk-factors/ (accessed on 8 October 2018).
7. World Health Organization. *Commission on Ending Childhood Obesity*; Report of the Commission on Ending Childhood Obesity; WHO: Geneva, Switzerland, 2016; ISBN 9789241510066.
8. Ambrosini, G.L. Childhood dietary patterns and later obesity: A review of the evidence. *Proc. Nutr. Soc.* **2014**, *73*, 137–146. [CrossRef]
9. Estruch, R.; Martínez-González, M.A.; Corella, D.; Salas-Salvadó, J.; Ruiz-Gutiérrez, V.; Covas, M.I.; Fiol, M.; Gómez-Gracia, E.; López-Sabater, M.C.; Vinyoles, E.; et al. Effects of a Mediterranean-style diet on cardiovascular risk factors: A randomized trial. *Ann. Intern. Med.* **2006**, *145*, 1–11. [CrossRef] [PubMed]
10. Carvalho, K.; Ronca, D.; Michels, N.; Huybrechts, I.; Cuenca-Garcia, M.; Marcos, A.; Molnár, D.; Dallongeville, J.; Manios, Y.; Schaan, B.; et al. Does the Mediterranean Diet Protect against Stress-Induced Inflammatory Activation in European Adolescents? The HELENA Study. *Nutrients* **2018**, *10*, 1770. [CrossRef]

11. WHO. *Information Sheet: Global Recommendations on Physical Activity for Health 5–17 Years Old*; WHO: Geneva, Switzerland, 2015.
12. Physical activity and young people. Available online: http://www.who.int/dietphysicalactivity/factsheet_young_people/en/ (accessed on 8 October 2018).
13. Cole, T.J.; Bellizzi, M.C.; Flegal, K.M.; Dietz, W.H. Establishing a standard definition for child overweight and obesity worldwide: International survey. *BMJ* **2000**, *320*, 1240–1243. [CrossRef]
14. Valerio, G.; Maffeis, C.; Saggese, G.; Ambruzzi, M.A.; Balsamo, A.; Bellone, S.; Bergamini, M.; Bernasconi, S.; Bona, G.; Calcaterra, V.; et al. Diagnosis, treatment and prevention of pediatric obesity: Consensus position statement of the Italian Society for Pediatric Endocrinology and Diabetology and the Italian Society of Pediatrics. *Ital. J. Pediatr.* **2018**, *44*, 88. [CrossRef] [PubMed]
15. Morandi, A.; Miraglia del Giudice, E.; Martino, F.; Martino, E.; Bozzola, M.; Maffeis, C. Anthropometric Indices Are Not Satisfactory Predictors of Metabolic Comorbidities in Obese Children and Adolescents. *J. Pediatr.* **2014**, *165*, 1178.e2–1183.e2. [CrossRef]
16. Sharma, A.K.; Metzger, D.L.; Daymont, C.; Hadjiyannakis, S.; Rodd, C.J. LMS tables for waist-circumference and waist-height ratio Z-scores in children aged 5–19 y in NHANES III: Association with cardio-metabolic risks. *Pediatr. Res.* **2015**, *78*, 723–729. [CrossRef] [PubMed]
17. Stergiou, G.S.; Yiannes, N.G.; Rarra, V.C. Validation of the Omron 705 IT oscillometric device for home blood pressure measurement in children and adolescents: The Arsakion School Study. *Blood Press. Monit.* **2006**, *11*, 229–234. [CrossRef]
18. National High Blood Pressure Education Program Working Group on High Blood Pressure in Children and Adolescents. The fourth report on the diagnosis, evaluation, and treatment of high blood pressure in children and adolescents. *Pediatrics* **2004**, *114*, 555–576. [CrossRef]
19. Lurbe, E.; Agabiti-Rosei, E.; Cruickshank, J.K.; Dominiczak, A.; Erdine, S.; Hirth, A.; Invitti, C.; Litwin, M.; Mancia, G.; Pall, D.; et al. 2016 European Society of Hypertension guidelines for the management of high blood pressure in children and adolescents. *J. Hypertens.* **2016**, *34*, 1887–1920. [CrossRef]
20. Stabouli, S.; Printza, N.; Zervas, C.; Dotis, J.; Chrysaidou, K.; Maliahova, O.; Antza, C.; Papachristou, F.; Kotsis, V. Comparison of the SphygmoCor XCEL device with applanation tonometry for pulse wave velocity and central blood pressure assessment in youth. *J. Hypertens.* **2018**, *37*, 30–36. [CrossRef] [PubMed]
21. Elmenhorst, J.; Hulpke-Wette, M.; Barta, C.; Dalla Pozza, R.; Springer, S.; Oberhoffer, R. Percentiles for central blood pressure and pulse wave velocity in children and adolescents recorded with an oscillometric device. *Atherosclerosis* **2015**, *238*, 9–16. [CrossRef]
22. Reusz, G.S.; Cseprekal, O.; Temmar, M.; Kis, É.; Cherif, A.B.; Thaleb, A.; Fekete, A.; Szabó, A.J.; Benetos, A.; Salvi, P. Reference Values of Pulse Wave Velocity in Healthy Children and Teenagers. *Hypertension* **2010**, *56*, 217–224. [CrossRef] [PubMed]
23. Rapi, S.; Bazzini, C.; Tozzetti, C.; Sbolci, V.; Modesti, P.A. Point-of-care testing of cholesterol and triglycerides for epidemiologic studies: Evaluation of the multicare-in system. *Transl. Res.* **2009**, *153*, 71–76. [CrossRef]
24. Lockyer, M.G.; Fu, K.; Edwards, R.M.; Collymore, L.; Thomas, J.; Hill, T.; Devaraj, S. Evaluation of the Nova StatStrip glucometer in a pediatric hospital setting. *Clin. Biochem.* **2014**, *47*, 840–843. [CrossRef]
25. Rockett, H.R.H.; Breitenbach, M.; Frazier, A.L.; Witschi, J.; Wolf, A.M.; Field, A.E.; Colditz, G.A. Validation of a Youth/Adolescent Food Frequency Questionnaire. *Prev. Med.* **1997**, *26*, 808–816. [CrossRef]
26. Manios, Y.; Androutsos, O.; Moschonis, G.; Birbilis, M.; Maragkopoulou, K.; Giannopoulou, A.; Argyri, E.; Kourlaba, G. Criterion validity of the Physical Activity Questionnaire for Schoolchildren (PAQ-S) in assessing physical activity levels: The Healthy Growth Study. *J. Sports Med. Phys. Fitness* **2013**, *53*, 502–508.
27. Kowalski, K.C.; Crocker, P.R.E.; Faulkner, R.A. Validation of the Physical Activity Questionnaire for Older Children. *Pediatr. Exerc. Sci.* **1997**, *9*, 174–186. [CrossRef]
28. Hu, F.B. Dietary pattern analysis: A new direction in nutritional epidemiology. *Curr. Opin. Lipidol.* **2002**, *13*, 3–9. [CrossRef]
29. Tucker, K.L. Dietary patterns, approaches, and multicultural perspective. *Appl. Physiol. Nutr. Metab.* **2010**, *35*, 211–218. [CrossRef]
30. Moeller, S.M.; Reedy, J.; Millen, A.E.; Dixon, L.B.; Newby, P.K.; Tucker, K.L.; Krebs-Smith, S.M.; Guenther, P.M. Dietary Patterns: Challenges and Opportunities in Dietary Patterns Research. *J. Am. Diet. Assoc.* **2007**, *107*, 1233–1239. [CrossRef] [PubMed]

31. Esmaillzadeh, A.; Kimiagar, M.; Mehrabi, Y.; Azadbakht, L.; Hu, F.B.; Willett, W.C. Dietary patterns, insulin resistance, and prevalence of the metabolic syndrome in women. *Am. J. Clin. Nutr.* **2007**, *85*, 910–918. [CrossRef]
32. IPAQ Research Committee. Guidelines for data Processing and Analysis of the International Physical Activity Questionnaire (IPAQ)—Short and Long Form Scoring. Available online: https://sites.google.com/site/theipaq/ (accessed on 14 November 2018).
33. Ainsworth, B.E.; Haskell, W.L.; Herrmann, S.D.; Meckes, N.; Bassett, D.R., Jr.; Tudor-Locke, C.; Greer, J.L.; Vezina, J.; Whitt-Glover, M.C.; Leon, A.S.; et al. 2011 Compendium of Physical Activities: A second update of codes and MET values. *Med. Sci. Sports Exerc.* **2011**, *43*, 1575–1581. [CrossRef] [PubMed]
34. Cura, A.; Nardone, D.P.; Spinelli, A.; Buoncristiano, M.; Lauria, L.; Pierannunzio, D.; Galeone, D. *IL Sistema di sorveglianza OKkio alla SALUTE: Risultati 2016*; Istituto Superiore di Sanità: Roma, Italy, 2016.
35. Saladini, F.; Palatini, P. Isolated Systolic Hypertension in Young Individuals: Pathophysiological Mechanisms, Prognostic Significance, and Clinical Implications. *High Blood Press. Cardiovasc. Prev.* **2017**, *24*, 133–139. [CrossRef] [PubMed]
36. Dionne, J.M. Updated Guideline May Improve the Recognition and Diagnosis of Hypertension in Children and Adolescents; Review of the 2017 AAP Blood Pressure Clinical Practice Guideline. *Curr. Hypertens. Rep.* **2017**, *19*, 84. [CrossRef] [PubMed]
37. Menghetti, E.; Strisciuglio, P.; Spagnolo, A.; Carletti, M.; Paciotti, G.; Muzzi, G.; Beltemacchi, M.; Concolino, D.; Strambi, M.; Rosano, A. Hypertension and obesity in Italian school children: The role of diet, lifestyle and family history. *Nutr. Metab. Cardiovasc. Dis.* **2015**, *25*, 602–607. [CrossRef] [PubMed]
38. Orlando, A.; Cazzaniga, E.; Giussani, M.; Palestini, P.; Genovesi, S. Hypertension in Children: Role of Obesity, Simple Carbohydrates, and Uric Acid. *Front. Public Health* **2018**, *6*, 129. [CrossRef]
39. Prasad, M.; Takkinen, H.-M.; Uusitalo, L.; Tapanainen, H.; Ovaskainen, M.-L.; Alfthan, G.; Erlund, I.; Ahonen, S.; Åkerlund, M.; Toppari, J.; et al. Carotenoid Intake and Serum Concentration in Young Finnish Children and Their Relation with Fruit and Vegetable Consumption. *Nutrients* **2018**, *10*, 1533. [CrossRef]
40. Wall, C.; Stewart, A.; Hancox, R.; Murphy, R.; Braithwaite, I.; Beasley, R.; Mitchell, E.; Group, T.I.P.T.S.; Wall, C.R.; Stewart, A.W.; et al. Association between Frequency of Consumption of Fruit, Vegetables, Nuts and Pulses and BMI: Analyses of the International Study of Asthma and Allergies in Childhood (ISAAC). *Nutrients* **2018**, *10*, 316. [CrossRef] [PubMed]
41. Braithwaite, I.; Stewart, A.W.; Hancox, R.J.; Beasley, R.; Murphy, R.; Mitchell, E.A.; ISAAC Phase Three Study Group. Fast-food consumption and body mass index in children and adolescents: An international cross-sectional study. *BMJ Open* **2014**, *4*, e005813. [CrossRef] [PubMed]
42. Hughes, A.R.; Henderson, A.; Ortiz-Rodriguez, V.; Artinou, M.L.; Reilly, J.J. Habitual physical activity and sedentary behaviour in a clinical sample of obese children. *Int. J. Obes.* **2006**, *30*, 1494–1500. [CrossRef] [PubMed]
43. Thompson, A.M.; Thompson, A.M.; Campagna, P.D.; Durant, M.; Murphy, R.J.L.; Rehman, L.A.; Wadsworth, L.A. Are overweight students in Grades 3, 7, and 11 less physically active than their healthy weight counterparts? *Int. J. Pediatr. Obes.* **2009**, *4*, 28–35. [CrossRef]
44. Schwarzfischer, P.; Weber, M.; Gruszfeld, D.; Socha, P.; Luque, V.; Escribano, J.; Xhonneux, A.; Verduci, E.; Mariani, B.; Koletzko, B.; et al. BMI and recommended levels of physical activity in school children. *BMC Public Health* **2017**, *17*, 595. [CrossRef]
45. Janssen, I.; LeBlanc, A.G. Systematic review of the health benefits of physical activity and fitness in school-aged children and youth. *Int. J. Behav. Nutr. Phys. Act.* **2010**, *7*, 40. [CrossRef]
46. Aatola, H.; Koivistoinen, T.; Hutri-Kähönen, N.; Juonala, M.; Mikkilä, V.; Lehtimäki, T.; Viikari, J.S.A.; Raitakari, O.T.; Kähönen, M. Lifetime Fruit and Vegetable Consumption and Arterial Pulse Wave Velocity in Adulthood. *Circulation* **2010**, *122*, 2521–2528. [CrossRef] [PubMed]
47. Rodríguez-Martin, C.; Alonso-Domínguez, R.; Patino-Alonso, M.C.; Gómez-Marcos, M.A.; Maderuelo-Fernández, J.A.; Martin-Cantera, C.; García-Ortiz, L.; Recio-Rodríguez, J.I. The EVIDENT diet quality index is associated with cardiovascular risk and arterial stiffness in adults. *BMC Public Health* **2017**, *17*, 305. [CrossRef]
48. Lydakis, C.; Stefanaki, E.; Stefanaki, S.; Thalassinos, E.; Kavousanaki, M.; Lydaki, D. Correlation of blood pressure, obesity, and adherence to the Mediterranean diet with indices of arterial stiffness in children. *Eur. J. Pediatr.* **2012**, *171*, 1373–1382. [CrossRef]
49. Freeman, A.M.; Morris, P.B.; Barnard, N.; Esselstyn, C.B.; Ros, E.; Agatston, A.; Devries, S.; O'Keefe, J.; Miller, M.; Ornish, D.; et al. Trending Cardiovascular Nutrition Controversies. *J. Am. Coll. Cardiol.* **2017**, *69*, 1172–1187. [CrossRef] [PubMed]

50. Wang, P.-Y.; Fang, J.-C.; Gao, Z.-H.; Zhang, C.; Xie, S.-Y. Higher intake of fruits, vegetables or their fiber reduces the risk of type 2 diabetes: A meta-analysis. *J. Diabetes Investig.* **2016**, *7*, 56–69. [CrossRef] [PubMed]
51. de Souza, R.G.M.; Schincaglia, R.M.; Pimentel, G.D.; Mota, J.F.; de Souza, R.G.M.; Schincaglia, R.M.; Pimentel, G.D.; Mota, J.F. Nuts and Human Health Outcomes: A Systematic Review. *Nutrients* **2017**, *9*, 1311. [CrossRef]
52. Freeman, A.M.; Morris, P.B.; Aspry, K.; Gordon, N.F.; Barnard, N.D.; Esselstyn, C.B.; Ros, E.; Devries, S.; O'Keefe, J.; Miller, M.; et al. A Clinician's Guide for Trending Cardiovascular Nutrition Controversies: Part II. *J. Am. Coll. Cardiol.* **2018**, *72*, 553–568. [CrossRef]
53. Bonafini, S.; Tagetti, A.; Gaudino, R.; Cavarzere, P.; Montagnana, M.; Danese, E.; Benati, M.; Ramaroli, D.A.; Raimondi, S.; Giontella, A.; et al. Individual fatty acids in erythrocyte membranes are associated with several features of the metabolic syndrome in obese children. *Eur. J. Nutr.* **2018**. [CrossRef]
54. Freisling, H.; Noh, H.; Slimani, N.; Chajès, V.; May, A.M.; Peeters, P.H.; Weiderpass, E.; Cross, A.J.; Skeie, G.; Jenab, M.; et al. Nut intake and 5-year changes in body weight and obesity risk in adults: Results from the EPIC-PANACEA study. *Eur. J. Nutr.* **2018**, *57*, 2399–2408. [CrossRef]
55. Henriksson, P.; Cuenca-García, M.; Labayen, I.; Esteban-Cornejo, I.; Henriksson, H.; Kersting, M.; Vanhelst, J.; Widhalm, K.; Gottrand, F.; Moreno, L.A.; et al. Diet quality and attention capacity in European adolescents: The Healthy Lifestyle in Europe by Nutrition in Adolescence (HELENA) study. *Br. J. Nutr.* **2017**, *117*, 1587–1595. [CrossRef]
56. Hinnig, P.; Monteiro, J.; de Assis, M.; Levy, R.; Peres, M.; Perazi, F.; Porporatti, A.; Canto, G. Dietary Patterns of Children and Adolescents from High, Medium and Low Human Development Countries and Associated Socioeconomic Factors: A Systematic Review. *Nutrients* **2018**, *10*, 436. [CrossRef]
57. Boucher, J.L. Mediterranean Eating Pattern. *Diabetes Spectr.* **2017**, *30*, 72–76. [CrossRef]
58. Salas-Salvadó, J.; Becerra-Tomás, N.; García-Gavilán, J.F.; Bulló, M.; Barrubés, L. Mediterranean Diet and Cardiovascular Disease Prevention: What Do We Know? *Prog. Cardiovasc. Dis.* **2018**, *61*, 62–67. [CrossRef]
59. Bonafini, S.; Antoniazzi, F.; Maffeis, C.; Minuz, P.; Fava, C. Beneficial effects of ω-3 PUFA in children on cardiovascular risk factors during childhood and adolescence. *Prostaglandins Other Lipid Mediat.* **2015**, *120*, 72–79. [CrossRef] [PubMed]
60. Malakou, E.; Linardakis, M.; Armstrong, M.; Zannidi, D.; Foster, C.; Johnson, L.; Papadaki, A. The Combined Effect of Promoting the Mediterranean Diet and Physical Activity on Metabolic Risk Factors in Adults: A Systematic Review and Meta-Analysis of Randomised Controlled Trials. *Nutrients* **2018**, *10*, 1577. [CrossRef]
61. Lind, L.; Carlsson, A.C.; Siegbahn, A.; Sundström, J.; Ärnlöv, J. Impact of physical activity on cardiovascular status in obesity. *Eur. J. Clin. Investig.* **2017**, *47*, 167–175. [CrossRef]
62. Zimmer, P.; Bloch, W. Physical exercise and epigenetic adaptations of the cardiovascular system. *Herz* **2015**, *40*, 353–360. [CrossRef]
63. Gerage, A.M.; Benedetti, T.R.B.; Farah, B.Q.; da S. Santana, F.; Ohara, D.; Andersen, L.B.; Ritti-Dias, R.M. Sedentary Behavior and Light Physical Activity Are Associated with Brachial and Central Blood Pressure in Hypertensive Patients. *PLoS ONE* **2015**, *10*, e0146078. [CrossRef] [PubMed]
64. Müller, J.; Meyer, J.; Elmenhorst, J.; Oberhoffer, R. Body Weight and Not Exercise Capacity Determines Central Systolic Blood Pressure, a Surrogate for Arterial Stiffness, in Children and Adolescents. *J. Clin. Hypertens.* **2016**, *18*, 762–765. [CrossRef]
65. Raitakari, O.T.; Porkka, K.V.; Taimela, S.; Telama, R.; Räsänen, L.; Viikari, J.S. Effects of persistent physical activity and inactivity on coronary risk factors in children and young adults. The Cardiovascular Risk in Young Finns Study. *Am. J. Epidemiol.* **1994**, *140*, 195–205. [CrossRef] [PubMed]
66. Sirard, J.R.; Pate, R.R. Physical Activity Assessment in Children and Adolescents. *Sports Med.* **2001**, *31*, 439–454. [CrossRef]
67. Ruiz, J.R.; Castro-Pinero, J.; Artero, E.G.; Ortega, F.B.; Sjostrom, M.; Suni, J.; Castillo, M.J. Predictive validity of health-related fitness in youth: A systematic review. *Br. J. Sports Med.* **2009**, *43*, 909–923. [CrossRef]
68. Galan-Lopez, P.; Ries, F.; Gisladottir, T.; Domínguez, R.; Sánchez-Oliver, A.; Galan-Lopez, P.; Ries, F.; Gisladottir, T.; Domínguez, R.; Sánchez-Oliver, A.J. Healthy Lifestyle: Relationship between Mediterranean Diet, Body Composition and Physical Fitness in 13 to 16-Years Old Icelandic Students. *Int. J. Environ. Res. Public Health* **2018**, *15*, 2632. [CrossRef]

10

Effects and Mechanisms of Tea Regulating Blood Pressure: Evidences and Promises

Daxiang Li [1,2,†], Ruru Wang [1,2,†], Jinbao Huang [1,2], Qingshuang Cai [1,2], Chung S. Yang [2,3], Xiaochun Wan [1,2] and Zhongwen Xie [1,2,*]

1 State Key Laboratory of Tea Plant Biology and Utilization, School of Tea and Food Sciences and Technology, Anhui Agricultural University, Hefei 230036, China; dxli@ahau.edu.cn (D.L.); wrr@ahau.edu.cn (R.W.); jinbaohuang@ahau.deu.cn (J.H.); qingshuang@ahau.edu.cn (Q.C.); xcwan@ahau.edu.cn (X.W.)

2 International Joint Laboratory on Tea Chemistry and Health Effects of Ministry of Education, Anhui Agricultural University, Hefei 230036, China; csyang@pharmacy.rutgers.edu

3 Department of Chemical Biology, Ernest Mario School of Pharmacy, Rutgers, The State University of New Jersey, Piscataway, NJ 08854-8020, USA

* Correspondence: zhongwenxie@ahau.edu.cn

† These authors contributed equally to this work.

Abstract: Cardiovascular diseases have overtaken cancers as the number one cause of death. Hypertension is the most dangerous factor linked to deaths caused by cardiovascular diseases. Many researchers have reported that tea has anti-hypertensive effects in animals and humans. The aim of this review is to update the information on the anti-hypertensive effects of tea in human interventions and animal studies, and to summarize the underlying mechanisms, based on ex-vivo tissue and cell culture data. During recent years, an increasing number of human population studies have confirmed the beneficial effects of tea on hypertension. However, the optimal dose has not yet been established owing to differences in the extent of hypertension, and complicated social and genetic backgrounds of populations. Therefore, further large-scale investigations with longer terms of observation and tighter controls are needed to define optimal doses in subjects with varying degrees of hypertensive risk factors, and to determine differences in beneficial effects amongst diverse populations. Moreover, data from laboratory studies have shown that tea and its secondary metabolites have important roles in relaxing smooth muscle contraction, enhancing endothelial nitric oxide synthase activity, reducing vascular inflammation, inhibiting rennin activity, and anti-vascular oxidative stress. However, the exact molecular mechanisms of these activities remain to be elucidated.

Keywords: tea secondary metabolites; hypertension; endothelial function; inflammation

---

1. Introduction

Cardiovascular diseases (CVDs) are a group of diseases of the heart and blood vessels that include coronary heart disease, cerebrovascular disease, peripheral arterial disease, rheumatic heart disease, congenital heart disease and deep vein thrombosis [1]. During recent years, CVDs have overtaken cancer as the leading cause of deaths worldwide [2]. However, most CVDs can be prevented by modifying risk factors such as imbalanced diet, physical inactivity, diabetes, elevated lipids and high blood pressure [3]. Of these risk factors, high blood pressure is the most dangerous factor linked to CVDs death events [4]. It is estimated that high blood pressure is a comorbid factor in 69% of people who have their first heart attack, and 75% of those with chronic heart failure [5]. Clinical data shows that a 5 mmHg blood pressure reduction can reduce the risk of stroke and ischemic heart disease by 34 and 21%, respectively [6,7].

High blood pressure, or hypertension, is diagnosed when an individual has a systolic blood pressure (SBP) of 130–139 mmHg or a diastolic blood pressure (DBP) of 80–89 mmHg (Stage 1) and a systolic blood pressure (SBP) of ≥140 mmHg and/or a diastolic blood pressure (DBP) of ≥90 mmHg (Stage 2). [8] A significant prevalence of high blood pressure among adults aged 25 years and older exists, with a worldwide incidence of 40% [5]. Aging, dietary factors (for example alcohol consumption, excessive salt intake, and insufficient fruit and vegetable consumption), lifestyle factors (such as smoking and physical inactivity), and genetic predisposition have all been implicated in developing hypertension [9]. It has been estimated that hypertension affects one billion people and causes 9.4 million deaths every year globally [3]. This toll continues to increase as the incidence of hypertension rises sharply in low- and middle-income countries, where the social and economic costs associated with the disease are expected to place an especially heavy burden on socioeconomic development [10].

Tea is a beverage prepared by pouring hot or boiling water over the cured leaves or leaf buds of the tea plant *Camellia sinensis*. Based on the degree of fermentation, tea can also be classified into three major types: unfermented green tea, fermented black tea, and semi-fermented Oolong tea [11]. Tea is the second most consumed beverage after water and is thought to have a variety of health benefits [11,12]. It contains characteristic polyphenolic compounds known as catechins, namely (-)-epicatechin (EC), (-)-epigallocatechin (EGC), (-)-epicatechin gallate (ECG), (-)-epigallocatechin gallate (EGCG), (+)-catechin (C), and (+)-gallocatechin (GC), plus a small amount of (-)-catechin gallate (CG) and (-)-gallocatechin gallate (GCG). [13] A number of studies have shown that consumption of both green and black teas is linked to reductions in the risk of CVDs and some forms of cancers, to improved oral health, weight gain control and cognition in the elderly, and to increased antibacterial and antiviral activity and bone density [14,15]. These health benefits are often attributed to tea being rich in a class of polyphenolic compounds called flavonoids [16]. Diet plays an important role in the treatment and control of high blood pressure [17,18]. A survey showed that flavonoids can play an important role in the treatment and control of high blood pressure [19]. Anti-hypertension effects of drinking tea have become a hot topic for molecular nutrition and food research. In order to better understand the research achievements in this field, we summarized the role of tea in lowering blood pressure in clinical studies, as well as animal and cell experiments. The molecular mechanisms of tea hypotension effects were updated in this review.

2. Tea Regulating Blood Pressure in Human Intervention Studies

2.1. Hypotension Effects of Tea in Human Population Studies by Meta-analysis

In China, there is a long history of people drinking tea, made by collecting leaves from old tea plants to treat high blood pressure. Both in East Asian and western countries, lowering blood pressure by drinking tea has been reported in human population studies. Due to differences (genetic backgrounds, body composition, dietary habits, and amount and type of tea consumed) between different populations, the results of tea consumption in lowering blood pressure may not be consistent. However, during recent years, with improvements in experimental design and statistic software, great advances have been made in understanding the effect of tea consumption on blood pressure. Khalesi et al. [20] systematically reviewed randomized controlled trials that examined the effect of green tea consumption on blood pressure using meta-analysis. Based on their selected criteria, they collected papers from ProQuest, PubMed, Scopus and Cochrane Library published from 1995 to 2013. Thirteen studies were included for meta-analysis. The results showed that consumption of green tea significantly reduced SBP by 2.08 mmHg and DBP by 1.71 mmHg. In addition, subgroup analysis suggested a greater reduction in both SBP and DBP in participants whose baseline mean systolic blood pressure was ≥130 mmHg. Peng et al. [21] also investigated the effect of green tea consumption on blood pressure based on a meta-analysis of 13 randomized controlled trials across several countries, which were published in PubMed, Embase and Cochrane Library (up to March 2014).

Thirteen trials containing 1,367 subjects were included for the meta-analysis. The results indicated that consumption of green tea significantly reduced SBP level by 1.98 mmHg. Compared with the control group, green tea also showed a significant lowering effect on DBP in the treatment group (1.92 mmHg). Subgroup analyses further suggested that the positive effect of green tea polyphenols on blood pressure occurred with a low dose of green tea polyphenols (<582.8 mg/day) with long-term duration (≥12 weeks), whilst ruling out the confounding effects of caffeine. This analysis also supports the premise that green tea consumption has a favorable effect of decreasing blood pressure. Black tea is more popular than green tea in western countries. Greyling et al. [22] investigated the effect of black tea consumption on blood pressure based on a meta-analysis of 11 randomized controlled trials. The literature was systematically collected from Medline, Biosis, Chemical Abstracts and EMBASE databases through July 2013. Eleven studies (12 intervention arms, 378 subjects, dose of 4–5 cups of tea) were included for analysis. The SBP and DBP were decreased 1.8 mmHg ($P = 0.0013$) and 1.3 mmHg ($P < 0.0001$), respectively, by regular tea ingestion. Liu et al. [23] evaluated the effect of both green and black tea intake on blood pressure by a meta-analysis of randomized controlled trials. A systematic search was conducted in MEDLINE, EMBASE and the Cochrane Controlled Trials Register up to May 2014. The weighted mean difference was calculated for net changes in systolic and diastolic BP using fixed-effects or random-effects models. A total of twenty-five eligible studies with 1476 subjects were selected. The analysis showed that the acute intake of tea had no effects on SBP and DBP. However, after long-term tea intake, the pooled mean SBP and DBP were lower by 1.8 and 1.4 mmHg, respectively. When stratified by type of tea, green tea significantly reduced SBP by 2.1 mmHg and decreased DBP by 1.7 mmHg, and black tea showed a reduction in SBP of 1.4 mmHg and a decrease in DBP of 1.1 mmHg. The subgroup analyses showed that the BP-lowering effect was apparent in subjects who consumed tea more than 12 weeks (SBP – 2.6 mmHg and DBP – 2.2 mmHg, both $P < 0.001$). These data suggest that long-term (≥12 weeks) ingestion of tea could result in a significant reduction in SBP and DBP.

Tea is thought to have an anti-hypertension effect in people with elevated blood pressure. Yarmolinsky et al. [24] evaluated the effects of tea on blood pressure in hypertensive individuals. They searched the CENTRAL, PubMed, Embase, and Web of Science databases for relevant studies published from 1946 to September 27, 2013. The selection criteria included: randomized controlled trials of adults with pre-hypertension or hypertension subjected to intervention with green or black tea; controls consisting of placebo, minimal tea intervention, or no intervention; a follow-up period of at least two months. Meta-analyses of 10 trials (834 participants) revealed statistically significant reductions in SBP (2.36 mmHg) and DBP (1.77 mmHg) with tea consumption. Therefore, consumption of green or black tea can reduce blood pressure in individuals within pre-hypertensive and hypertensive ranges, although studies of longer duration and stronger methodological quality are warranted to confirm these findings.

Obesity is known to be one of the most important risk factors for the development of hypertension [25]. Obese individuals have a more than threefold increased likelihood of developing hypertension [26]. Li et al. [27] performed a systematic review and meta-analysis to clarify the efficacy of green tea or green tea extract (GTE) on the blood pressure of overweight and obese adults. They systematically searched electronic databases, conference proceedings including parallel and cross-over randomized controlled trials (RCTs) that examined the effectiveness of green tea or GTE on blood pressure. Data was meta-analyzed using a random effects model, to compare the mean differences in blood pressure changes from baseline in the intervention and placebo groups. Based on the selected criteria, 14 RCTs with a total of 971 participants (47% women) were pooled for analysis. Of the 14 studies, five were conducted in Asia (two Japanese and three Chinese), six in Europe (three in UK, two in Poland, and one in Netherlands), two in USA and one in Australia. All the studies were published between 2006 and 2014. Green tea or GTE produced a significant reduction in both SBP (mean difference of 1.42 mmHg) and DBP (mean difference 1.25 mmHg), compared with the placebo group. Similar results were found in the subgroup and sensitivity analyses. The results demonstrated that green tea or GTE supplementation evokes a small but significant reduction in blood pressure in overweight and obese adults. The data also indicated a strong beneficial effect of green tea or GTE supplementation in this group.

2.2. Interventional Trials for General Population

In a long-term follow-up study, Tong et al. [28] recruited 1,109 Chinese men (n = 472) and women (n = 637) who had participated in the Jiangsu Nutrition Study (JIN). Blood pressure was measured in 2002 and 2007. Tea (green, black and total tea) consumption was quantitatively assessed at the follow-up survey in 2007. Their results showed that total tea and green tea consumption were inversely associated with five-year DBP but not SBP. In the multivariable analysis, those with a daily total tea consumption of at least 10 g had DBP readings 2.41 mmHg (Total) and 3.68 mmHg (green) lower than those who consumed no tea. There was a significant interaction between smoking and total tea/green tea consumption, and diastolic blood pressure change. Green tea consumption was inversely associated with DBP change only in non-smokers and those without central obesity. The authors concluded that the consumption of green tea is inversely associated with five-year blood pressure change in Chinese adults, an effect diminished by smoking. Yang et al. [29] also examined the long-term effects of tea drinking on the risk of hypertension. The study was carefully designed and used a large number of people (1,507 subjects of 711 men and 796 women), and detailed information on tea consumption and other lifestyle and dietary factors associated with hypertension risk. The result showed that those who drank at least 120 mL/day (half a cup) of moderate-strength green or oolong tea for a year, had a 46% lower risk of developing hypertension than the non-tea drinkers. Amongst those who drank 120 to 599 mL/day (two and a half cups), the risk of high blood pressure was reduced by 65%. They concluded that habitual moderate-strength green or oolong tea consumption of at least 120 mL/day for one year significantly reduces the risk of developing hypertension in the Chinese population. Additionally, in a double-blind trial of 111 healthy volunteers, Nantz et al. [30] compared the effects of a standardized capsule containing 200 mg of decaffeinated catechin green tea extract with a placebo. The volunteers consumed a standardized capsule of *Camellia sinensis* compounds twice a day. After three weeks, SBP and DBP was lowered by 5 and 4 mmHg, respectively. After three months, SBP remained significantly lower.

The relation of tea consumption to cholesterol level and SBP was studied by Stensvold et al. [31], who recruited 9,856 men and 10,233 women (35–49 years of age) from the county of Oppland, Norway. Mean serum cholesterol decreased with an increase in black tea consumption. SBP was inversely related to tea consumption with differences of 2.1 mmHg in men and 3.5 mmHg in women. The data suggested that black tea consumption was associated with a lower systolic blood pressure in Norwegian men and women. Hodgson et al. [32] conducted a randomized controlled trial into the effects of black tea consumption on blood pressure regulation in Australia. A total of 95 men and women aged 35 to 75 years who were regular tea drinkers with a daytime ambulatory SBP between 115 and 150 mmHg, were recruited from the general population. Participants consumed 3 cups/d of regular tea for a four-week run-in period. After 6 months, participants then consumed 3 cups/d of either 1,493 mg powdered black tea solids containing 429 mg of polyphenols and 96 mg of caffeine, or a placebo matched in flavor and caffeine content, but containing no tea solids. The 24 h ambulatory blood pressure was measured at baseline, 3 months, and 6 months. Compared with the placebo, regular ingestion of black tea over 6 months resulted in lower 24 h SBP and DBP. The mean reductions in 24 h SBP were 2.7 mmHg at 3 months and 2.0 mmHg at 6 months. Similarly, the mean reductions in 24 h DBP were 2.3 mmHg at 3 months and 2.1 mmHg at 6 months. Significant differences in blood pressure were also observed for daytime and nighttime measurements, but effects on the overall 24 h blood pressure were mainly driven by daytime blood pressure. The results showed that regular consumption of 3 cups/day of black tea over 6 months, supplying approximately 429 mg/day of polyphenols, resulted in reductions in SBP and DBP of between 2 and 3 mmHg.

Arteries play an important role in cardiovascular function, including abnormalities in blood pressure. Since the aorta has a limited capacity, pressure increases during systole and is partially maintained during diastole by the rebounding of the expanded arterial walls. When arterial stiffness increases, the cushioning function is impaired, leading to a higher SBP and lower DBP. Stiffening of the arterial walls is a very important determinant of the development of hypertension [33–36]. Therefore, improvement in arterial elasticity is another mechanism for prevention of hypertension. To explore the relationship between habitual tea consumption and arterial stiffness, Lin et al. [37] performed a cross-sectional, epidemiological survey of 6,589 male and female residents aged 40–75 years, in Wuyishan, Fujian Province, China. The results showed that the levels of brachial-ankle pulse wave velocity (ba-PWV) were lowest amongst subjects who consumed tea habitually for more than 10 years, compared with the other 3 subgroups (nonhabitual, 1–5 year, and 6–10 year habitual tea drinkers). In addition, the levels of ba-PWV were lower in subjects who consumed 10–20 and >20 g/day tea habitually, than nonhabitual tea drinkers. As the duration and daily amount of tea consumption increased, the average ba-PWV decreased. Multiple logistic regression models revealed that habitual tea consumption was a positive predictor for ba-PWV. These results indicate that long-term habitual tea consumption may have a protective effect against arterial stiffness.

2.3. *Interventional Trials for Obese and/or Hypertensive Populations*

Nagao et al. [38] ran a double-blind parallel multicenter trial on the effect of green tea extract on body fat and hypertension in 240 Japanese women and men with visceral fat-type obesity. After a two-week diet run-in period, a 12-week trial was undertaken. The subjects ingested green tea containing 583 mg of catechins (catechin group) or 96 mg of catechins (control group) per day. The results showed that a greater decrease in SBP was observed in the catechin group than the control group for subjects whose initial SBP was 130 mmHg or higher. Low-density lipoprotein (LDL) cholesterol also decreased more in the catechin group. No adverse effect was found. Brown et al. [39] also ran a randomized controlled trial to investigate the effect of dietary supplementation with EGCG on insulin resistance, and associated metabolic risk factors including high blood pressure, in obese man. Overweight or obese male subjects, aged 40–65 years, were randomly assigned to take 400 mg capsules of EGCG ($n = 46$) or the placebo lactose ($n = 42$), twice a day for eight weeks. Oral glucose tolerance testing and measurement of metabolic risk factors (BMI, waist circumference, percentage body fat, blood pressure, total cholesterol, LDL-cholesterol and HDL-cholesterol) were performed pre- and post-intervention. The results showed that EGCG treatment had no effect on insulin sensitivity, insulin secretion or glucose tolerance, but did reduce DBP (mean change: placebo −0·058 mmHg; EGCG -2·68 mmHg). Significant changes in the other metabolic risk factors were not observed. EGCG treatment also had a positive effect on the mood of the participant. Recently, Nogueira et al. [40] ran a crossover randomized clinical trial investigating the short-term effects of green tea on blood pressure and endothelial function in obese pre-hypertensive women. Participants were randomly allocated to receive daily three capsules containing either 500 mg of GTE or a matching placebo for four weeks, with a washout period of two weeks between treatments. After four weeks of GTE supplementation, there was a significant decrease in SBP in comparison with the placebo over 24 h (3.61 vs. 1.05 mmHg), in the daytime (3.61 vs. 0.80 mmHg), and at night (3.94 vs. 1.90 mmHg). Differences in DBP and all other parameters were not significant between the GTE and placebo groups. The data suggests that in obese pre-hypertensive women, short-term daily intake of GTE may decrease blood pressure. Bogdanski et al. [41] examined the effects of GTE with insulin resistance and associated cardiovascular risk factors in obese, hypertensive patients. In this double-blind, placebo-controlled trial, 56 obese, hypertensive subjects were randomized to receive a daily supplement of 1 capsule that contained either 379 mg of GTE or a matching placebo, for 3 months. At baseline and after 3 months of treatment, the anthropometric parameters, blood pressure, plasma lipid levels, glucose levels, creatinine levels, and insulin levels were assessed. After three months of supplementation, both SBP and DBP had significantly decreased in the GTE group as compared with the placebo group ($P < 0.01$).

Black tea accounts for 78% of the world's tea production and is consumed worldwide. Therefore, it is important to determine whether black tea has an anti-hypertension effect. Grassi et al. [42]

investigated the effect of black tea on blood pressure and vessel wave reflections before and after fat consumption in hypertensive patients. In a randomized, double-blind, controlled, cross-over study, 19 patients were assigned to consume black tea (129 mg flavonoids) or a placebo twice a day for eight days (13-day wash-out period). Digital volume pulse and BP were measured before and 1, 2, 3 and 4 h after tea consumption. Measurements were performed in a fasted state and after a fat load. The authors found that fat consumption led to increase wave reflection, which was counteracted by tea. The results indicate that black tea consumption decreases SBP and DBP by 3.2 mmHg and 2.6 mmHg, respectively, and prevented blood pressure increase after a fat consumption. These findings indicate that regular consumption of black tea may play an important role in cardiovascular protection.

2.4. *Interventional Trials for Diabetic Populations*

High blood pressure is more common in people with diabetes. It was estimated that two-thirds of patients with type 2 diabetes have high blood pressure [43]. Mozaffari et al. [44] conducted a randomized clinical trial in which 100 mildly (equal to Stage 1 hypertension of new guideline) hypertensive patients with diabetes were randomly assigned into a green tea treatment group. The patients were instructed to drink green tea infusion three times a day, 2 h after each meal for four weeks. Blood pressure was measured at days one and 15, and at the end of the study. The results showed that the SBP of the green tea group was lower at the end of the study (from 119.4 to 114.8 mmHg). The DBP was also lower by the end of the study (from 78.9 to 75.3 mmHg). The therapeutic effectiveness of tea by the end of the intervention was 39.6% in the green tea group. This data indicates that mildly hypertensive type 2 diabetic individuals who drink green tea daily show significantly lower SBP and DBP. Another study [45] was conducted in Japan with 60 volunteers who had fasting blood glucose levels of ≥6.1 mmol/L or non-fasting blood glucose levels of ≥7.8 mmol/L. The intervention group consumed a packet of GTE containing 544 mg polyphenols (456 mg catechins) daily for the first two months, and then entered a two-month nonintervention period. Supplementation of GTE powder led to a significant reduction in DBP, but no significant changes in SBP.

2.5. *Intervention Trials for Aging Populations*

Hypertension generally increases with age [34]. Hodgson et al. [32] evaluated the effect of long-term regular ingestion of tea on blood pressure in older women. A total of 218 women over 70 years of age was included in this cross-sectional study. The results indicate that tea intake is associated with significantly lower SBP and DBP. Furthermore, a 250 mL/day (one cup) increase in tea intake was associated with a 2.2 mmHg lower SBP and a 0.9 mmHg lower DBP. This suggests that regular tea consumption may have a favorable effect on blood pressure in older women. Recently, Yin et al. conducted a cross-sectional study of blood pressure and tea consumption an elderly population in Jiangsu, China [35]. A total of 4579 older adults aged 60 years or older participated in this study. And a linear regression model was applied for analysis of association between tea consumption and risk of hypertension. The results showed that higher tea consumption frequency was found to be associated with lower systolic BP values, after adjusting for the effect of age, sex, education level, lifestyle-related factors, and cardiometabolic confounding factors in overall ($P = 0.0003$), normotensive ($P = 0.017$) and participants without anti-hypertensive treatment ($P = 0.027$). Significant inverse association between diastolic BP and frequency of tea consumption was also observed in the overall subjects ($P = 0.003$). In multivariate logistic analyses, habitual tea drinking was inversely associated with presence of hypertension ($P = 0.011$).

The main clinical studies of blood pressure-lowering effects by tea in humans are summarized in Table 1.

Table 1. Blood pressure-lowering effects of tea in human interventions.

No.	Methods of Study	Selected Participants	Tea or Dosage & Duration	Test Site	Primary Outcomes and Comments	Year (Citation)
1	Meta-analysis	13 studies	Green tea	Australia	Significantly reduced SBP by 2.08 mmHg and DBP by 1.71 mmHg. Good methodology analysis and trusted results	2014 [20]
2	Meta-analysis	13 randomized controlled trials across, 1367 subjects	Green tea polyphenols (<582.8 mg/day), ≥12 weeks	Several countries	Significantly reduced SBP level by 1.98 mmHg and DBP by 1.92 mmHg. Good methodology analysis, a large population and trusted results	2014 [21]
3	Meta-analysis	11 randomized controlled trials, 378 subjects	4–5 cups of black tea	Netherland	The SBP and DBP were decreased by 1.8 mmHg and 1.3 mmHg. Good methodology, and trusted results	2014 [22]
4	Meta-analysis	25 eligible studies, 1476 subjects	Both green and black tea intake,≥ 12 weeks	USA	Long-term (≥12 weeks) ingestion of tea could result in a significant Reduction in SBP and DBP Good methodology, a large population analysis and trusted results	2014 [23]
5	Meta-analysis	10 trials (834 participants) hypertensive individuals	Tea regular consumption	UK	Significant reductions in SBP (2.36 mmHg) and DBP (1.77 mmHg). Good methodology and trusted results.	2015 [24]
6	Meta-analysis	971 overweight and obese adult participants (47% women)	Green tea or green tea extract	China	Significant reduction in both SBP (1.42 mmHg) and DBP (1.25 mmHg). Good methodology and trusted results.	2015 [27]
7	Multivariable analysis	472 men and 637 women	Tea (green, black and mixed teas) consumption	China	The consumption of green tea is inversely associated with five-year BP change in Chinese adults, an effect was diminished by smoking. Long term study and trusted results.	2014 [28]
8	Meta-analysis	711 men and 796 women	120 mL/day (half a cup)green or oolong tea, a year	China	Significantly reduces the risk of developing hypertension. A large special population, and trusted results.	2004 [29]
9	Meta-analysis	9,856 men and 10,233 women (35–49 years of age)	Black tea regular consumption	Norway	SBP was inversely related to tea consumption with differences of 2.1 mmHg in men and 3.5 mmHg in women. Good methodology, a large population analysis and trusted results.	1992 [31]
10	Randomized controlled trial	95 men and women aged 35 to 75 who were regular tea drinkers	3 cups/d of regular black tea consumption, ≥ 6 months	Australia	Reductions in SBP and DBP of between 2 and 3 mmHg. A small population trial, and a reasonable result.	2012 [32]
11	Double-blind parallel multicenter trial	240 Japanese women and men with visceral fat-type obesity	583 mg of catechins or 96 mg of catechins per day, green tea	Japan	Catechin group decreased initial SBP that is 130 mmHg or higher. A small population trial, and a reasonable result.	2007 [38]

Table 1. *Cont.*

No.	Methods of Study	Selected Participants	Tea or Dosage & Duration	Test Site	Primary Outcomes and Comments	Year (Citation)
12	Randomized controlled trial	Overweight or obese male subjects, aged 40–65 years	400 mg capsules of EGCG (n = 46) or the placebo lactose (n = 42), twice a day for eight weeks.	UK	EGCG treatment did reduce DBP (mean change: placebo -0·058 mmHg; EGCG -2·68 mmHg). A small population trial, and a reasonable result.	2009 [39]
13	Randomized clinical trial	Obese pre-hypertensive women	500 mg of GTE or a matching placebo consumption, four weeks	Brazil	Short-term daily intake of GTE may decrease BP in obese pre-hypertensive women. A small population, short term trial, and a reasonable result.	2016 [40]
14	Double-blind	56 obese, hypertensive subjects	Daily supplement 379 mg of GTE or a matching placebo, 3 months	Poland	Both SBP and DBP had significantly decreased compared with the placebo group. A small population trial, and a reasonable result.	2012 [41]
15	Randomized, double-blind	19 patients	Black tea (129 mg flavonoids) or a placebo twice a day for eight days.	Italy	Black tea consumption decreases SBP and DBP by 3.2 mmHg and 2.6 mmHg, respectively, and prevented BP increase after a fat consumption. A small population trial may results in bias result.	2015 [42]
16	Randomized clinical trial	100 stage1 hypertensive patients with diabetes	Drink green tea infusion three times a day 2 hours after each meal, four weeks	Iran	Stage1 hypertensive type 2 diabetic individuals who drink green tea daily show significantly lower SBP and DBP. A small population trial, and a reasonable result.	2013 [44]
17	Cross-sectional study	60 volunteers, fasting blood glucose levels of ≥6.1 mmol/L or non-fasting blood glucose levels of ≥7.8 mmol/L	544 mg polyphenols (456 mg catechins) daily consumption, 3 months	Japan	Supplementation of GTE powder led to a significant reduction in DBP, but no significant changes in SBP. A small population trial, and a reasonable result.	2008 [45]
18	Cross-sectional study	218 women over 70 years old	250 mL/day (one cup)	Australia	Regular tea consumption may have a favorable effect on BP in older women. A small population trial, and a reasonable result.	2003 [32]
19	Cross-sectional study	4579 adults aged 60 years or older	tea consumption questionnaire	China	Higher tea consumption frequency was associated with lower systolic BP. A large population trial, and a reasonable result.	2017 [35]

3. Tea Metabolites Regulating Blood Pressure in Animal Studies

A growing number of reports indicate that tea has beneficial effects on blood pressure in various animal models. As early as 1984, Henry et al. [46] investigated the effect of decaffeinated tea on chronic psychosocial hypertension in CBA mice. They found that tea polyphenols (not caffeine) reduced blood pressure from 150 to 133 mmHg. Negishi et al. [47] evaluated the hypotensive effect of black and green tea polyphenols by using a stroke-prone spontaneously hypertensive (SHR) rat model. The male rats were divided into three groups: the control group consumed tap water (30 mL/d); the black tea polyphenol group (BTP) consumed water containing 3.5g/L thearubigins, 0.6 g/L theaflavins, 0.5 g/L flavonols and 0.4 g/L catechins; and the green tea polyphenol group (GTP) consumed water containing 3.5 g/L catechins, 0.5 g/L flavonols and 1 g/L polymetric flavonoids. The telemetry system was used to measure blood pressure, which was recorded continuously every 5 min for 24 h. During the daytime, SBP and DBP were significantly lower in the BTP and GTP groups than in the controls. As the amounts of polyphenols used in this experiment correspond to daily consumption of tea consumers, regular consumption of black and green tea may provide some protection against hypertension in humans.

EGCG is a polyphenol that makes up approximate 30% of the solids in green tea [48]. Potenza et al. [49] studied the effect of EGCG treatment on cardiovascular and metabolic function using a SHR rat model. In acute studies, EGCG (1–100 μM) elicited dose-dependent vasodilation in mesenteric vascular beds (MVB) isolated (ex vivo) from SHR. In chronic studies, nine-week-old SHR were treated by gavage for 3 weeks with EGCG (200 mg/kg/day), enalapril (30 mg/kg/day), or vehicle. They found that both EGCG and enalapril therapy significantly lowered SBP in the SHR rat. Using the Goto-Kakizaki rat model, Igarashi et al. [50] also demonstrated that a diet containing 0.2% tea catechins tended to maintain SBP (in the latter stages of a 76-day feeding period) at lower levels than in subjects not receiving dietary catechins.

Tea plant has a characterized amino acid, theanine. Yasuhiko et al. [51] investigated the effect of green tea, rich inγaminobutyric acid, on blood pressure in young and old Dahl salt-sensitive rats. For therapeutic effect, 11-month-old rats were fed a 4% NaC1 diet for 3 weeks, then were given water (group W), an ordinary tea solution (group T), or a GABA-rich tea solution (group G) for 4 weeks. After this treatment, blood pressure was significantly decreased in group G (176 mmHg) compared with group W (207 mmHg) or group T (193mmHg). For the preventive experiment, 5-week-old rats were fed a 4% NaCI diet and divided into groups W, T, and G. After 4 weeks of treatment, although blood pressure was comparable in groups W and T (165 vs. 164 mmHg), it was significantly lower in group G (142 mmHg). Therefore, GABA-rich tea seems to decrease the established high blood pressure and prevent the development of hypertension in Dahl rats fed a high salt diet. Yokogoshi et al. [52] also studied the hypotensive effect of γ-glutamylmethylamide glutamic acid (GMA) and theanine in SHR rats. Glutamic acid (2000 mg/kg) did not alter the rat blood pressure but the same dose of theanine decreased rat blood pressure significantly. GMA administration to SHR also reduced the blood pressure significantly, and its hypotensive action was more effective than that of theanine only administration.

Tannic acid is a water-soluble polyphenol that is present in tea. Turgut et al. [53] evaluated the effect of tannic acid on SBP in a L-NNA-induced essential hypertension rat model. Tannic acid was intraperitoneally injected at a dose of 50 mg/kg for 15 days. Compared with the hypertension group, tannic acid administration significantly decreased blood pressure values after 20 and 30 days. Sagesaka-Mitane et al. [54] investigated the effect of tea-leaf saponin on blood pressure using SHR rats. Tea-leaf saponin led to a time- and dose-dependent reduction in blood pressure when it was administered orally to young SHR (7 weeks old) for 5 days. Oral administration of tea-leaf saponin (100 mg/kg) to older SHR (15 weeks old) for 5 days decreased the mean blood pressure by 29.2 mmHg, compared to the control group. Single administration of tea-leaf saponin at 50 mg/kg showed a long-lasting hypotensive effect which was as potent as that of enalapril maleate at 3 mg/kg. Their data proved that both tannic acid and tea-leaf saponin have the effect of lowering blood pressure in hypertensive rats.

4. Molecular Mechanisms of Tea Regulating Blood Pressure

A growing body of evidence indicates that oxidative stress and the inactivation of NO by vascular superoxide anion play critical roles in the development of hypertension [55]. Vascular superoxide anion is enhanced in angiotensin II (Ang II)-induced hypertension, mainly attributable to nicotinamide adenine dinucleotide phosphate (NADPH) oxidase activation by Ang II [56,57]. In addition, an excess of vascular superoxide anion production has also been found in spontaneously hypertensive and deoxycorticosterone acetate (DOCA) salt hypertension [58], and in mineralocorticoid hypertensive rats [59]. Antonello et al. [60] investigated the preventative effects of GTE on Ang II-induced blood pressure increases using the Sprague-Dawley (SD) rat model. Male SD rats were randomly assigned to drinking water with or without GTE (6 mg/mL) and received (by osmotic mini-pumps) a vehicle, high (700 μg/kg/day) or low (350 μg/kg/day) dose of Ang II for 13 days. Night-time and daytime SBP and DBP were recorded with telemetry. By day two of infusion, the AngII group showed significantly higher SBP and DBP during the day and night, compared to all other groups. Moreover, GTE significantly lowered both SBP and DBP throughout the study period, compared with the AngII group. In addition, GTE blunted the increase in HO-1, p22phox, and SOD-1 mRNA in the aorta caused by Ang II. The data suggests that GTE prevented hypertension induced by a high Ang II dose, possible by the prevention or scavenging of superoxide anion generation. GTE consists of both catechins and caffeine. In order to remove the caffeine contribution, Ihm et al. [61] studied the effect of decaffeinated GTE on hypertension and insulin resistance in an Otsuka Long-Evans Tokushima Fatty (OLETF) rat model of metabolic syndrome (MetS). OLETF rats were randomized into a saline-treated group and a group treated with decaffeinated-GTE (25 mg/kg/day). They found that decaffeinated-GTE significantly reduced BP (130 vs. 121 mmHg). In addition, decaffeinated-GTE significantly reduced vascular reactive oxygen species (ROS) formation and NADPH oxidase activity, and improved endothelium-dependent relaxation in the thoracic aorta of OLETF rats. Decaffeinated-GTE also suppressed the expression of p47 and p22phox in the immunohistochemical staining and stimulated phosphorylation of endothelial nitric oxide synthase (eNOS) and Akt in immunoblotting of the aortas. These results revealed that decaffeinated-GTE reduced the formation of ROS and NADPH oxidase activity and stimulated phosphorylation of eNOS and Akt in the aorta of a rat model of MetS, which resulted in improved endothelial function and eventually in lower blood pressure.

Gómez-Guzmán et al. [62] studied the effects of chronic treatment with epicatechin on blood pressure, endothelial function, and oxidative status using the DOCA-salt-induced hypertensive rat model. The rats were treated for 5 weeks with (-)-epicatechin at 2 or 10 mg/kg/day. The higher dose of epicatechin prevented the increase in SBP induced by DOCA-salt. The authors found that aortic superoxide levels were elevated in the DOCA-salt group and abolished by both doses of epicatechin. However, only epicatechin at 10 mg/kg/day reduced the DOCA-salt-induced increase in aortic NADPH oxidase activity, and p47phox and p22phox gene overexpression. They also showed that epicatechin increased the transcription of nuclear factor-E2-related factor-2 (Nrf2) and Nrf2 target genes in the aortas of control rats. Furthermore, epicatechin improved the impaired endothelium-dependent relaxation response to acetylcholine and increased the phosphorylation of both Akt and eNOS in aortic rings. Epicatechin also induced a decrease in ET-1 release, systemic and vascular oxidative stress, and inhibition of NADPH oxidase activity. Galleano et al. [63] used a SHR rat to investigate the effects of dietary consumption of (-)-epicatechin on blood pressure regulation. They found that consumption of 0.3% (-)-epicatechin for 2 and 6 days significantly deceased SBP by 27 and 23 mmHg, respectively. They also studied the mechanism relating to decreased blood pressure and observed a 173% increase in nitric synthase (NOS) activity in the aorta of (-)-epicatechin SHR on day six, compared with non-supplemented SHR. These findings infer that (-)-epicatechin can modulate blood pressure in hypertensive rats by increasing NO levels in the vasculature. Litterio et al. [64] also investigated the effects of (-)-epicatechin on blood pressure in No-nitro-L-arginine methyl ester (L-NAME)-treated rats. The administration of (-)-epicatechin prevented the 42 mmHg increase in blood pressure associated with the inhibition of NO production in a dose-dependent manner (0.2–4.0 g/kg diet). This blood pressure effect was associated with a reduction in L-NAME-mediated increases in the indexes of oxidative stress, and with a restoration of the NO concentration. At the vascular level, none of the treatments modified NOS expression, but (-)-epicatechin administration alleviated the L-NAME-mediated decrease in eNOS activity and increase in both superoxide anion production and NOX subunit p47phox expression. In summary, (-)-epicatechin prevented the increase in blood pressure and oxidative stress and restored NO bioavailability.

It is well known that sympathetic nerve activity plays a pivotal role in blood pressure regulation. Tanida et al. [65] reported the effects of oolong tea (OT) on renal sympathetic nerve activity (RSNA) and spontaneous hypertension in SHR rats. They found that intraduodenal injection of OT in urethane-anesthetized rats suppressed RSNA and decreased blood pressure. In addition, pretreatment with the histaminergic H3-receptor-antagonist thioperamide or bilateral subdiaphragmatic vagotomy eliminated the effects of OT on RSNA and blood pressure. Furthermore, drinking OT for 14 weeks reduced blood pressure elevation in SHR rats. These results suggest that OT may exert its hypotensive action through changes in autonomic neurotransmission via an afferent neural mechanism. The authors also found that intraduodenal injections of decaffeinated OT lowered RSNA and blood pressure to the same degree as caffeinated OT, indicating that substances other than caffeine may function as effective modulators of RSNA and blood pressure. Han et al. [66] provided additional evidence that EGCG counteracts caffeine-induced increases in arterial pressure, adrenaline and noradrenaline levels in the blood, and heart rate. The authors suggested that EGCG may exhibit these properties by decreasing the levels of catecholamines in the blood.

The stimulatory effects of caffeine may be reduced by the amount of EGCG in green tea. Recently, Garcia et al. [67] investigated the effects of green tea on blood pressure and sympathoexcitation in a L-NAME-induced hypertensive rat model. They found that L-NAME-treated rats exhibited an increase in blood pressure (165 mmHg) compared with control rats (103 mmHg), and that green tea-treatment reduced hypertension (119 mmHg). Hypertensive rats showed a higher renal sympathetic nerve activity (161± 12 spikes/second) than the control group (97 ± 2 spikes/second); green tea also decreased this parameter in the hypertensive treated group (125 ± 5 spikes/second). Arterial baroreceptor function and vascular and systemic oxidative stress were improved in hypertensive rats after green tea treatment. Taken together, short-term green tea treatment improved cardiovascular function in a hypertension model characterized by sympathoexcitation, possible due to its antioxidant properties.

Blood vessels are able to self-regulate tone and adjust blood flow in response to changes to the local environment, due to their capacity to respond to physical and chemical stimuli in the lumen. Endothelium is an inner layer of blood vessels, which directly sense the physical and chemical stimuli. Endothelial-dependant vasodilation contributes to the maintenance of an adequate blood flow to cells and tissues. Therefore, the endothelium plays a key role in the control of vascular tone by releasing several vasorelaxing factors including nitric oxide (NO) and endothelium-derived hyperpolarizing factor (EDHF). The calcium signal is a pivotal pathway leading to the activation of eNOS. The phosphatidylinositol 3-kinase/Akt (PI3-kinase/Akt) pathway is another significant signal pathway in the activation of eNOS.

Anter et al. [68] found that when porcine aortic endothelial cells are exposed to components of black tea, the polyphenol fraction acutely enhanced nitric oxide bioactivity. This effect involved eNOS phosphorylation at Ser-1177 (activator site) and dephosphorylation at Thr-495 (an inhibitor site), consistent with increased eNOS activity. Furthermore, they demonstrated that black tea polyphenol-induced eNOS activation was dependent upon the PI3-kinase/Akt pathway. These stimulatory effects were found to be calcium-dependent, and involved both intracellular and extracellular calcium, and the p38 mitogen-activated protein kinase (p38 MAPK) upstream of the PI3-kinase/Akt pathway. Caveolin-1 is a major negative regulator of eNOS activity. Green tea polyphenols down-regulate caveolin-1 gene expression in a time- and dose-dependent manner, via the activation of extracellular signal-regulated kinase 1/2 (ERK 1/2), and inhibition of p38 MAPK signaling pathways, in bovine aortic endothelial cells (thereby increasing eNOS activation) [69]. However, using Ca2+-deprived endothelial cells, Ramirez-Sanchez et al. [70] found that (-)-epicatechin induced calcium-independent eNOS activation. The results demonstrated that (-)-epicatechin induced a partial AKT/HSP90 migration from the cytoplasm to the caveolar membrane fraction where HSP90, AKT, and eNOS physically associated. Thus, under Ca2+ free conditions, (-)-epicatechin stimulates NO synthesis via the formation of an active complex between eNOS, AKT, and HSP90. Moreover, Fyn (a member of the Src family), mediates the EGCG -induced PI3-kinase/Akt-mediated activation of eNOS [71]. In addition, another study showed that transient receptor potential vanilloid type 1(TRPV1) is pivotal for EGCG-mediated activation of eNOS [72]. The results indicate that EGCG may trigger activation of TRPV1-Ca2+ signaling, which leads to phosphorylation of Akt, AMPK, and CaMKII, and further eNOS activation and NO production.

Vascular smooth muscle is a main component of vascular vessels. The contraction and relaxation of vascular smooth muscle determine vascular tone, and play a pivotal role in the regulation of blood pressure. The effects of GTE on arterial blood pressure and contractile responses of isolated aortic strips were assessed in normotensive rats [73]. Phenylephrine -induced contractile responses were significantly inhibited in the presence of GTE (0.3–1.2 mg/mL) in a dose-dependent fashion. Also, high potassium-induced contractile responses were depressed in the presence of 0.6–1.2 mg/mL of GTE, but not affected in low concentrations (0.3 mg/mL). Interestingly, the infusion of a moderate dose of GTE (10 mg/kg/30 min) caused a significant reduction in pressor responses induced by intravenous norepinephrine, although EGCG (1 mg/kg/30 min) did not affect them. The authors further demonstrated that dose-dependent depressor action of GTE is (at least) partly due to the inhibition of adrenergic αl-receptors. GTE also promoted a relaxation in the isolated aortic strips of rats via the blockade of adrenergic α1-receptors. These findings suggest that there is a big difference in the vascular effect of GTE and EGCG.

Renin also plays a pivotal role in the development of hypertension. Patients with low renin (i.e., salt-sensitive hypertension) represent approximately 30% of the essential hypertensives, and show a poor therapeutic response to angiotensin-converting enzyme inhibitors and angiotensin receptor blockers [74]. Renin inhibitory activities of three tea products have been investigated [75] and strong inhibition was observed with water extracts from fermented oolong and black tea. The authors demonstrated that theasinensin B, theasinensin C, strictinin, and a hexose sulfate with a galloyl moiety, exhibited IC50 values (against renin activity) of 19.33, 40.21, 311.09 and 50.16 μM, respectively. Moreover, the potent inhibitor theasinensin B was present only in black tea, and monomeric catechins did not contribute significantly to the renin inhibitory activities. These results suggest another potential pathway through which tea consumption helps to control hypertension.

Hypertension may be caused by vascular inflammation and remodeling [76,77]. Inflammation may play a role in the pathogenesis of hypertension or it may characterize a functional state of the vessel wall due to high blood pressure. IL-6 (a proinflammatory molecule) and MMP enzymes have important functions in vessel remodeling in vasculature. Mahajan et al. [78] demonstrated significant induction of IL-6 and MMP-9 expression in THP-1 macrophages by normocholesterolaemic hypertensive sera. Also, green tea polyphenols were found to significantly attenuate this induced expression in vitro. Their study revealed the existence of a potential causal relationship between hypertension, inflammation and vascular remodeling. Monocyte chemotactic protein-1 (MCP-1) plays a pivotal role in the recruitment of monocytes and amplifies inflammatory responses. Ahn et al. [79] studied the mechanisms by which EGCG inhibits tumor necrosis factor-α (TNF-α)-induced MCP-1 production in bovine coronary artery endothelial cells. The data showed that EGCG inhibited TNF-α-induced MCP-1 production, but it blunted Akt phosphorylation and TNF-α activation of TNFR1, which subsequently resulted in reduced MCP-1 production.

Endothelin-1 (ET-1) is the most potent vasoconstrictor produced in the blood vessel wall and has been shown to contribute to the pathogenesis of salt-sensitive hypertension in animals and humans [80]. ET-1 also augments vascular superoxide anion production, at least in part, via the ETA/NADPH oxidase pathway, leading to endothelial dysfunction and hypertension [81,82]. Nicholson et al. [83] reported that EGCG inhibited both eNOS and ET-1 mRNA expression at the physiological concentration (0.1 μM). These observed effects on gene expression should result in vasodilation and subsequent reduction in blood pressure. Reiter et al. [84] found that the phosphatidylinositol 3-kinase-dependent transcription factor FOXO1 mediates the effects of EGCG in the regulation of ET-1 expression in endothelial cells. EGCG treatment (10 μM for 8 h) of human aortic endothelial cells reduced expression of ET-1 mRNA, protein, and ET-1 secretion. A further study indicated that EGCG decreases ET-1 expression and secretion from endothelial cells, partly via Akt- and AMPK-stimulated FOXO1 regulation of the ET-1 promoter. This finding highlights another potential mechanism for the inhibition of vascular ET-1 release, due to ECGC in tea, which facilitates the protection of endothelial function and lowering of blood pressure.

The underlying mechanisms of tea regulating blood pressure using cell culture and animal models are illustrated in the Figure 1.

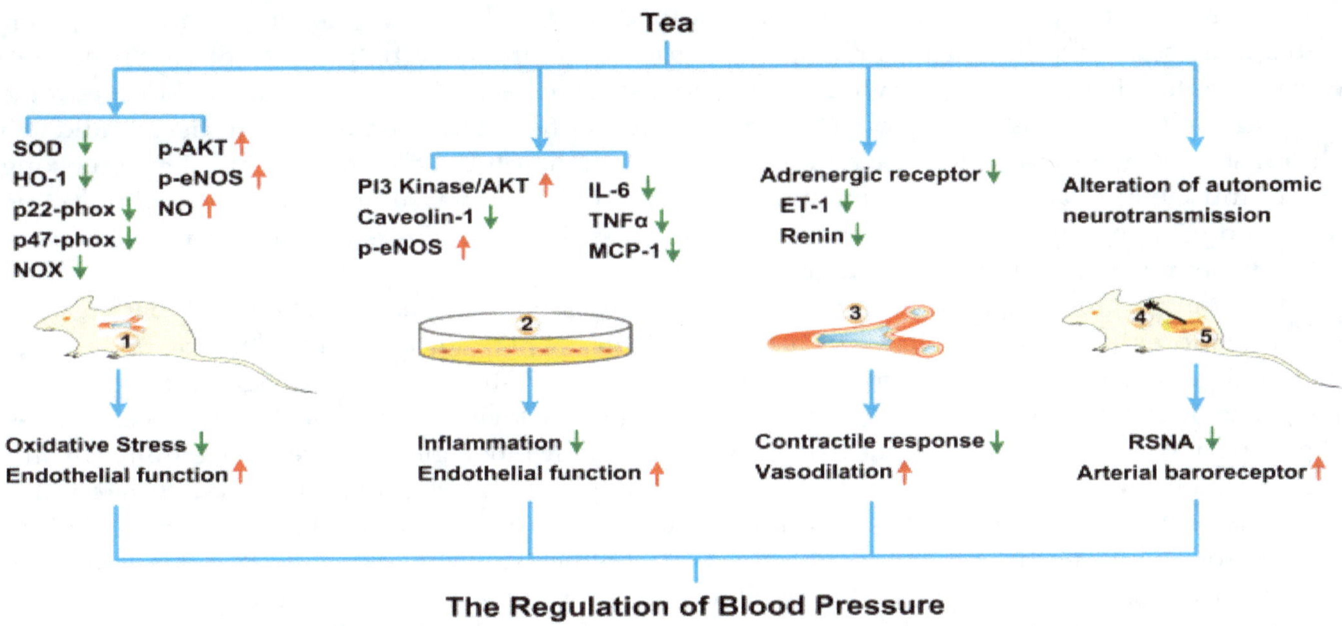

Figure 1. The underlying mechanisms of tea regulating blood pressure using animal, tissue and cell line models. After intake or adding into cell cultures, tea and its bioactive ingredients can alter several blood pressure regulating processes, including ① alleviation of the oxidative stress and improvement of the endothelial function in the aortas in vivo; ② mitigation of the inflammation and amelioration of the endothelial function in the aortic epithelial cell lines in vitro; ③ suppression of contractile response and improvement of vasodilation in the aortic tissues in vitro; ④,⑤ inhibition of renal sympathetic nerve activity and amelioration of arterial baroreceptor. Abbreviation: SOD, superoxide dismutase; HO-1, heme oxygenase 1; NOX, NADPH oxidase; p-AKT, phosphorylated protein kinase B; p-eNOS, phosphorylated endothelial nitric oxide synthase; NO, nitric oxide; PI3 Kinase, phosphatidylinositol 3 kinase; IL6, Interleukin 6; TNFα, Tumor necrosis factor α; MCP-1, Monocyte chemotactic protein-1; ET-1, Endothelin-1; RSNA, renal sympathetic nerve activity.

5. Discussion and Prospective

In conclusion, the bulk of evidence suggests that consumption of both green and black tea is associated with reductions in blood pressure, despite the negative results of some studies [85,86]. Many factors may influence the effect of tea consumption on blood pressure in human population studies. For example, the duration of tea consumption has an important impact on blood pressure. In a cohort of Norwegian men and women, higher consumption of black tea was associated with lower SBP [26]. However, in a four-week randomized, controlled, crossover trial in normotensive men and women, drinking six mugs of tea daily had no significant effect on clinic-measured blood pressure [87]. Other human intervention studies investigating the short-term effects of tea consumption on blood pressure also failed to achieve a positive outcome [88,89]. Differences in the origin of the tea and its secondary metabolites are further variables that occur between studies. In addition to flavonoids, tea contains caffeine, which causes a short-term increase in blood pressure [90]. These increases in blood pressure should be considered in the design of research projects. Hodgson [91] observed an increase in blood pressure 30 min after the ingestion of green or black tea in normotensive men; this increase was not evident after 60 min. Interestingly, the increase in blood pressure was greater than that induced by an equivalent dose of caffeine alone, suggesting that tea or tea polyphenols may also promote acute increases in blood pressure. Consumption of either black or green tea for seven days had no effect on 24 h ambulatory blood pressure in the same population. The same study showed that the acute hypertensive effect of tea consumption was blunted when tea was consumed with food [30]. The initial blood pressure is another factor that should be considered. Some case studies examined normotensive populations and those already well-controlled by anti-hypertensive therapy. In this situation, it is difficult to demonstrate a blood pressure lowering effect of tea intervention. Further large-scale investigations with longer terms of observation and tighter controls, are needed to determine optimal doses in subjects with varying degrees of hypertensive risk factors, and to determine differences in beneficial effects amongst diverse populations. Moreover, data from tissues and cell cultural studies have shown that tea and its secondary metabolites have important roles in relaxing smooth muscle contraction, enhancing eNOS activity, reducing vascular inflammation, inhibiting rennin and ET-1 activity and anti-vascular oxidative stress. However, the exact molecular mechanisms of these activities remain to be elucidated.

According to previous research, hypertension is more common in diabetic patients. Hypertension is present in more than 50% of patients with diabetes mellitus [92]. Recently, a systematic review and meta-analysis of randomized controlled trials involved in 27 studies (1898 participants) suggested that green tea may reduce fasting blood glucose (FBG) levels compared with placebo/water. Subgroup analysis showed that the effect of green tea on fasting blood glucose levels was significant only in studies with a mean age of < 55-years-old or Asian-based studies [93]. Previous researches reported that the potential beneficial effect of green tea on glucose metabolism may be mediated by EGCG, the most abundant catechin present in green tea [94]. Waltner-Law et al. reported that EGCG reduces hepatic glucose production by increasing tyrosine phosphorylation of the insulin receptor and insulin receptor substrate-1 in H4IIE rat hepatoma cell [95]. Recent studies have also suggested that green tea and yellow tea increase insulin sensitivity and glucose metabolism, preventing progress of type 2 diabetes [96]. Ortsäter et al. also reported that EGCG preserves islet structure and enhances glucose tolerance in db/db mice [97]. Therefore, teas decrease diabetes-related hypertension might mediate by ameliorating diabetes complication, which prevents high glucose induced damages of vascular endothelial and smooth muscle cells and maintain normal dilation and contraction of vascular system. The exact mechanisms of teas preventing diabetes-related hypertension need further investigation.

Clinical data shows that a 5-mmHg blood pressure reduction can reduce the risk of stroke and ischemic heart disease by 34 and 21%, respectively [6,7]. Although no clinical data available to demonstrate CVD outcome of 1-3 mmHg reduction of SBP and DBP, such small reductions of BP may benefit Stage 1 hypertension patients to control BP at range. Based on animal models, teas treatment significantly decreased SBP and DBP. There is a huge disparity between blood pressure lowering effects of tea in animal studies and human intervention. This difference may due to simplicity of animal studies and complicity of human intervention. In animal experiment, genetic background (same strain), living environment (standard facility), dosage and duration of treatment can be strictly controlled. Therefore, it is easy to see BP lowing effect by teas. For human population studies, complicated social and genetic backgrounds, varying degrees of hypertensive, dietary intaking and physical activity all can affect BP lowing effect of teas. Therefore, tighter controls are needed to determine BP lowing effects of tea in human populations.

6. Conclusions

In summary, human interventions and animal studies have confirmed that both tea and tea metabolites have anti-hypertensive effects although some controversial reports existed. The underlying mechanisms include relaxing smooth muscle contraction, enhancing endothelial nitric oxide synthase activity, reducing vascular inflammation, inhibiting rennin activity, and anti-vascular oxidative stress based on ex-vivo tissue and in vitro cell culture studies.

Author Contributions: Conceptualization, Z.X.; Methodology, D.L., R.W., J.H., and Q.C.; Review Process, C.S.Y., X.W., and Z.X.; Original Draft Preparation, D.L., R.W. and Z.X.; Review and Editing of Final Manuscript, D.L., R.W., and Z.X.; and Supervision, C.S.Y., and X.W.

References

1. Mendis, S.; Puska, P.; Norrving, B. *Global Atlas on Cardiovascular Disease Prevention and Control*; Geneva World Health Organizationn: Geneva, Switzerland, 2011.
2. Townsend, N.; Wilson, L.; Bhatnagar, P.; Wickramasinghe, K.; Rayner, M.; Nichols, M. Cardiovascular disease in Europe: Epidemiological update 2016. *Eur. Heart J.* **2016**, *37*, 3232–3245. [CrossRef] [PubMed]
3. Lim, S.S.; Vos, T.; Flaxman, A.D. A comparative risk assessment of burden of disease and injury attributable to 67 risk factor clusters in 21 regions, 1990–2010: A systematic analysis for the global Burden of Disease Study 2010. *Lancet* **2012**, *380*, 2224–2260. [CrossRef]
4. Conti, C.R. Diabetes, hypertension, and cardiovascular disease. *Clin. Cardiol.* **2001**, *24*, 1. [PubMed]
5. Horst-Meyer, H.Z. Report on the World Health Organization Global Observatory for eHealth Strategic Planning Workshop. *Meth. Inf. Med.* **2008**, *47*, 381–387.
6. Law, M.; Wald, N.; Morris, J. Lowering blood pressure to prevent myocardial infarction and stroke: A new preventive strategy. *Int. J. Technol. Assess. Health Care* **2005**, *21*, 145. [CrossRef]
7. Qureshi, A.; Sapkota, B.L. Blood Pressure Reduction in Secondary Stroke Prevention. *Continuum* **2011**, *17*, 1233–1241. [CrossRef]
8. Whelton, P.K.; Carey, R.M.; Aronow, W.S.; Casey Jr, D.E.; Collins, K.J.; Himmelfarb, C.D.; DePalma, S.M.; Gidding, S.; Jamerson, K.A.; Jones, D.W.; et al. 2017 ACC/AHA/AAPA/ABC/ACPM/AGS/APhA/ASH/ASPC/NMA/PCNA Guideline for the Prevention, Detection, Evaluation, and Management of High Blood Pressure in Adults: Executive Summary: A Report of the American College of Cardiology/American Heart Association Task Force on Clinical Practice Guidelines. *Hypertension* **2017**, *19*, 213–221.
9. Mozaffarian, D.; Benjamin, E.J.; Go, A.S.; Arnett, D.K.; Blaha, M.J.; Cushman, M.; Das, S.R.; de Ferranti, S.; Després, J.P.; Fullerton, H.J. Heart Disease and stroke statistics-2016 update a report from the American Heart Association. *Circulation* **2016**, *133*, e38–e48. [PubMed]
10. World Health Organization. *A Global Brief on Hypertension: Silent Killer, Global Public Health Crisis*; Geneva World Health Organization: Geneva, Switzerland, 2013.
11. Macfarlane, A.; Macfarlane, I. *The Empire of Tea*; Overlook Press: New York, NY, USA, 2004.
12. Heinrich, U.; Moore, C.E.; De Spirt, S.; Hagen, T.; Wilhelm, S. Green tea polyphenols provide photoprotection, increase microcirculation, and modulate skin properties of women. *J. Nutr.* **2012**, *141*, 1202–1208. [CrossRef]
13. Cabrera, C.; Artacho, R.; Gimenez, R. Beneficial effects of green tea—A review. *J. Am. Coll. Nutr.* **2006**, *25*, 79–99.
14. Hodgson, J.M.; Croft, K.D. Tea flavonoids and cardiovascular health. *Mol. Asp. Med.* **2010**, *31*, 495–502. [CrossRef] [PubMed]
15. Chobanian, A.V.; Bakris, G.L.; Black, H.R.; Cushman, W.; Green, L.; Izzo, J.; Jones, D.; Materson, B.; Oparil, S.; Wright, J. Seven report of the joint national committee on prevention, detection, and treatment of high blood pressure. *Hypertension* **2003**, *42*, 1206–1252. [CrossRef]
16. Hooper, L.; Kroon, P.A.; Rimm, E.B.; Cohn, J.S.; Harvey, I.; Kathryn, A.; Cornu, L.; Jonathan, J.R.; Hall, W.L.; Cassidy, A. Flavonoids, flavonoid-rich foods, and cardiovascular risk: A meta-analysis of randomized controlled trials. *Am. J. Clin. Nutr.* **2008** *88*, 38–50. [CrossRef]

17. Yang, C.S.; Hong, J. Prevention of chronic diseases by tea: Possible mechanisms and human relevance. *Annu. Rev. Nutr.* **2013**, *33*, 161–181. [CrossRef]
18. Sang, S.; Lambert, J.D.; Ho, C.T.; Yang, C.S. The chemistry and biotransformation of tea constituents. *Pharmacol. Res.* **2011**, *64*, 87–99. [CrossRef] [PubMed]
19. Zhang, L.; Zhang, Z.Z.; Zhou, Y.B.; Ling, T.J.; Wan, X.C. Chinese dark teas: Postfermentation, chemistry and biological activities. *Food Res. Int.* **2013**, *53*, 600–607. [CrossRef]
20. Khalesi, S.; Sun, J.; Buys, N.; Jamshidi, A.; Nikbakht-Nasrabadi, E.; Khosravi-Boroujeni, H. Green tea catechins and blood pressure: A systematic review and meta-analysis of randomized controlled trials. *Eur. J. Nutr.* **2014**, *53*, 1299–1311. [CrossRef] [PubMed]
21. Peng, X.; Zhou, R.; Wang, B.; Yu, X.; Yang, X.; Liu, K.; Mi, M. Effect of green tea consumption on blood pressure: A meta-analysis of 13 randomized controlled trials. *Sci. Rep.* **2014**, *4*, 6251. [CrossRef]
22. Greyling, A.; Ras, R.T.; Zock, P.L.; Lorenz, M.; Hopman, M.T.; Thijssen, D.H.; Draijer, R. The effect of black tea on blood pressure: A systematic review with meta-analysis of randomized controlled trials. *PLoS ONE* **2014**, *9*, e103247. [CrossRef] [PubMed]
23. Liu, G.; Mi, X.N.; Zheng, X.X.; Xu, Y.L.; Lu, J.; Huang, X.H. Effects of tea intake on blood pressure: A meta-analysis of randomised controlled trials. *Br. J. Nutr.* **2014**, *112*, 1043–1054. [CrossRef]
24. Yarmolinsky, J.; Gon, G.; Edwards, P. Effect of tea on blood pressure for secondary prevention of cardiovascular disease: A systematic review and meta-analysis of randomized controlled trials. *Nutr. Rev.* **2015**, *73*, 236–246. [CrossRef] [PubMed]
25. Kotsis, V.; Nilsson, P.; Grassi, G.; Mancia, G.; Redon, J.; Luft, F.; Schmieder, R.; Engeli, S.; Stabouli, S.; Antza, C.; et al. New developments in the pathogenesis of obesity-induced hypertension. *J. Hypertens.* **2015**, *33*, 1499–1508. [CrossRef] [PubMed]
26. Hall, J.E.; do Carmo, J.M.; da Silva, A.A.; Wang, Z.; Hall, M.E. Obesity-induced hypertension: Interaction of neurohumoral and renal mechanisms. *Circ. Res.* **2015**, *116*, 991–1006. [CrossRef]
27. Li, G.W.; Zhang, Y.; Thabane, L.; Liu, A.; Levine, M.A.; Holbrook, A. Effect of green tea supplementation on blood pressure among overweight and obese adults: A systematic review and meta-analysis. *J. Hypertens.* **2015**, *33*, 243–254. [CrossRef]
28. Tong, X.; Taylor, A.; Giles, L.; Wittert, G.A.; Shi, Z. Tea consumption is inversely related to 5-year blood pressure change among adults in Jiangsu, China: A cross-sectional study. *Nutr. J.* **2014**, *13*, 98. [CrossRef]
29. Yang, Y.C.; Lu, F.H.; Wu, J.S.; Chang, C.J. The protective effect of habitual tea consumption on hypertension. *Arch. Intern. Med.* **2004**, *164*, 1534–1540. [CrossRef] [PubMed]
30. Nantz, M.P.; Rowe, C.A.; Bukowski, J.F.; Percival, S.S. Standardized capsule of Camellia sinensis lowers cardiovascular risk factors in a randomized, double-blind, placebo-controlled study. *Nutrition* **2009**, *25*, 147–154. [CrossRef] [PubMed]
31. Stensvold, I.; Tverdal, A.; Solvoll, K.; Foss, O.P. Tea consumption, relationship to cholesterol, blood pressure and coronary and total mortality. *Prev. Med.* **1992**, *21*, 546–553. [CrossRef]
32. Hodgson, J.M.; Puddey, I.B.; Woodman, R.J.; Mulder, T.P.; Fuchs, D.; Scott, K.; Croft, K.D. Effects of black tea on blood pressure: A randomized controlled trial. *Arch. Intern. Med.* **2012**, *172*, 186–188. [CrossRef] [PubMed]
33. Pinto, E. Blood pressure and aging. *Postgrad. Med. J.* **2007**, *83*, 109–114. [CrossRef]
34. Hodgson, J.M.; Devine, A.; Puddey, I.B.; Chan, S.Y.; Beilin, L.J.; Prince, R.L. Tea intake is inversely related to blood pressure in older women. *J. Nutr.* **2003**, *133*, 2883–2886. [CrossRef]
35. Yin, J.Y.; Duan, S.Y.; Liu, F.C.; Yao, Q.K.; Tu, S.; Xu, Y.; Pan, C.W. Blood Pressure Is Associated with Tea Consumption: A Cross-sectional Study in a Rural, Elderly Population of Jiangsu China. *J. Nutr. Health Aging* **2017**, *21*, 1151–1159. [CrossRef] [PubMed]
36. Liao, D.; Arnett, D.; Tyroler, H.; Riley, W.A.; Chambless, L.E.; Szklo, M.; Heiss, G. Arterial Stiffness and the Development of Hypertension The ARIC Study. *Hypertension* **1999**, *34*, 201–206. [CrossRef]
37. Lin, Q.F.; Qiu, C.S.; Wang, S.L.; Huang, L.F.; Chen, Z.Y.; Chen, Y.; Chen, G. A Cross-sectional Study of the Relationship Between Habitual Tea Consumption and Arterial Stiffness. *J. Am. Coll. Nutr.* **2016**, *35*, 354–361. [CrossRef] [PubMed]
38. Nagao, T.; Hase, T.; Tokimitsu, I. A green tea extract high in catechins reduces body fat and cardiovascular risks in humans. *Obesity (Silver Spring)* **2007**, *15*, 1473–1483. [CrossRef] [PubMed]

39. Brown, A.L.; Lane, J.; Coverly, J.; Stocks, J.; Jackson, S.; Stephen, A.; Bluck, L.; Coward, A.; Hendrickx, H. Effects of dietary supplementation with the green tea polyphenol epigallocatechin-3-gallate on insulin resistance and associated metabolic risk factors: Randomized controlled trial. *Br. J. Nutr.* **2009**, *101*, 886–894. [CrossRef] [PubMed]
40. Nogueira, L.P.; Nogueira Neto, J.F.; Klein, M.R.; Sanjuliani, A.F. Short-term Effects of Green Tea on Blood Pressure, Endothelial Function, and Metabolic Profile in Obese Prehypertensive Women: A Crossover Randomized Clinical Trial. *J. Am. Coll. Nutr.* **2017**, *36*, 108–115. [CrossRef]
41. Bogdanski, P.; Suliburska, J.; Szulinska, M.; Stepien, M.; Pupek-Musialik, D.; Jablecka, A. Green tea extract reduces blood pressure, inflammatory biomarkers, and oxidative stress and improves parameters associated with insulin resistance in obese, hypertensive patients. *Nutr. Res.* **2012**, *32*, 421–427. [CrossRef]
42. Grassi, D.; Draijer, R.; Desideri, G.; Mulder, T.; Ferri, C. Black tea lowers blood pressure and wave reflections in fasted and postprandial conditions in hypertensive patients: A randomized study. *Nutrients* **2015**, *7*, 1037–1051. [CrossRef]
43. Ferrannini, E.; Cushman, W.C. Diabetes and hypertension: The bad companions. *Lancet* **2012**, *380*, 601–610. [CrossRef]
44. Mozaffari-Khosravi, H.; Ahadi, Z.; Barzegar, K. The effect of green tea and sour tea on blood pressure of patients with type 2 diabetes: A randomized clinical trial. *J. Diet. Suppl.* **2013**, *10*, 105–115. [CrossRef] [PubMed]
45. Fukino, Y.; Ikeda, A.; Maruyama, K.; Aoki, N.; Okubo, T.; Iso, H. Randomized controlled trial for an effect of green tea-extract powder supplementation on glucose abnormalities. *Eur. J. Clin. Nutr.* **2008**, *62*, 953–960. [CrossRef] [PubMed]
46. Henry, J.P.; Stephenes-Larson, P. Reduction of chronic psychosocial hypertension in mice by decaffeinated tea. *Hypertension* **1984**, *6*, 437–444. [CrossRef]
47. Negishi, H.; Xu, J.W.; Ikeda, K.; Njelekela, M.; Nara, Y.; Yamori, Y. Black and Green Tea Polyphenols Attenuate Blood Pressure Increases in Stroke-Prone Spontaneously Hypertensive Rats. *J. Nutr.* **2004**, *134*, 38–42. [CrossRef] [PubMed]
48. Yang, C.S.; Chen, L.; Lee, M.J.; Balentine, D.; Kuo, M.C.; Schantz, S.P. Blood and urine levels of tea catechins after ingestion of different amounts of green tea by human volunteers. *Cancer Epidemiol. Biomark. Prev.* **1998**, *7*, 351–354.
49. Potenza, M.A.; Marasciulo, F.L.; Tarquinio, M.; Tiravanti, E.; Colantuono, G.; Federici, A.; Kim, J.A.; Quon, M.J.; Montagnani, M. EGCG, a green tea polyphenol, improves endothelial function and insulin sensitivity, reduces blood pressure, and protects against myocardial I/R injury in SHR. *Am. J. Physiol. Endocrinol. Metab.* **2007**, *292*, E1378–E1387. [CrossRef] [PubMed]
50. Igarashi, K.; Honma, K.; Yoshinari, O.; Nanjo, F.; Hara, Y. Effects of dietary catechins on glucose tolerance, blood pressure and oxidative status in Goto-Kakizaki rats. *J. Nutr. Sci. Vitaminol. (Tokyo)* **2007**, *53*, 496–500. [CrossRef] [PubMed]
51. Yasuhiko, A.; Satoshi, U.; Koh-Ichi, S.; Hirawa, N.; Kato, Y.; Yokoyama, N.; Yokoyama, T.; Iwai, J.; Ishii, M. Effect of green tea rich in γ-aminobutyric acid on blood pressure of Dahl salt-sensitive rats. *Am. J. Hypertens.* **1995**, *8*, 74–79.
52. Yokogoshi, H.; Kobayashi, M. Hypotensive effect of γ-glutamylmethylamide glutamic acid in spontaneously hypertensive rats. *Life Sci.* **1998**, *62*, 1065–1068. [CrossRef]
53. Coşan, D.T.; Saydam, F.; Özbayer, C.; Doğaner, F.; Soyocak, A.; Güneş, H.V.; Değirmenci, İ.; Kurt, H.; Üstüner, M.C.; Bal, C. Impact of tannic acid on blood pressure, oxidative stress and urinary parameters in L-NNA-induced hypertensive rats. *Cytotechnology* **2015**, *67*, 97–105. [CrossRef] [PubMed]
54. Sagesaka-Mitane, Y.; Sugiura, T.; Miwa, Y.; Yamaguchi, K.; Kyuki, K. Effect of tea-leaf saponin on blood pressure of spontaneously hypertensive rats. *Yakugaku Zasshi* **1996**, *116*, 388–395. [CrossRef]
55. Griendling, K.K.; Alexander, R.W. Oxidative stress and cardiovascular disease. *Circulation* **1997**, *96*, 3264–3265. [PubMed]
56. Rajagopalan, S.; Kurz, S.; Munzel, T.; Tarpey, M.; Freeman, B.A.; Griendling, K.K.; Harrison, D.G. Angiotensin II-mediated hypertension in the rat increases vascular superoxide production via membrane NADH/NADPH oxidase activation: Contribution to alterations of vasomotor tone. *J. Clin. Investig.* **1996**, *97*, 1916–1923. [CrossRef] [PubMed]

57. Pagano, P.J.; Clark, J.K.; Cifuentes-Pagano, M.E.; Clark, S.M.; Callis, G.M.; Quinn, M.T. Localization of a constitutively active, phagocyte-like NADPH oxidase in rabbit aortic adventitia: Enhancement by angiotensin II. *Proc. Natl. Acad. Sci. USA* **1997**, *94*, 14483–14488. [CrossRef]
58. Wu, R.; Millette, E.; Wu, L.; de Champlain, J. Enhanced superoxide anion formation in vascular tissues from spontaneously hypertensive and desoxycorticosterone acetate-salt hypertensive rats. *J. Hypertens.* **2001**, *19*, 741–748. [CrossRef]
59. Beswick, R.A.; Dorrance, A.M.; Leite, R.; Webb, R.C. NADH/NADPH oxidase and enhanced superoxide production in the mineralocorticoid hypertensive rat. *Hypertension* **2001**, *38*, 1107–1111. [CrossRef]
60. Antonello, M.; Montemurro, D.; Bolognesi, M.; Di, P.M.; Piva, A.; Grego, F.; Sticchi, D.; Giuliani, L.; Garbisa, S.; Rossi, G.P. Prevention of hypertension, cardiovascular damage and endothelial dysfunction with green tea extracts. *Am. J. Hypertens.* **2007**, *20*, 1321–1328. [CrossRef]
61. Ihm, S.H.; Jang, S.W.; Kim, O.R.; Chang, K.; Oak, M.H.; Lee, J.O.; Lim, D.Y.; Kim, J.H. Decaffeinated green tea extract improves hypertension and insulin resistance in a rat model of metabolic syndrome. *Atherosclerosis* **2012**, *224*, 377–383. [CrossRef]
62. Gómez-Guzmán, M.; Jiménez, R.; Sánchez, M.; Zarzuelo, M.J.; Galindo, P.; Quintela, A.M.; López-Sepúlveda, R.; Romero, M.; Tamargo, J.; Vargas, F.; et al. Epicatechin lowers blood pressure, restores endothelial function, and decreases oxidative stress and endothelin-1 and NADPH oxidase activity in DOCA-salt hypertension. *Free Radic. Biol. Med.* **2012**, *52*, 70–79. [CrossRef] [PubMed]
63. Galleano, M.; Bernatova, I.; Puzserova, A.; Balis, P.; Sestakova, N.; Pechanova, O.; Fraga, C.G. (-)-Epicatechin reduces blood pressure and improves vasorelaxation in spontaneously hypertensive rats by NO-mediated mechanism. *IUBMB Life* **2013**, *65*, 710–715. [CrossRef]
64. Litterio, M.C.; Jaggers, G.; Celep, G.S.; Adamo, A.M.; Costa, M.A.; Oteiza, P.I.; Fraga, C.G.; Galleano, M. Blood pressure-lowering effect of dietary (-)-epicatechin administration in L-NAME-treated rats is associated with restored nitric oxide levels. *Free Radic. Biol. Med.* **2012**, *53*, 1894–1902. [CrossRef]
65. Tanida, M.; Tsuruoka, N.; Shen, J.; Kiso, Y.; Nagai, K. Effects of oolong tea on renal sympathetic nerve activity and spontaneous hypertension in rats. *Metabolism* **2008**, *57*, 526–534. [CrossRef]
66. Han, J.Y.; Kim, C.S.; Lim, K.H.; Kim, J.H.; Kim, S.; Yun, Y.P.; Hong, J.T.; Oh, K.W. Increases in blood pressure and heart rate induced by caffeine are inhibited by (-)-epigallocatechin-3-O-gallate: Involvement of catecholamines. *J. Cardiovasc. Pharmacol.* **2011**, *58*, 446–449. [CrossRef] [PubMed]
67. Garcia, M.L.; Pontes, R.B.; Nishi, E.E.; Ibuki, F.K.; Oliveira, V.; Sawaya, A.C.; Carvalho, P.O.; Nogueira, F.N.; Franco, M.D.; Campos, R.R.; et al. The antioxidant effects of green tea reduces blood pressure and sympathoexcitation in an experimental model of hypertension. *J. Hypertens.* **2017**, *35*, 348–354. [CrossRef] [PubMed]
68. Anter, E.; Thomas, S.R.; Schulz, E.; Shapira, O.M.; Vita, J.A.; Keaney, J.F. Activation of endothelial nitric-oxide synthase by the p38 MAPK in response to black tea polyphenols. *J. Biol. Chem.* **2004**, *279*, 46637–46643. [CrossRef] [PubMed]
69. Li, Y.; Ying, C.; Zuo, X.; Yi, H.; Yi, W.; Meng, Y.; Ikeda, K.; Ye, X.; Yamori, Y.; Sun, X. Green tea polyphenols down-regulate caveolin-1 expression via ERK1/2 and p38MAPK in endothelial cells. *J. Nutr. Biochem.* **2009**, *20*, 1021–1027. [CrossRef]
70. Ramirez-Sanchez, I.; Aguilar, H.; Ceballos, G.; Villarreal, F. (-)-Epicatechin-induced calcium independent eNOS activation: Roles of HSP90 and AKT. *Mol. Cell. Biochem.* **2012**, *370*, 141–150. [CrossRef] [PubMed]
71. Kim, J.A.; Formoso, G.; Li, Y.; Potenza, M.A.; Marasciulo, F.L.; Montagnani, M.; Quon, M.J. Epigallocatechin gallate, a green tea polyphenol, mediates NO-dependent vasodilation using signaling pathways in vascular endothelium requiring reactive oxygen species and Fyn. *J. Biol. Chem.* **2007**, *282*, 13736–13745. [CrossRef] [PubMed]
72. Guo, B.C.; Wei, J.; Su, K.H.; Chiang, A.N.; Zhao, J.F.; Chen, H.Y.; Shyue, S.K.; Lee, T.S. Transient receptor potential vanilloid type 1 is vital for (-)-epigallocatechin-3-gallate mediated activation of endothelial nitric oxide synthase. *Mol. Nutr. Food Res.* **2015**, *59*, 646–657. [CrossRef]
73. Lim, D.Y.; Lee, E.S.; Park, H.G.; Kim, B.C.; Hong, S.P.; Lee, E.B. Comparison of Green Tea Extract and Epigallocatechin Gallate on Blood Pressure and Contractile Responses of Vascular Smooth Muscle of Rats. *Arch. Pharm. Res.* **2003**, *26*, 214–223. [CrossRef]
74. Letizia, C.; Cerci, S.; De Toma, G.; D'Ambrosio, C.; De Ciocchis, A.; Coassin, S.; Scavo, D. High plasma endothelin-1 levels in hypertensive patients with low renin essential hypertension. *J. Hum Hypertens.* **1997**, *11*, 447–451. [CrossRef] [PubMed]

75. Li, F.; Ohnishi-Kameyama, M.; Takahashi, Y.; Yamaki, K. Tea polyphenols as novel and potent inhibitory substances against renin activity. *J Agric. Food Chem.* **2013**, *61*, 9697–9704. [CrossRef]
76. Soltani, S.; Chitsazi, M.J.; Salehi-Abargouei, A. The effect of dietary approaches to stop hypertension (DASH) on serum inflammatory markers: A systematic review and meta-analysis of randomized trials. *Clin. Nutr.* **2018**, *37*, 542–550. [CrossRef]
77. Savoia, C.; Schiffrin, E.L. Vascular inflammation in hypertension and diabetes: Molecular mechanisms and therapeutic interventions. *Clin. Sci.* **2007**, *112*, 375–384. [CrossRef] [PubMed]
78. Mahajan, N.; Dhawan, V.; Sharma, G.; Jain, S.; Kaul, D. Induction of inflammatory gene expression by THP-1 macrophages cultured in normocholesterolaemic hypertensive sera and modulatory effects of green tea polyphenols. *J. Hum. Hypertens.* **2008**, *22*, 141–143. [CrossRef]
79. Ahn, H.Y.; Xu, Y.; Davidge, S.T. Epigallocatechin-3-O-gallate inhibits TNFalpha-induced monocyte chemotactic protein-1 production from vascular endothelial cells. *Life Sci.* **2008**, *82*, 964–968. [CrossRef] [PubMed]
80. Elijovich, F.; Laffer, C.L.; Amador, E.; Gavras, H.; Bresnahan, M.R.; Schiffrin, E.L. Regulation of plasma endothelin by salt in salt-sensitive hypertension. *Circulation* **2001**, *103*, 263–268. [CrossRef]
81. Li, L.; Fink, G.D.; Watts, S.W.; Northcott, C.A.; Galligan, J.J.; Pagano, P.J.; Chen, A.F. Endothelin-1 increases vascular superoxide via endothelin(A)–NADPH oxidase pathway in low-renin hypertension. *Circulation* **2003**, *107*, 1053–1058. [CrossRef] [PubMed]
82. Jiménez, R.; López-Sepúlveda, R.; Kadmiri, M.; Romero, M.; Vera, R.; Sánchez, M.; Vargas, F.; O'Valle, F.; Zarzuelo, A.; Dueñas, M.; et al. Polyphenols restore endothelial function in DOCA-salt hypertension: Role of endothelin-1 and NADPH oxidase. *Free Radic. Biol. Med.* **2007**, *43*, 462–473. [CrossRef]
83. Nicholson, S.K.; Tucker, G.A.; Brameld, J.M. Physiological concentrations of dietary polyphenols regulate vascular endothelial cell expression of genes important in cardiovascular health. *Br. J. Nutr.* **2010**, *103*, 1398–1403. [CrossRef]
84. Reiter, C.E.; Kim, J.A.; Quon, M.J. Green tea polyphenol epigallocatechin gallate reduces endothelin-1 expression and secretion in vascular endothelial cells: Roles for AMP-activated protein kinase, Akt, and FOXO1. *Endocrinology* **2010**, *151*, 103–114. [CrossRef] [PubMed]
85. Hodgson, J.M.; Puddey, I.B.; Burke, V.; Beilin, L.J.; Jordan, N. Effects on blood pressure of drinking green and black tea. *J Hypertens.* **1999**, *17*, 457–463. [CrossRef] [PubMed]
86. Rakic, V.; Beilin, L.J.; Burke, V. Effect of coffee and tea drinking on postprandial hypotension in older men and women. *Clin. Exp. Pharmacol. Physiol.* **1996**, *23*, 559–563. [CrossRef]
87. Bingham, S.A.; Vorster, H.; Jerling, J.C.; Magee, E.; Mulligan, A.; Runswick, S.A.; Cummings, J.H. Effect of black tea drinking on blood lipids, blood pressure and aspects of bowel habit. *Br. J. Nutr.* **1997**, *78*, 41–55. [CrossRef] [PubMed]
88. Hodgson, J.M.; Puddey, I.B.; Burke, V.; Watts, G.F.; Beilin, L.J. Regular ingestion of black tea improves brachial artery vasodilator function. *Clin. Sci. (Lond.)* **2002**, *102*, 195–201. [CrossRef] [PubMed]
89. Quinlan, P.; Lane, J.; Aspinall, L. Effects of hot tea, coffee and water ingestion on physiological responses and mood: The role of caffeine, water and beverage type. *Psychopharmacology (Berl.)* **1997**, *134*, 164–173. [CrossRef]
90. Hodgson, J.M.; Burke, V.; Puddey, I.B. Acute effects of tea on fasting and postprandial vascular function and blood pressure in humans. *J. Hypertens.* **2005**, *23*, 47–54. [CrossRef]
91. Hodgson, J.M.; Woodman, R.J.; Puddey, I.B.; Mulder., T.; Fuchs, D.; Croft, K.D. Short-term effects of polyphenol-rich black tea on blood pressure in men and women. *Food Funct.* **2013**, *4*, 111–115. [CrossRef]
92. Lastra, G.; Syed, S.; Kurukulasuriya, L.R.; Manrique, C.; Sowers, J.R. Type 2 diabetes mellitus and hypertension: An update. *Endocrinol. Metab. Clin. N. Am.* **2014**, *43*, 103–122. [CrossRef]
93. Kondo, Y.; Goto, A.; Noma, H.; Iso, H.; Hayashi, K.; Noda, M. Effects of Coffee and Tea Consumption on Glucose Metabolism: A Systematic Review and Network Meta-Analysis. *Nutrients* **2018**, *11*, 48. [CrossRef]
94. Eng, Q.Y.; Thanikachalam, P.V.; Ramamurthy, S. Molecular understanding of Epigallocatechin gallate (EGCG) in cardiovascular and metabolic diseases. *J. Ethnopharmacol.* **2018**, *210*, 296–310. [CrossRef] [PubMed]
95. Waltner-Law, M.E.; Wang, X.L.; Law, B.K.; Hall, R.K.; Nawano, M.; Granner, D.K. Epigallocatechin gallate, a constituent of green tea, represses hepatic glucose production. *J. Biol. Chem.* **2002**, *277*, 34933–34940. [CrossRef] [PubMed]

96. Teng, Y.; Li, D.; Guruvaiah, P.; Xu, N.; Xie, Z. Dietary Supplement of Large Yellow Tea Ameliorates Metabolic Syndrome and Attenuates Hepatic Steatosis in db/db Mice. *Nutrients* **2018**, *10*, 75. [CrossRef] [PubMed]
97. Ortsater, H.; Grankvist, N.; Wolfram, S.; Kuehn, N.; Sjoholm, A. Diet supplementation with green tea extract epigallocatechin gallate prevents progression to glucose intolerance in db/db mice. *Nutr. Metab.* **2012**, *9*, 11. [CrossRef] [PubMed]

11

Hesperidin Prevents Nitric Oxide Deficiency-Induced Cardiovascular Remodeling in Rats via Suppressing TGF-β1 and MMPs Protein Expression

Putcharawipa Maneesai [1,2], Sarawoot Bunbupha [3], Prapassorn Potue [1], Thewarid Berkban [3], Upa Kukongviriyapan [1,2], Veerapol Kukongviriyapan [4], Parichat Prachaney [2,5] and Poungrat Pakdeechote [1,2,*]

1 Department of Physiology, Faculty of Medicine, Khon Kaen University, Khon Kaen 40002, Thailand; putcma@kku.ac.th (P.M.); pairpassorn@gmail.com (P.P.); upa_ku@kku.ac.th (U.K.)
2 Cardiovascular Research Group, Khon Kaen University, Khon Kaen 40002, Thailand; parpra@kku.ac.th
3 Faculty of Medicine, Mahasarakham University, Maha Sarakham 44000, Thailand; bugvo@hotmail.com (S.B.); no_ng_pt@hotmail.com (T.B.)
4 Department of Pharmacology, Faculty of Medicine, Khon Kaen University, Khon Kaen 40002, Thailand; veerapol@kku.ac.th
5 Department of Anatomy, Faculty of Medicine, Khon Kaen University, Khon Kaen 40002, Thailand
* Correspondence: ppoung@kku.ac.th

Abstract: Hesperidin is a major flavonoid isolated from citrus fruits that exhibits several biological activities. This study aims to evaluate the effect of hesperidin on cardiovascular remodeling induced by N-nitro L-arginine methyl ester (L-NAME) in rats. Male Sprague-Dawley rats were treated with L-NAME (40 mg/kg), L-NAME plus hesperidin (15 mg/kg), hesperidin (30 mg/kg), or captopril (2.5 mg/kg) for five weeks (n = 8/group). Hesperidin or captopril significantly prevented the development of hypertension in L-NAME rats. L-NAME-induced cardiac remodeling, i.e., increases in wall thickness, cross-sectional area (CSA), and fibrosis in the left ventricular and vascular remodeling, i.e., increases in wall thickness, CSA, vascular smooth muscle cells, and collagen deposition in the aorta were attenuated by hesperidin or captopril. These were associated with reduced oxidative stress markers, tumor necrosis factor-alpha (TNF-α), transforming growth factor-beta 1 (TGF-β1), and enhancing plasma nitric oxide metabolite (NOx) in L-NAME treated groups. Furthermore, up-regulation of tumor necrosis factor receptor type 1 (TNF-R1) and TGF- β1 protein expression and the overexpression of matrix metalloproteinase-2 (MMP-2) and matrix metalloproteinase-9 (MMP-9) was suppressed in L-NAME rats treated with hesperidin or captopril. These data suggested that hesperidin had cardioprotective effects in L-NAME hypertensive rats. The possible mechanism may involve antioxidant and anti-inflammatory effects.

Keywords: hesperidin; L-NAME; cardiovascular remodeling; oxidative stress; inflammation

---

1. Introduction

Nitric oxide (NO) is a crucial vasodilator derived from vascular endothelium to regulate vascular tone [1]. A reduction of NO production results in increased vascular resistance and high blood pressure. N^{ω}-nitro L-arginine methyl ester (L-NAME), an L-arginine analogue, is widely used as an inhibitor of nitric oxide synthase (NOS) activity to represent an animal model of hypertension. It has been reported that L-NAME-induced hypertension in rats is characterized by insufficient NO production, increased systemic oxidative stress, inflammation, and endothelial dysfunction [2]. Furthermore, L-NAME-induced hypertension and cardiovascular remodeling have also been reported in rats. For example, the administration of L-NAME (40 mg/kg) for four or five weeks causes high blood pressure and cardiovascular remodeling, including left ventricular hypertrophy, myocardial fibrosis, and thickening of the vascular wall [3–5]. It is generally known that the main sequel of cardiovascular remodeling is heart failure, which is the major cause of death worldwide [6].

The initial stage of cardiac remodeling is myocardial hypertrophy because of the adaptive response to a high-pressure load to preserve cardiac function and obtain normal cardiac work. In addition, the cardiac remodeling process in L-NAME-treated rats is involved in the production of myocardial fibrosis [7]. There are substantial data to show the molecular mechanism of extensive areas of cardiac fibrosis which is associated with the activation of various downstream inflammatory [8] and oxidative stress initiatives [9,10]. For example, a high level of tumor necrosis factor (TNF-α), a pro-inflammatory cytokine, developed in response to oxidative stress in L-NAME-induced hypertension has been reported [4,11]. These inflammatory responses subsequently activate the profibrotic mediator of the transforming growth factor β1 (TGF-β1) [11]. It is well-established that TGF-β1 plays a key role in fibrogenesis by activating apoptosis, collagen, and matrix protein synthesis [12–14]. For vascular structural changes in hypertension, it is known to be an adaptive response to an increase in wall tension [15]. This response is also related to the extracellular matrix degradation of elastic fibers since the up-regulation of matrix metalloproteinase-2 (MMP-2) and matrix metalloproteinase-9 (MMP-9) expression in vessel tissue has been confirmed in animal models of hypertension. Several lines of evidence have indicated that the activation of MMP-2/9 protein expression found in the vascular remodeling process is mediated by the inflammatory cytokine, TNF-α [16–18]. Thus, it is noteworthy that natural products with high antioxidant and anti-inflammatory activities might be useful for alleviating cardiovascular alterations induced by nitric oxide deficiency.

Captopril is an angiotensin-converting enzyme (ACE) inhibitor and is commonly used as an anti-hypertensive drug [19]. Its mechanism of action has been well-documented to reduce angiotensin II production, which subsequently suppresses the renin-angiotensin-aldosterone system (RAAS) [19]. Other possible anti-hypertensive mechanisms include increased bradykinin and prostaglandins levels [20], the inhibition of superoxide production [21], and the free radical scavenging effect [22]. Many studies have already reported on the cardiovascular effects of captopril in nitric oxide-deficient hypertensive rats, i.e., lowering high blood pressure, improving vascular function [21], and preventing cardiovascular remodeling [23]. In L-NAME hypertensive rats, there is evidence showing the up-regulation of angiotensin II receptor type 1 (AT1R) which mediates nicotinamide adenine dinucleotide phosphate (NADPH) oxidase expression and superoxide formation [10]. This study used captopril as a positive control agent because the L-NAME hypertension model is also involved in the activation of the RAAS, where captopril inhibits the RAAS.

Hesperidin is a flavanone glycoside, a subclass of flavonoids, abundantly found in citrus fruits such as lemon or orange peels or juices [24]. Numerous beneficial effects of hesperidin have been published. For example, the antioxidant effect of hesperidin has been reported to be able to sequester 1,1-diphenyl-2-picrylhydrazyl (DPPH) and protect cell injury-induced by paraquat and hydrogen peroxide [25], reduce plasma levels of lipid peroxidation markers, and increase antioxidant enzyme activities in heart tissue in experimentally ischemic myocardial rats [26]. Hesperidin has also exhibited an anti-inflammatory effect by reducing circulating inflammatory markers, i.e., TNF-α, interleukin 6 (IL-6), and a high-sensitivity C-reactive protein (hs-CRP), in patients with type 2 diabetes [27] and suppressed inflammatory responses in lipopolysaccharide-induced RAW 264.7 cells [28]. Subsequently, a clinical study revealed that a combination of hesperidin, diosmin, and troxerutin was effective in relieving the symptoms of acute hemorrhoidal disease [29]. Recently, the current authors have demonstrated an anti-hypertensive effect of hesperidin in renovascular hypertensive rats that involved the suppression of the renin-angiotensin system [30]. This study was intended to further explore whether hesperidin could prevent L-NAME-induced hypertension and cardiovascular remodeling in rats.

2. Materials and Methods

2.1. Drugs and Chemicals

Hesperidin (purity ≥ 98%) was purchased from Chem Faces Company (Wuhan, Hubei, China). N(G)-Nitro-L-arginine methyl ester hydrochloride (L-NAME) and captopril were purchased from Sigma-Aldrich Corp (St. Louis, MO, USA). All the other chemicals used in this study were obtained from standard companies and were of analytical grade quality.

2.2. Animals and Experimental Protocols

Male Sprague-Dawley rats (body weight 220–250 g) were supplied by Nomura Siam International Co., Ltd., Bangkok, Thailand. The animals were housed in a Heating, Ventilation and Air-Conditioning (HVAC) System (25 ± 2 °C) facility and maintained on a 12 h light and 12 h dark cycle with free access to a standard rat diet and water at the Northeast Laboratory Animal Center, Khon Kaen University. All the experimental protocols in this study were in accordance with the standards for the care and use of experimental animals and approval for all the experiments was obtained from the Animal Ethics Committee of Khon Kaen University, Khon Kaen, Thailand (AEKKU-NELAC 37/2559).

After a seven-day acclimatization period, the rats were randomly assigned to 5 groups (8/group). The control group animals received tap water and were orally administrated propylene glycol (PG, 1.5 mL/Kg) as a vehicle. L-NAME treated rats received L-NAME (40 mg/kg/day) in their drinking water and were further divided into the following 4 groups; L-NAME plus PG, L-NAME plus hesperidin at a dose of 15 mg/kg (L-NAME + H15 group), L-NAME plus hesperidin 30 mg/kg (L-NMAE + H30 group), L-NAME group plus captopril at a dose of 2.5 mg/kg (L-NAME + Cap group). Additionally, normal rats (n = 5) were orally treated with hesperidin (30 mg/kg) for 5 weeks to test the hypotensive effect of hesperidin. Hesperidin and captopril were dissolved in vehicle and intragastrically administered once daily for five weeks. The doses of hesperidin and captopril used in this study were influenced by previous studies in this laboratory [10,30].

2.3. Blood Pressure Measurements

To monitor blood pressure changes throughout the experimental period, systolic blood pressure (SP) was obtained in awake rats once a week for 5 weeks using tail-cuff plethysmography (IITC/Life Science Instrument model 229 and model 179 amplifier; Woodland Hills, CA, USA). At the end of the final experimental day, the rats were anesthetized with pentobarbital sodium (60 mg/kg, ip.). Then, the femoral artery was cannulated and connected to a pressure transducer for monitoring the baseline values of SP, diastolic blood pressure (DP), mean arterial pressure (MAP), and heart rate (HR) using the Acknowledge Data Acquisition software (Biopac Systems Inc., Santa Barbara, CA, USA).

2.4. Collection of Blood and Organs

After the blood pressure measurement, the rats were sacrificed by exsanguination and blood samples were collected from abdominal aortas into Ethylenediaminetetraacetic acid (EDTA) or heparin tubes for assays of oxidative stress and inflammatory markers. The carotid arteries were rapidly excised for analysis of superoxide ($O_2^{\bullet-}$) production. The thoracic aortas and heart tissues were collected for western blotting and morphometric analysis.

2.5. Assays of Vascular $O_2^{\bullet-}$ Production, Plasma Malondialdehyde (MDA), Plasma Nitric Oxide Metabolite (Nitrate/Nitrite, NOx), Plasma TNF-α and Plasma TGF- β1 Levels

The carotid arteries were cleaned of connective tissues, cut into 0.5 cm lengths, and incubated with 1 mL oxygenated Krebs-KCl solution at pH 7.4, 37 °C for 30 min. The production of $O_2^{\bullet-}$ in the carotid arteries was determined by lucigenin-enhanced chemiluminescence, as previously described [31], with some modifications [32]. Plasma NOx was assayed using an enzymatic conversion method [33], with some modifications [32]. The concentrations of plasma TNF-α and TGF-β1 were measured using enzyme-immunoassay assay (ELISA) kits (eBioscienc, Inc., San Diego, CA, USA and ab119557, Abcam Plc, Cambridge, UK).

2.6. *Morphometric Analysis of Thoracic Aorta and Heart Tissue*

Heart weight (HW) and left ventricular weight (LVW) were measured, and calculated as an LVW/BW ratio. Thereafter, the left ventricles and thoracic aortas were fixed with 4% paraformaldehyde and then embedded in paraffin and cut into serial 5-μm-thick sections. Each section was stained with hematoxylin and eosin (H&E) and/or Picrosirius Red. Sections were captured with a Digital sight DS-2MV light microscope (Nikon, Tokyo, Japan) or a stereoscope (Nikon SMZ745T with NIS-elements D 3.2, Tokyo, Japan). Morphometric evaluations of the sections were performed with Image J software (National Institutes of Health, Bethesda, MD, USA).

2.7. *Western Blot Analysis of Tumor Necrosis Factor Receptor 1 (TNF-R1), TGF- β1, MMP-2 and MMP-9 Protein Expressions in Cardiac and Aortic Tissues*

Protein samples were prepared through the homogenization of cardiac and aortic tissues in a lysis buffer (Cell Signaling Technology Inc., Danvers, MA, USA). The proteins were then electrophoresed on a sodium dodecylsulfate polyacrylamide gel electrophoresis system and transferred to a polyvinylidene fluoride membrane (Millipore Corporation, Bedford, MA, USA). The membranes were blocked with 5% skimmed milk in Tris-buffered saline (TBS) with 0.1% Tween 20 for 2 h at room temperature before overnight incubation at 4 °C with primary antibodies against TNF-R1, TGF-β1, MMP-2, MMP-9, or β-actin (Santa Cruz Biotechnology, Inc., Santa Cruz, CA, USA). Thereafter, the membranes were washed three times with TBS and then incubated for 2 h at room temperature with a horseradish peroxidase conjugated secondary antibody. The protein bands were detected using Luminata™ Forte horseradish peroxidase (HRP) detection reagent (Merck KGaA, Darmstadt, Germany) and the densitometric analysis was performed using ImageQuantTM 400 (GE Healthcare Life Sciences, Piscataway, NJ, USA). The intensity of each band was normalized to that of β-actin, and data were expressed as a percentage of the values determined in the control group from the same gel.

2.8. *Statistical Analysis*

Data are expressed as mean ± S.E.M. The differences among the treatment groups were analyzed through a one-way analysis of variance (ANOVA) followed by Bonferini's post-hoc test. A *p*-value of less than 0.05 was considered as statistically significant.

3. Results

3.1. *Effects of Hesperidin and Captopril on Blood Pressure in Conscious Rats*

There were no significant differences in the systolic blood pressure of all the rats at the beginning of the study. The administration of L-NAME caused a gradual increase in the SP of all the rats compared to the control rats (SP at 5th week, 200.21 ± 6.52 vs. 122.14 ± 1.75 mmHg, $p < 0.01$, Figure 1). The co-administration of L-NAME and hesperidin at doses of 15 or 30 mg/kg (2.5 mg/kg) partially prevented L-NAME-induced high blood pressure in a dose-dependent manner compared to that of untreated rats (SP at 5th week, 177.50 ± 3.91 and 162.74 ± 2.82 mmHg, $p < 0.05$). Captopril also partially alleviated L-NAME-induced hypertension (152.19 ± 5.01 mmHg) compared to untreated rats ($p < 0.05$). In addition, captopril produced a greater preventive effect on SP than hesperidin (15 and 30 mg/kg).

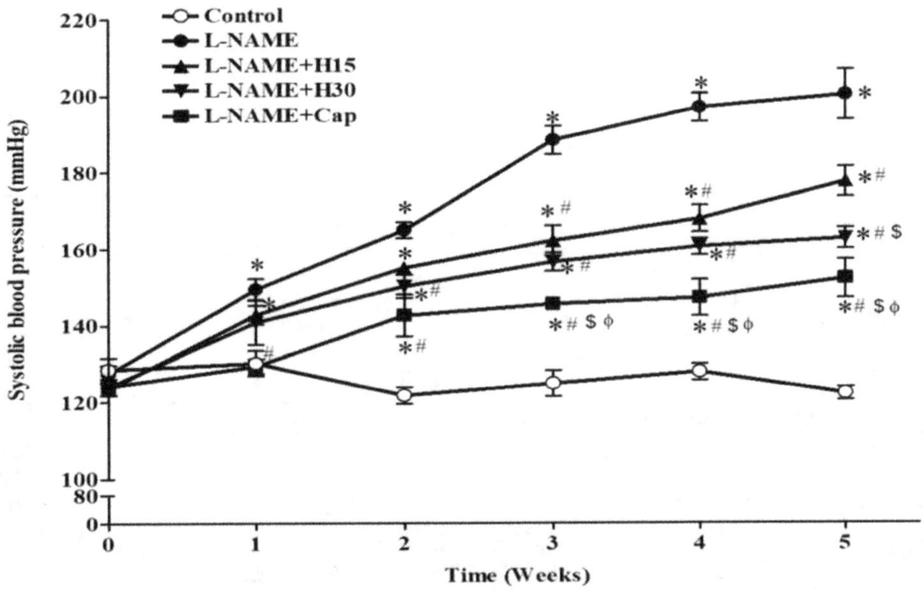

Figure 1. Time-course changes in systolic blood pressures of all experimental groups. Data are expressed as mean ± S.E.M (n = 7–8/group), * $p < 0.05$ vs. control, # $p < 0.05$ vs. L-NAME, $ $p < 0.05$ vs. L-NAME + hesperidin (15 mg/kg), Φ $p < 0.05$ vs. L-NAME + hesperidin (30 mg/kg) group.

3.2. Effects of Hesperidin and Captopril on SP, DP, MAP, and HR in Anesthetized Rats

The blood pressure data obtained using the indirect blood pressure measurement method were consistent with the values from the direct method since L-NAME treated rats exhibited high blood pressure, including high SP, DP, MAP, and high HR compared to those of control rats ($p < 0.05$, Table 1). Hesperidin at doses of 15 and 30 mg/kg significantly decreased SP, DP, and MAP in a dose-dependent manner compared to the untreated group ($p < 0.05$). Similarly, captopril reduced the development of hypertension induced by L-NAME compared to untreated rats ($p < 0.05$). Hesperidin at a dose 30 mg/kg, however, also affected the elevation of HR compared to untreated rats ($p < 0.05$, Table 1). Furthermore, hesperidin had no effect on blood pressure in normotensive rats (SP = 122.29 ± 4.05 mmHg, n =4).

Table 1. Effects of hesperidin and captopril on blood pressure and heart rate in anesthetized rats.

Parameters	Control	L-NAME	L-NAME + H15	L-NAME + H30	L-NAME + Cap
SP (mmHg)	120.92 ± 2.27	205.88 ± 3.19 *	179.38 ± 16.51 *,#	154.07 ± 4.88 *,#,$	140.14 ± 7.06 #,$
DP (mmHg)	72.68 ± 3.31	141.65 ± 5.73 *	114.13 ± 16.57 *,#	86.89 ± 5.74 *,#,$	91.48 ± 7.36 #,$
MAP (mmHg)	88.76 ± 2.47	161.41 ± 4.01 *	135.88 ± 16.00 *,#	109.28 ± 5.39 *,#,$	107.70 ± 6.27 #,$
HR (beat/min)	367.86 ± 11.90	419.30 ± 11.96 *	391.93 ± 14.35	351.44 ± 13.47 #,$	384.28 ± 17.31

SP: systolic blood pressure; DP: diastolic blood pressure; MAP: mean arterial pressure; HR: heart rate. Values are mean ± S.E.M (n = 7–8/group), * $p < 0.05$ vs. control, # $p < 0.05$ vs. L-NAME, $ $p < 0.05$ vs. L-NAME + H15.

3.3. Effects of Hesperidin and Captopril on Left Ventricular (LV) Morphometry and Fibrosis

Rat body weights did not differ among all experimental groups. After 5 weeks of L-NAME administration, the HW, LVW, and LVW/BW ratios were significantly increased compared to those of control rats. The co-administration of L-NAME and hesperidin or captopril significantly decreased those values when compared to the untreated group (Table 2). Morphometric analysis of hearts showed that the chronic administration of L-NAME significantly increased LV wall thickness and LV muscle fiber cross-sectional area (CSA) compared to the normal control group ($p < 0.05$, Table 2). Hypertensive rats that received hesperidin or captopril had significantly reduced wall thicknesses and CSA of the LV compared to untreated rats ($p < 0.05$) (Table 2, Figure 2A). LV fibrosis was significantly increased in the L-NAME-treated rats compared to the normal control rats ($p < 0.05$). Hesperidin or captopril treatment significantly prevented L-NAME-induced LV fibrosis compared to the untreated rats ($p < 0.05$) (Figure 2B).

Table 2. Effect of hesperidin and captopril on the cardiac mass indices and cardiovascular structural modifications in left ventricle and thoracic aorta.

Cardiac Mass Indices			
Groups	**Body Weight (g)**	**Heart Weight/BW (mg/g)**	**LVW/BW (mg/g)**
Control	434 ± 6.8	3.14 ± 0.17	2.06 ± 0.10
L-NAME	413 ± 16.9	4.21 ± 0.26 *	3.04 ± 0.18 *
L-NAME + H30	406 ± 9.7	3.11 ± 0.23 #	2.23 ± 0.17 #
L-NAME + Cap	401 ± 9.7	3.12 ± 0.18 #	2.07 ± 0.12 #
Left Ventricle			
Groups	**LV Wall Thickness (mm)**	**LV CSA (mm²)**	**LV Fibrosis (%)**
Control	2.72 ± 0.05	57.58 ± 1.05	0.69 ± 0.04
L-NAME	3.28 ± 0.04 *	72.42 ± 0.51 *	2.72 ± 0.15 *
L-NAME + H30	2.90 ± 0.06 #	61.12 ± 1.75 #	0.92 ± 0.09 #
L-NAME + Cap	2.79 ± 0.09 #	59.87 ± 1.63 #	1.00 ± 0.06 #

Thoracic Aorta Structural Modifications				
Groups	**Wall Thickness (μm)**	**CSA (×10³ μm²)**	**VSMCs (cells/CSA)**	**Collagen Deposition (% Area Fraction)**
Control	106.39 ± 1.02	579.00 ± 15.16	1298.00 ± 73.64	15.78 ± 0.70
L-NAME	150.58 ± 2.09 *	810.50 ± 18.64 *	2013.71 ± 51.62 *	31.32 ± 1.00 *
L-NAME + H30	127.11 ± 2.90 *,#	617.95 ± 18.65 #	1540.16 ± 46.88 *,#	24.84 ± 0.69 *,#
L-NAME + Cap	129.91 ± 6.50 *,#	658.38 ± 40.22 #	1671.78 ± 24.90 *,#	23.68 ± 0.63 *,#

LV: left ventricular, LVW: left ventricular weight, BW: body weight, CSA: cross-sectional area, VSMCs: vascular smooth muscle cells. Values are expressed as mean ± S.E.M, ($n = 6$/group). * $p < 0.05$ when compared to the control group, and # $p < 0.05$ when compared to the L-NAME group.

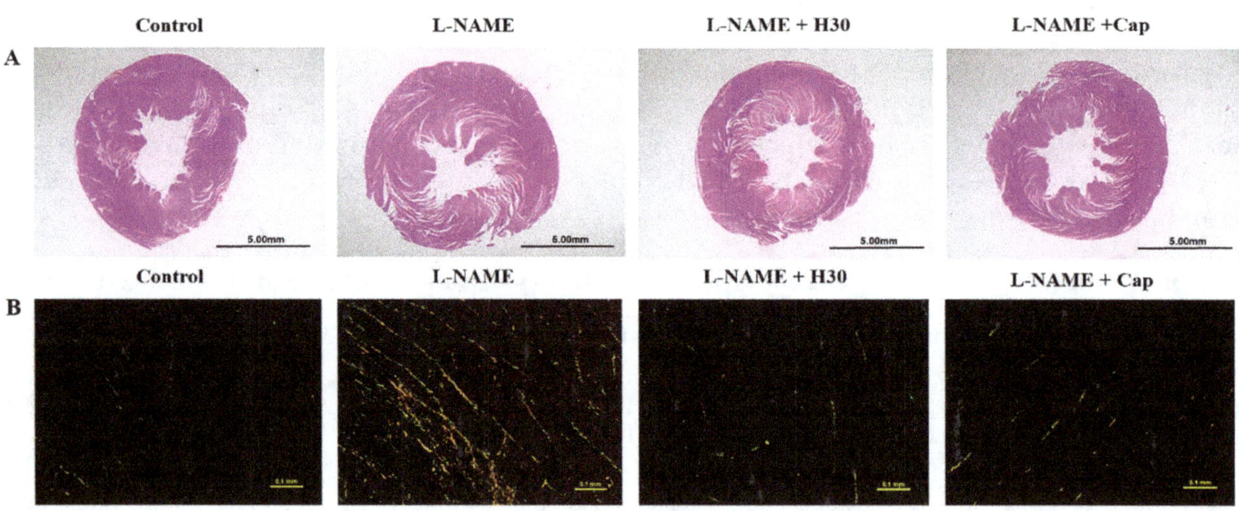

Figure 2. The histology and morphology of LV from control, L-NAME, L-NAME + hesperidin (30 mg/kg) and L-NAME + captopril (2.5 mg/kg) groups. Representative images of LV sections, (**A**) stained with hematoxylin and eosin under stereomicroscopes, and (**B**) stained with picrosirius red under a polarized light microscope using a 20× objective lens.

3.4. Effect of Hesperidin and Captopril on Vascular Morphology

Vascular wall hypertrophy was observed in thoracic aortas collected from L-NAME hypertensive rats (Figure 3A) with significant increases in vascular wall thickness, CSA, and smooth muscle cells numbers compared to those of the control rats ($p < 0.05$; Table 2, Figure 3A). Moreover, the relative amounts of collagen depositions (Figure 3B) in the aortic walls of L-NAME hypertensive rats were also clearly observed ($p < 0.05$; Table 2, Figure 3B). Hesperidin or captopril treatment partially prevented the vascular structural abnormalities in aortas induced by L-NAME ($p < 0.05$).

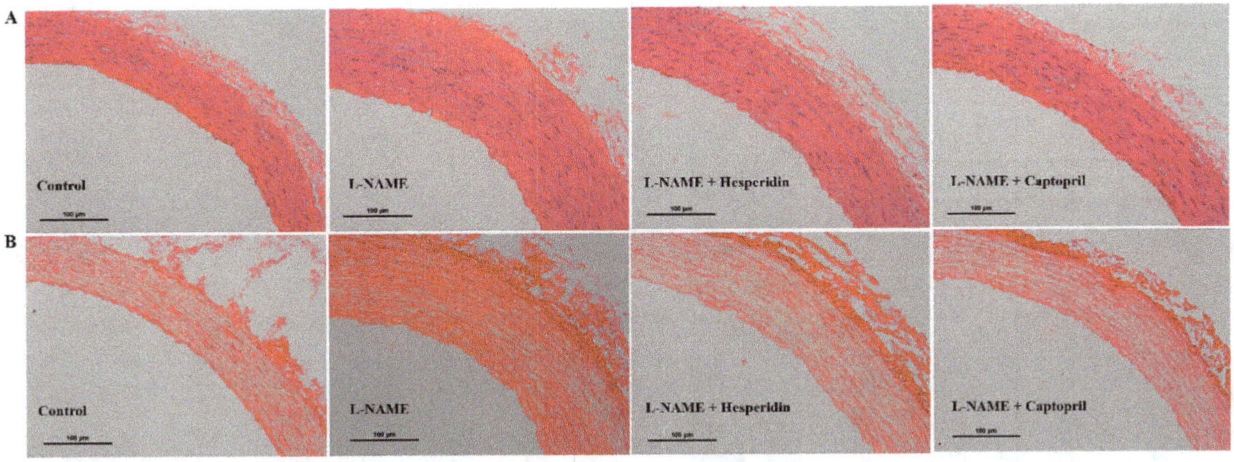

Figure 3. The histology and morphology of thoracic aorta from control, L-NAME, L-NAME + hesperidin (30 mg/kg), and L-NAME + captopril (2.5 mg/kg) groups. Representative images of aortic sections, (**A**) stained with hematoxylin and eosin and (**B**) stained with picrosirius red under a light microscope using a 20× objective lens.

3.5. Effects of Hesperidin and Captopril Supplementation on Oxidative Stress Markers, Plasma Nitric Oxide Metabolites (NOx) Levels in L-NAME Treated Rats

L-NAME treated rats showed a significant increase in the production of vascular $O_2^{\bullet-}$ (263.26 ± 11.20 vs. 71.42 ± 15.97 count/mg dry wt/min, $p < 0.001$) and plasma MDA levels compared to the control groups (10.24 ± 0.4 vs. 3.11 ± 0.27 μM, $p < 0.05$). When treated with hesperidin or captopril, the elevations of vascular $O_2^{\bullet-}$ and plasma MDA were mitigated compared to those of untreated rats (7.91 ± 0.92, 4.83 ± 0.74 and 3.88 ± 0.25 count/mg dry wt/min and 138.86 ± 28.75, 97.28 ± 16.67 and 92.14 ± 12.90 μM, $p < 0.05$) (Figure 4A,B). In addition, low levels of plasma NOx were found in L-NAME hypertensive rats compared to control rats (3.49 ± 1.0 vs. 10.17 ± 0.95 μM, $p < 0.05$). These low levels of plasma NOx were improved by hesperidin or captopril supplementation (4.38 ± 1.15, 7.48 ± 1.03 and 8.48 ± 1.21 μM, $p < 0.05$) (Figure 4C).

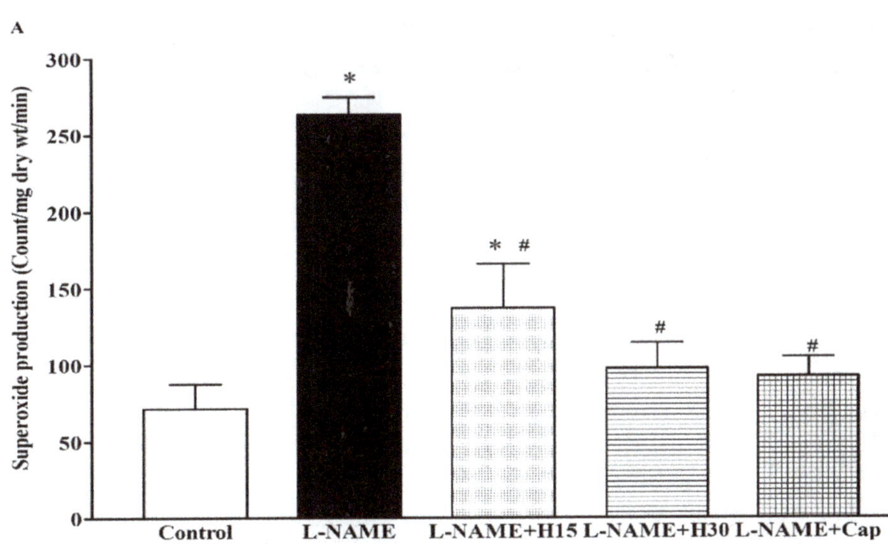

Figure 4. *Cont.*

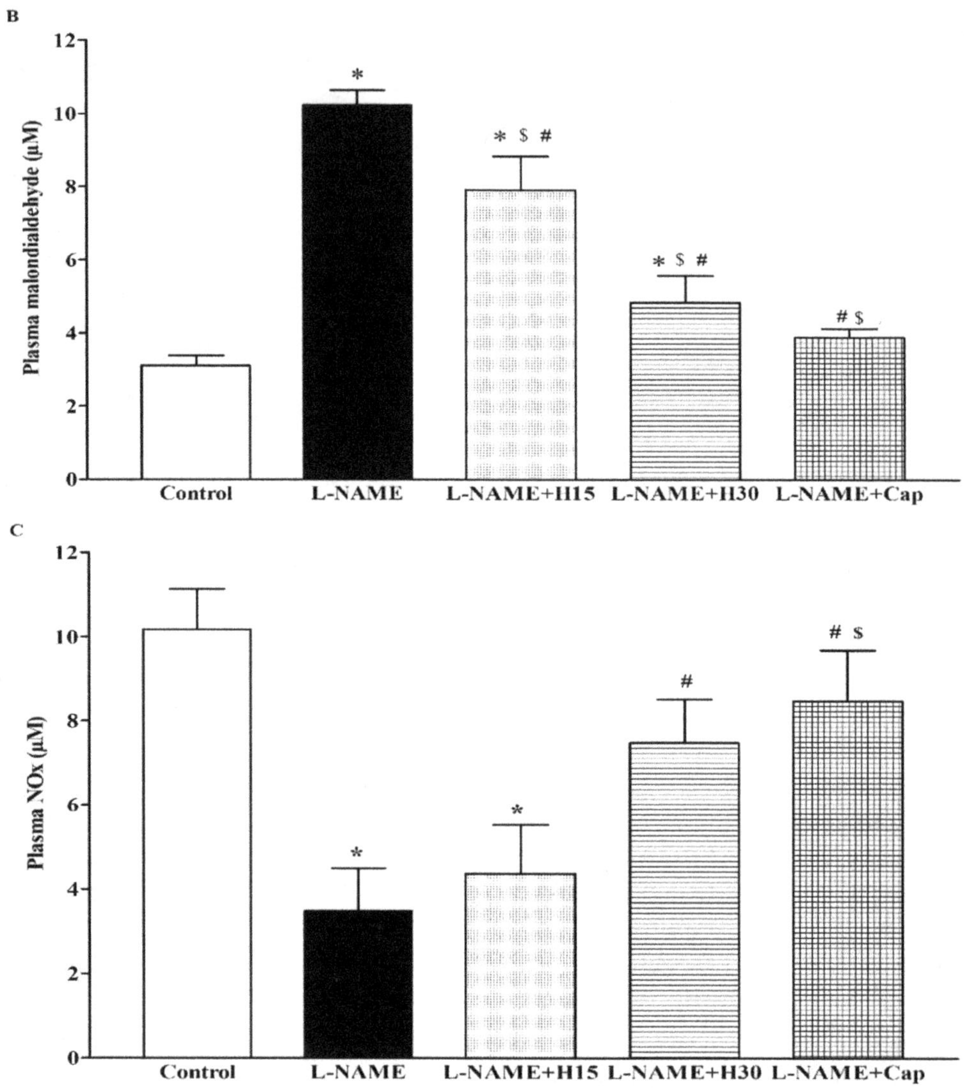

Figure 4. Effects of hesperidin and captopril supplementation on vascular $O_2^{\bullet -}$ production, (**A**) plasma MDA (**B**) and plasma NOx (**C**) levels in control, L-NAME, L-NAME + hesperidin (15 mg/kg), L-NAME + hesperidin (30 mg/kg) and L-NAME + captopril (5 mg/kg) groups. Data are expressed as mean ± S.E.M (n = 7–8/group), * $p < 0.05$ vs. control, # $p < 0.05$ vs. L-NAME group, $ $p < 0.05$ vs. L-NAME + H15.

3.6. Effects of Hesperidin and Captopril on Protein Expression of TNF-R1 and TGF-β1 in Heart Tissues and Concentrations of TNF-α and TGF-β1 in Plasma

Over-expressions of TNF-R1 and TGF-β1 proteins were found in heart tissues collected from the hypertensive group compared to the control group ($p < 0.001$). Interestingly, supplementation with hesperidin and captopril partially reversed these protein up-regulations ($p < 0.01$; Figure 5A,B). These results were consistent with the results in that high levels of plasma TNF-α and TGF-β1 were observed in L-NAME hypertensive rats compared to those of control rats (168.49 ± 13.05 vs. 24.21 ± 8.51 pg/mL and 23.54 ± 3.91 vs. 4.90 ± 0.50 ng/mL, $p < 0.01$). The administration of hesperidin or captopril attenuated these high levels of plasma TNF-α (58.23 ± 14.71 or 20.97 ± 6.97 pg/mL) and TGF-β1 (5.23 ± 0.32 or 4.79 ± 0.55 ng/mL, $p < 0.05$) in hypertensive rats (Figure 5C,D).

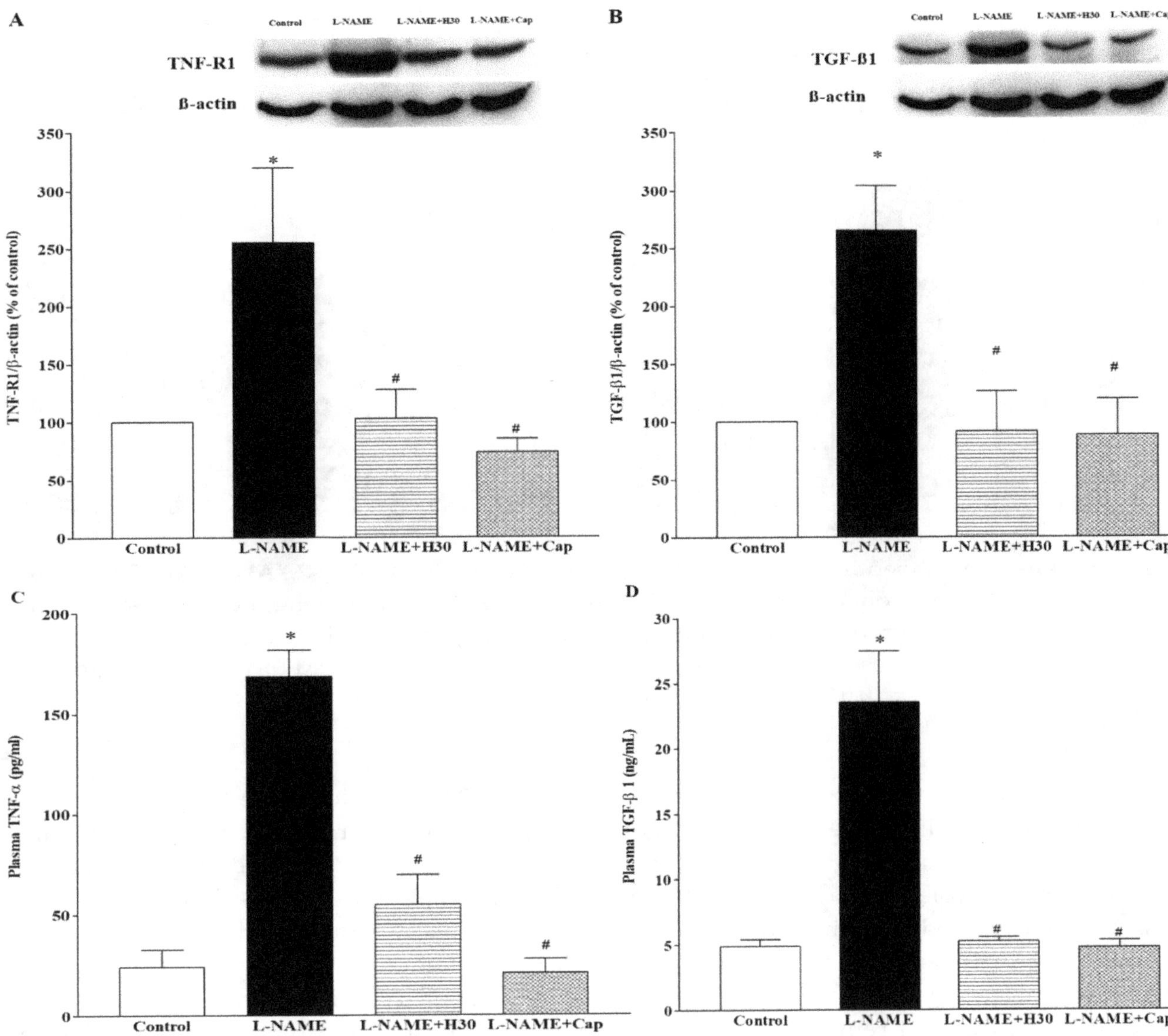

Figure 5. Effects of hesperidin and captopril on protein expression of TNF-R1, (**A**) and TGF-β1, (**B**) in heart tissue and on concentrations of plasma TNF-α, (**C**) and TGF-β1, (**D**) collected from control, L-NAME, L-NAME + hesperidin (30 mg/kg) and L-NAME + captopril (2.5 mg/kg) groups. The top panel shows the representative bands of TNF-R1, (**A**) and TGF-β1, (**B**) protein expression in heart tissues. Values are mean ± S.E.M ($n = 4$ for each group), * $p < 0.05$ vs. control, # $p < 0.05$ vs. L-NAME group.

3.7. Effects of Hesperidin and Captopril on Protein Expression of MMP-2 and MMP-9 in Aortic Tissue

A significant increase in MMP-2 and MMP-9 protein expression was observed in thoracic aortic tissues collected from the hypertensive group compared to the control group (Figure 6A,B, $p < 0.05$). Hesperidin or captopril treatment significantly suppressed the level of MMP-2 and MMP-9 protein expression compared to untreated rats, ($p < 0.05$).

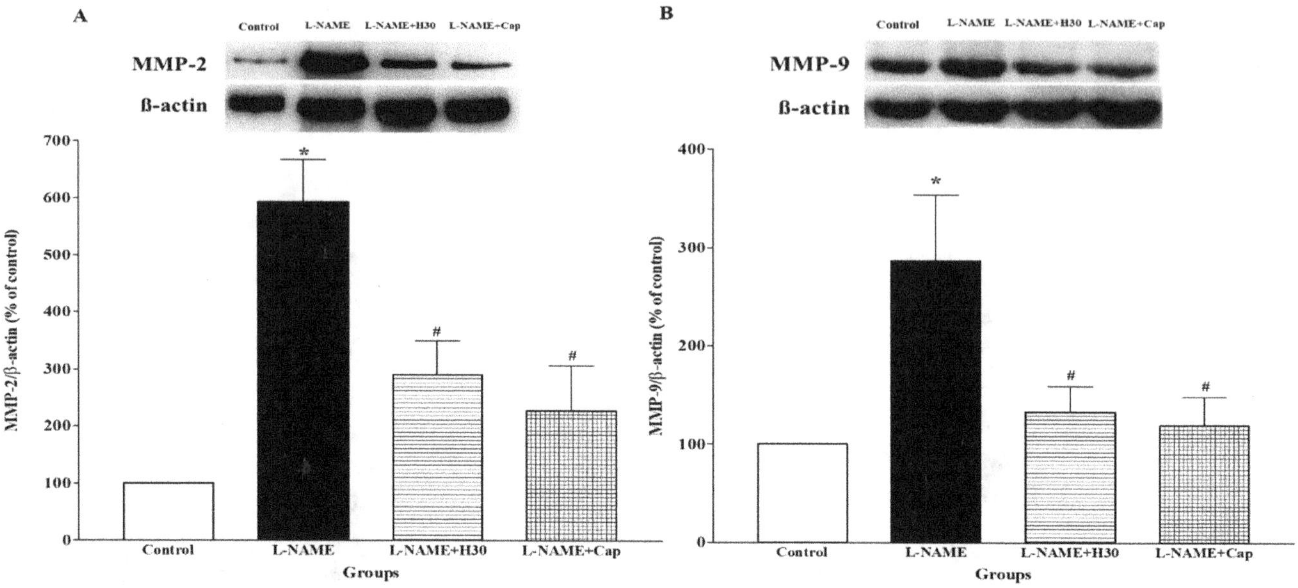

Figure 6. Effects of hesperidin and captopril on protein expression of MMP-2, (**A**) and MMP-9, (**B**) in aortic tissue collected from control, L-NAME, L-NAME + hesperidin (30 mg/kg) and L-NAME + captopril (2.5 mg/kg) groups. The top panels show the representative bands of MMP-2, (**A**) and MMP-9, (**B**) protein expression in thoracic aortas. Values are mean ± S.E.M (n = 4 for each group), * $p < 0.05$ vs. control, # $p < 0.05$ vs. L-NAME group.

4. Discussion

This study demonstrates that rats that received L-NAME developed hypertension and cardiovascular remodeling. Hesperidin mitigated high blood pressure and cardiac remodeling by reducing the left ventricular hypertrophy and fibrosis associated with down-regulations of TGF-β1 and TNF-R1 protein expression and a reduction of plasma TGF-β1 levels in L-NAME-induced hypertension in rats. Vascular remodeling, including vascular hypertrophy and increased collagen deposition, induced by L-NAME in rats was inhibited by hesperidin supplementation. This was consistent with the decreased protein expression of MMP-2 and MMP-9 in aortic tissue. Furthermore, hesperidin preventing cardiovascular remodeling induced by L-NAME in the present study was linked to the reduction of an inflammatory cytokine, oxidative stress markers, and enhanced NO availability.

It was found that chronic treatment of L-NAME led to the development of NO-deficient hypertension as well as cardiovascular remodeling. These remodelings included increases in LVW/HW ratio, LV wall thickness, LV CSA, LV fibrosis, aortic wall thickness, aortic cross-sectional areas, aortic smooth muscle cell numbers, and collagen deposition. It is well-accepted that the chronic inhibition of NO synthase using L-NAME results in NO depletion, increased vascular tone, and high blood pressure [34]. Several studies have demonstrated that cardiovascular remodeling occurs after chronic treatment with L-NAME (40 mg/kg) for five weeks [4,10,35]. The mechanisms involved in cardiac remodeling in an animal model of nitric oxide-deficient hypertension are still unclear; however, two possible mechanisms related to hemodynamics and non-hemodynamic aspects have been described [36]. Hemodynamic overload in hypertension provoked left ventricular hypertrophy because of the adaptive response to conserve cardiac output [37]. A reduction in NO is one of several non-hemodynamic factors that participate in cardiac remodeling because when NO is suppressed, hypertensive cardiac remodeling through the cyclic guanosine monophosphate/protein kinase G (cGMP/PKG) pathway is initiated to inhibit fibrotic synthesis [38]. It is well-documented that vascular remodeling in hypertension occurs in response to long-term modifications of hemodynamic conditions [39,40]. Furthermore, numerous studies have reported that vascular remodeling is characterized by increases in wall thickness, CSA, and smooth muscle cell numbers in L-NAME hypertensive rats [3,4,41]. In this study, hesperidin partially inhibited the development of hypertension as well as cardiovascular remodeling induced by chronic L-NAME treatment. These effects may have involved an increase in NO bioavailability, reductions of oxidative stress, and inflammation as further possibilities.

Oxidative stress is one of the important mechanisms of L-NAME-induced hypertension since L-arginine analogues activate eNOS uncoupling, leading to an overwhelming vascular superoxide generation [42]. Then, superoxide can rapidly react with nitric oxide to form peroxynitrite [43]. This reaction results in reducing nitric oxide bioavailability [44]. In the present study, increases in plasma MDA levels and vascular superoxide production were accompanied by decreased plasma NOx levels observed in the L-NAME hypertensive rats. Hesperidin alleviated L-NAME-induced oxidative stress and thus increased NO bioavailability with an increase in the plasma NOx level. Many studies have confirmed that hesperidin has a strong antioxidant activity [26,45]. Hesperidin exhibits its antioxidant properties with two main mechanisms, including directly scavenging reactive oxygen species [46], and boosting cellular antioxidant defense [25]. Thus, this is one of the possible mechanisms of the cardiovascular protective effects of hesperidin in this study that might have involved its antioxidant capability, resulting in increased NO bioavailability, which reduced vascular resistance.

There is substantial evidence to suggest that inflammation is one of pathologies that occurs in L-NAME hypertensive rats [47,48]. The results of this study proved that, as in the previous studies, there were increases in the levels of pro-inflammatory cytokine, TNF-α, in plasma and expression of TNF-α protein in the heart tissue of L-NAME hypertensive rats. Myocardial TGF-β protein expression was also observed in L-NAME hypertensive rats. It is well-established that TGF-β plays an important role in responses to inflammation to activate fibrogenesis, which is an important pathological process for cardiac remodeling [49,50]. The present study has also shown that hesperidin attenuated cardiac remodeling, accompanied by decreased systemic and heart inflammation in L-NAME hypertensive rats. The protein expression of TGF-β in cardiac tissue was also down-regulated in the hesperidin supplemented group. The anti-inflammatory effect of hesperidin has been clearly revealed in both cellular and animal models. In human umbilical vein endothelial cells, hesperidin significantly suppressed TNF-α [51]. Li and coworkers demonstrated that hesperidin decreased the production of IL-1β, IL-6, and TNF-α in a rat model of rheumatoid arthritis [52]. Thus, the current results confirmed that the cardiprotective effect of hesperidin was associated with its great anti-inflammatory effect.

Additionally, vascular remodeling with collagen deposition was associated with the overexpression of MMP-2 and MMP-9 in aortic tissue in L-NAME hypertensive rats, as shown in this study. Several studies report that MMPs play an important role in physiological processes that contribute to hypertension-induced maladaptive arterial changes and sustained hypertension [53,54]. The overexpression of MMP-mediated vascular remodeling was stimulated by oxidative stress and inflammatory cytokines [54]. Del Mauro and coworkers demonstrated that MMP-2 and MMP-9 activity was a pathologic process in L-NAME-induced morphometric alterations in the aorta [55]. Interestingly, the authors of the present study first reported L-NAME-induced hypertension and vascular remodeling in rats in which there was an up-regulation of MMP-2 and MMP-9 protein expression in response to oxidative stress. Hesperidin prevented vascular remodeling induced by L-NAME associated with the down-regulation of MMP-2 and MMP-9. This effect might be involved in its antioxidant and anti-inflammatory effects, which further inhibited MMP activation and collagen degradation.

Captopril was used as a positive control to prevent the development of hypertension and cardiovascular remodeling. These findings are supported by previous studies that found that captopril prevented high blood pressure, left ventricular hypertrophy, and vascular remodeling induced by L-NAME in rats [56,57]. Captopril also reduced oxidative stress and inflammatory markers and suppressed protein expressions of TNF-R1, TGF-β1, and MMPs. An antioxidative effect of captopril in the present study might be associated with two main mechanisms, direct and indirect effects. Captopril contains free sulfhydryl groups that directly scavenge oxygen free radicals [58], or it suppresses AT1R-mediated NADPH oxidase expression and superoxide production [10]. It has been demonstrated that captopril improved ventricular hypertrophy in rats by suppressing MMP-2 and MMP-9 expression [59]. In addition, an anti-inflammatory effect of captopril in the animal model of hypertension has been reported [60].

In conclusion, the findings of this study indicated that hesperidin had cardiovascular protective effects by preventing the L-NAME-induced development of hypertension and cardiovascular remodeling in rats. These effects were affirmed by reducing oxidative stress and inflammation.

Author Contributions: P.M. performed the majority of the experiments and wrote the manuscript; S.B., T.B., P.P. (Prapassorn Potue) and P.P. (Parichat Prachaney), U.K., V.K. contributed to the data analysis; P.P. (Poungrat Pakdeechote) designed and supervised the study, and checked the final manuscript.

Acknowledgments: We would like to thank James A. Will for editing this manuscript via the Publication Clinic, KKU, Thailand.

References

1. Furchgott, R.F.; Zawadzki, J.V. The obligatory role of endothelial cells in the relaxation of arterial smooth muscle by acetylcholine. *Nature* **1980**, *288*, 373–376. [CrossRef] [PubMed]
2. Bunbupha, S.; Pakdeechote, P.; Kukongviriyapan, U.; Prachaney, P.; Kukongviriyapan, V. Asiatic acid reduces blood pressure by enhancing nitric oxide bioavailability with modulation of eNOS and p47phox expression in L-NAME-induced hypertensive rats. *Phytother. Res.* **2014**, *28*, 1506–1512. [CrossRef] [PubMed]
3. Pechanova, O.; Bernatova, I.; Babal, P.; Martinez, M.C.; Kysela, S.; Stvrtina, S.; Andriantsitohaina, R. Red wine polyphenols prevent cardiovascular alterations in L-NAME-induced hypertension. *J. Hypertens.* **2004**, *22*, 1551–1559. [CrossRef] [PubMed]
4. Bunbupha, S.; Prachaney, P.; Kukongviriyapan, U.; Kukongviriyapan, V.; Welbat, J.U.; Pakdeechote, P. Asiatic acid alleviates cardiovascular remodelling in rats with L-NAME-induced hypertension. *Clin. Exp. Pharmacol. Physiol.* **2015**, *42*, 1189–1197. [CrossRef] [PubMed]
5. Bernatova, I.; Pechanova, O.; Babal, P.; Kysela, S.; Stvrtina, S.; Andriantsitohaina, R. Wine polyphenols improve cardiovascular remodeling and vascular function in NO-deficient hypertension. *Am. J. Physiol. Heart Circ. Physiol.* **2002**, *282*, H942–H948. [CrossRef] [PubMed]
6. Liu, L.; Eisen, H.J. Epidemiology of heart failure and scope of the problem. *Cardiol. Clin.* **2014**, *32*, 1–8. [CrossRef] [PubMed]
7. Babal, P.; Pechanova, O.; Bernatova, I.; Stvrtina, S. Chronic inhibition of NO synthesis produces myocardial fibrosis and arterial media hyperplasia. *Histol. Histopathol.* **1997**, *12*, 623–629. [PubMed]
8. Mir, S.A.; Chatterjee, A.; Mitra, A.; Pathak, K.; Mahata, S.K.; Sarkar, S. Inhibition of signal transducer and activator of transcription 3 (STAT3) attenuates interleukin-6 (IL-6)-induced collagen synthesis and resultant hypertrophy in rat heart. *J. Biol. Chem.* **2012**, *287*, 2666–2677. [CrossRef] [PubMed]
9. Siwik, D.A.; Pagano, P.J.; Colucci, W.S. Oxidative stress regulates collagen synthesis and matrix metalloproteinase activity in cardiac fibroblasts. *Am. J. Physiol. Cell Physiol.* **2001**, *280*, C53–C60. [CrossRef] [PubMed]
10. Boonprom, P.; Boonla, O.; Chayaburakul, K.; Welbat, J.U.; Pannangpetch, P.; Kukongviriyapan, U.; Kukongviriyapan, V.; Pakdeechote, P.; Prachaney, P. Garcinia mangostana pericarp extract protects against oxidative stress and cardiovascular remodeling via suppression of p47(phox) and iNOS in nitric oxide deficient rats. *Ann. Anat.* **2017**, *212*, 27–36. [CrossRef] [PubMed]
11. Ndisang, J.F.; Chibbar, R.; Lane, N. Heme oxygenase suppresses markers of heart failure and ameliorates cardiomyopathy in L-NAME-induced hypertension. *Eur. J. Pharmacol.* **2014**, *734*, 23–34. [CrossRef] [PubMed]
12. Cao, S.; Zheng, B.; Chen, T.; Chang, X.; Yin, B.; Huang, Z.; Shuai, P.; Han, L. Semen brassicae ameliorates hepatic fibrosis by regulating transforming growth factor-beta1/Smad, nuclear factor-kappaB, and AKT signaling pathways in rats. *Drug Des. Dev. Ther.* **2018**, *12*, 1205–1213. [CrossRef] [PubMed]
13. Bowen, T.; Jenkins, R.H.; Fraser, D.J. MicroRNAs, transforming growth factor beta-1, and tissue fibrosis. *J. Pathol.* **2013**, *229*, 274–285. [CrossRef] [PubMed]
14. Xu, F.; Liu, C.; Zhou, D.; Zhang, L. TGF-beta/SMAD pathway and its regulation in hepatic fibrosis. *J. Histochem. Cytochem.* **2016**, *64*, 157–167. [CrossRef] [PubMed]
15. Arribas, S.M.; Hinek, A.; Gonzalez, M.C. Elastic fibres and vascular structure in hypertension. *Pharmacol. Ther.* **2006**, *111*, 771–791. [CrossRef] [PubMed]

16. Moon, S.K.; Cha, B.Y.; Kim, C.H. ERK1/2 mediates TNF-alpha-induced matrix metalloproteinase-9 expression in human vascular smooth muscle cells via the regulation of NF-kappaB and AP-1: Involvement of the ras dependent pathway. *J. Cell. Physiol.* **2004**, *198*, 417–427. [CrossRef] [PubMed]
17. Arenas, I.A.; Xu, Y.; Lopez-Jaramillo, P.; Davidge, S.T. Angiotensin II-induced MMP-2 release from endothelial cells is mediated by TNF-alpha. *Am. J. Physiol. Cell Physiol.* **2004**, *286*, C779–C784. [CrossRef] [PubMed]
18. Li, H.; Liang, J.; Castrillon, D.H.; DePinho, R.A.; Olson, E.N.; Liu, Z.P. FoxO4 regulates tumor necrosis factor alpha-directed smooth muscle cell migration by activating matrix metalloproteinase 9 gene transcription. *Mol. Cell. Biol.* **2007**, *27*, 2676–2686. [CrossRef] [PubMed]
19. Wilson, T.W.; Dubois, M.P. New drugs for the treatment of hypertension: Where do they fit? *Can. Fam. Phys.* **1987**, *33*, 2583–2589.
20. Rodriguez-Garcia, J.L.; Villa, E.; Serrano, M.; Gallardo, J.; Garcia-Robles, R. Prostacyclin: Its pathogenic role in essential hypertension and the class effect of ACE inhibitors on prostaglandin metabolism. *Blood Press* **1999**, *8*, 279–284. [CrossRef] [PubMed]
21. Maneesai, P.; Prasarttong, P.; Bunbupha, S.; Kukongviriyapan, U.; Kukongviriyapan, V.; Tangsucharit, P.; Prachaney, P.; Pakdeechote, P. Synergistic Antihypertensive effect of *Carthamus tinctorius* L. extract and captopril in L-NAME-induced hypertensive rats via restoration of eNOS and AT(1)R expression. *Nutrients* **2016**, *8*, 122. [CrossRef] [PubMed]
22. Suzuki, S.; Sato, H.; Shimada, H.; Takashima, N.; Arakawa, M. Comparative free radical scavenging action of angiotensin-converting enzyme inhibitors with and without the sulfhydryl radical. *Pharmacology* **1993**, *47*, 61–65. [CrossRef] [PubMed]
23. Sonoda, K.; Ohtake, K.; Uchida, H.; Ito, J.; Uchida, M.; Natsume, H.; Tamada, H.; Kobayashi, J. Dietary nitrite supplementation attenuates cardiac remodeling in L-NAME-induced hypertensive rats. *Nitric Oxide* **2017**, *67*, 1–9. [CrossRef] [PubMed]
24. Emim, J.A.; Oliveira, A.B.; Lapa, A.J. Pharmacological evaluation of the anti-inflammatory activity of a citrus bioflavonoid, hesperidin, and the isoflavonoids, duartin and claussequinone, in rats and mice. *J. Pharm. Pharmacol.* **1994**, *46*, 118–122. [CrossRef] [PubMed]
25. Wilmsen, P.K.; Spada, D.S.; Salvador, M. Antioxidant activity of the flavonoid hesperidin in chemical and biological systems. *J. Agric. Food Chem.* **2005**, *53*, 4757–4761. [CrossRef] [PubMed]
26. Selvaraj, P.; Pugalendi, K.V. Hesperidin, a flavanone glycoside, on lipid peroxidation and antioxidant status in experimental myocardial ischemic rats. *Redox Rep.* **2010**, *15*, 217–223. [CrossRef] [PubMed]
27. Homayouni, F.; Haidari, F.; Hedayati, M.; Zakerkish, M.; Ahmadi, K. Blood pressure lowering and anti-inflammatory effects of hesperidin in type 2 diabetes; a randomized double-blind controlled clinical trial. *Phytother. Res.* **2018**, *32*, 1073–1079. [CrossRef] [PubMed]
28. Ren, H.; Hao, J.; Liu, T.; Zhang, D.; Lv, H.; Song, E.; Zhu, C. Hesperetin suppresses inflammatory responses in lipopolysaccharide-induced raw 264.7 cells via the inhibition of NF-kappaB and activation of Nrf2/HO-1 pathways. *Inflammation* **2016**, *39*, 964–973. [PubMed]
29. Giannini, I.; Amato, A.; Basso, L.; Tricomi, N.; Marranci, M.; Pecorella, G.; Tafuri, S.; Pennisi, D.; Altomare, D.F. Flavonoids mixture (diosmin, troxerutin, hesperidin) in the treatment of acute hemorrhoidal disease: A prospective, randomized, triple-blind, controlled trial. *Tech. Coloproctol.* **2015**, *19*, 665–666. [CrossRef] [PubMed]
30. Wunpathe, C.; Potue, P.; Maneesai, P.; Bunbupha, S.; Prachaney, P.; Kukongviriyapan, U.; Kukongviriyapan, V.; Pakdeechote, P. Hesperidin suppresses renin-angiotensin system mediated NOX2 over-expression and sympathoexcitation in 2K-1C hypertensive rats. *Am. J. Chin. Med.* **2018**, *46*, 751–767. [CrossRef]
31. Lu, F.J.; Lin, J.T.; Wang, H.P.; Huang, W.C. A simple, sensitive, non-stimulated photon counting system for detection of superoxide anion in whole blood. *Experientia* **1996**, *52*, 141–144. [CrossRef] [PubMed]
32. Luangaram, S.; Kukongviriyapan, U.; Pakdeechote, P.; Kukongviriyapan, V.; Pannangpetch, P. Protective effects of quercetin against phenylhydrazine-induced vascular dysfunction and oxidative stress in rats. *Food Chem. Toxicol.* **2007**, *45*, 448–455. [CrossRef] [PubMed]
33. Verdon, C.P.; Burton, B.A.; Prior, R.L. Sample pretreatment with nitrate reductase and glucose-6-phosphate dehydrogenase quantitatively reduces nitrate while avoiding interference by NADP+ when the Griess reaction is used to assay for nitrite. *Anal. Biochem.* **1995**, *224*, 502–508. [CrossRef] [PubMed]
34. Ribeiro, M.O.; Antunes, E.; de Nucci, G.; Lovisolo, S.M.; Zatz, R. Chronic inhibition of nitric oxide synthesis. A new model of arterial hypertension. *Hypertension* **1992**, *20*, 298–303. [CrossRef] [PubMed]

35. Paulis, L.; Zicha, J.; Kunes, J.; Hojna, S.; Behuliak, M.; Celec, P.; Kojsova, S.; Pechanova, O.; Simko, F. Regression of L-NAME-induced hypertension: The role of nitric oxide and endothelium-derived constricting factor. *Hypertens. Res.* **2008**, *31*, 793–803. [CrossRef] [PubMed]
36. Simko, F.; Simko, J. The potential role of nitric oxide in the hypertrophic growth of the left ventricle. *Physiol. Res.* **2000**, *49*, 37–46. [PubMed]
37. Simko, F. Physiologic and pathologic myocardial hypertrophy–physiologic and pathologic regression of hypertrophy? *Med. Hypotheses* **2002**, *58*, 11–14. [CrossRef] [PubMed]
38. Lee, D.I.; Kass, D.A. Phosphodiesterases and cyclic GMP regulation in heart muscle. *Physiology* **2012**, *27*, 248–258. [CrossRef] [PubMed]
39. Wolinsky, H. Response of the rat aortic media to hypertension: Morphological and chemical studies. *Circ. Res.* **1970**, *26*, 507–522. [CrossRef] [PubMed]
40. Gibbons, G.H.; Dzau, V.J. The emerging concept of vascular remodeling. *N. Engl. J. Med.* **1994**, *330*, 1431–1438. [PubMed]
41. Tronc, F.; Wassef, M.; Esposito, B.; Henrion, D.; Glagov, S.; Tedgui, A. Role of NO in flow-induced remodeling of the rabbit common carotid artery. *Arterioscler. Thromb. Vasc. Biol.* **1996**, *16*, 1256–1262. [CrossRef] [PubMed]
42. Leo, M.D.; Kandasamy, K.; Subramani, J.; Tandan, S.K.; Kumar, D. Involvement of inducible nitric oxide synthase and dimethyl arginine dimethylaminohydrolase in Nomega-nitro-L-arginine methyl ester (L-NAME)-induced hypertension. *Cardiovasc. Pathol.* **2015**, *24*, 49–55. [CrossRef] [PubMed]
43. Xia, Y.; Zweier, J.L. Superoxide and peroxynitrite generation from inducible nitric oxide synthase in macrophages. *Proc. Natl. Acad. Sci. USA* **1997**, *94*, 6954–6958. [CrossRef] [PubMed]
44. Pryor, W.A.; Squadrito, G.L. The chemistry of peroxynitrite: A product from the reaction of nitric oxide with superoxide. *Am. J. Physiol.* **1995**, *268*, L699–L722. [CrossRef] [PubMed]
45. Garg, A.; Garg, S.; Zaneveld, L.J.; Singla, A.K. Chemistry and pharmacology of the citrus bioflavonoid hesperidin. *Phytother. Res.* **2001**, *15*, 655–669. [CrossRef] [PubMed]
46. Kim, J.Y.; Jung, K.J.; Choi, J.S.; Chung, H.Y. Hesperetin: A potent antioxidant against peroxynitrite. *Free Radic. Res.* **2004**, *38*, 761–769. [CrossRef] [PubMed]
47. Gonzalez, W.; Fontaine, V.; Pueyo, M.E.; Laquay, N.; Messika-Zeitoun, D.; Philippe, M.; Arnal, J.F.; Jacob, M.P.; Michel, J.B. Molecular plasticity of vascular wall during N(G)-nitro-L-arginine methyl ester-induced hypertension: Modulation of proinflammatory signals. *Hypertension* **2000**, *36*, 103–109. [CrossRef] [PubMed]
48. Luvara, G.; Pueyo, M.E.; Philippe, M.; Mandet, C.; Savoie, F.; Henrion, D.; Michel, J.B. Chronic blockade of NO synthase activity induces a proinflammatory phenotype in the arterial wall: Prevention by angiotensin II antagonism. *Arterioscler. Thromb. Vasc. Biol.* **1998**, *18*, 1408–1416. [CrossRef] [PubMed]
49. Miguel-Carrasco, J.L.; Mate, A.; Monserrat, M.T.; Arias, J.L.; Aramburu, O.; Vazquez, C.M. The role of inflammatory markers in the cardioprotective effect of L-carnitine in L-NAME-induced hypertension. *Am. J. Hypertens.* **2008**, *21*, 1231–1237. [CrossRef] [PubMed]
50. Nyby, M.D.; Abedi, K.; Smutko, V.; Eslami, P.; Tuck, M.L. Vascular Angiotensin type 1 receptor expression is associated with vascular dysfunction, oxidative stress and inflammation in fructose-fed rats. *Hypertens. Res.* **2007**, *30*, 451–457. [CrossRef] [PubMed]
51. Nizamutdinova, I.T.; Jeong, J.J.; Xu, G.H.; Lee, S.H.; Kang, S.S.; Kim, Y.S.; Chang, K.C.; Kim, H.J. Hesperidin, hesperidin methyl chalone and phellopterin from Poncirus trifoliata (Rutaceae) differentially regulate the expression of adhesion molecules in tumor necrosis factor-alpha-stimulated human umbilical vein endothelial cells. *Int. Immunopharmacol.* **2008**, *8*, 670–678. [CrossRef] [PubMed]
52. Li, R.; Li, J.; Cai, L.; Hu, C.M.; Zhang, L. Suppression of adjuvant arthritis by hesperidin in rats and its mechanisms. *J. Pharm. Pharmacol.* **2008**, *60*, 221–228. [CrossRef] [PubMed]
53. Belo, V.A.; Guimaraes, D.A.; Castro, M.M. Matrix Metalloproteinase 2 as a potential mediator of vascular smooth muscle cell migration and chronic vascular remodeling in hypertension. *J. Vasc. Res.* **2015**, *52*, 221–231. [CrossRef] [PubMed]
54. Chen, Q.; Jin, M.; Yang, F.; Zhu, J.; Xiao, Q.; Zhang, L. Matrix metalloproteinases: Inflammatory regulators of cell behaviors in vascular formation and remodeling. *Mediat. Inflamm.* **2013**, *2013*, 928315. [CrossRef] [PubMed]

55. Del Mauro, J.S.; Prince, P.D.; Donato, M.; Fernandez Machulsky, N.; Moretton, M.A.; Gonzalez, G.E.; Bertera, F.M.; Carranza, A.; Gorzalczany, S.B.; Chiappetta, D.A.; et al. Effects of carvedilol or amlodipine on target organ damage in L-NAME hypertensive rats: Their relationship with blood pressure variability. *J. Am. Soc. Hypertens.* **2017** *11*, 227–240. [CrossRef] [PubMed]

56. Bernatova, I.; Pechanova, O.; Simko, F. Captopril prevents NO-deficient hypertension and left ventricular hypertrophy without affecting nitric oxide synthase activity in rats. *Physiol. Res.* **1996**, *45*, 311–316. [PubMed]

57. Bernatova, I.; Pechanova, O.; Simko, F. Effect of captopril in L-NAME-induced hypertension on the rat myocardium, aorta, brain and kidney. *Exp. Physiol.* **1999**, *84*, 1095–1105. [CrossRef] [PubMed]

58. Bartosz, M.; Kedziora, J.; Bartosz, G. Antioxidant and prooxidant properties of captopril and enalapril. *Free Radic. Biol. Med.* **1997**, *23*, 729–735. [CrossRef]

59. Okada, M.; Kikuzuki, R.; Harada, T.; Hori, Y.; Yamawaki, H.; Hara, Y. Captopril attenuates matrix metalloproteinase-2 and -9 in monocrotaline-induced right ventricular hypertrophy in rats. *J. Pharmacol. Sci.* **2008**, *108*, 487–494. [CrossRef] [PubMed]

60. Maneesai, P.; Bunbupha, S.; Kukongviriyapan, U.; Senggunprai, L.; Kukongviriyapan, V.; Prachaney, P.; Pakdeechote, P. Effect of asiatic acid on the Ang II-AT1R-NADPH oxidase-NF-kappaB pathway in renovascular hypertensive rats. *Naunyn Schmiedebergs Arch. Pharmacol.* **2017**, *390*, 1073–1083. [CrossRef] [PubMed]

12

Twelve-Week Protocatechuic Acid Administration Improves Insulin-Induced and Insulin-Like Growth Factor-1-Induced Vasorelaxation and Antioxidant Activities in Aging Spontaneously Hypertensive Rats

Kunanya Masodsai [1], Yi-Yuan Lin [2,3], Rungchai Chaunchaiyakul [4], Chia-Ting Su [5], Shin-Da Lee [2,6,7,†] and Ai-Lun Yang [1,*,†]

1 Institute of Sports Sciences, University of Taipei, Taipei 11153, Taiwan; kunanyamasodsai@gmail.com
2 Department of Occupational Therapy, Asia University, Taichung 41354, Taiwan; charlet8116@gmail.com (Y.-Y.L.); leeshinda@gmail.com (S.-D.L.)
3 Graduate Institute of Clinical Medical Science, China Medical University, Taichung 40402, Taiwan
4 College of Sports Science and Technology, Mahidol University, Nakhonpathom 73170, Thailand; gmrungchai@gmail.com
5 Department of Occupational Therapy, College of Medicine, Fu Jen Catholic University, New Taipei City 24205, Taiwan; chiatingsu@gmail.com
6 Department of Physical Therapy, Graduate Institute of Rehabilitation Science, China Medical University, Taichung 40402, Taiwan
7 School of Rehabilitation Science, Shanghai University of Traditional Chinese Medicine, Shanghai 201203, China
* Correspondence: yangailun@gmail.com or alyang@utaipei.edu.tw
† These authors contributed equally to this work.

Abstract: Protocatechuic acid (PCA), a strong antioxidant, has been reported for its cardiovascular-protective effects. This study aimed to investigate the effects of PCA administration on vascular endothelial function, mediated by insulin and insulin-like growth factor-1 (IGF-1), and antioxidant activities in aging hypertension. Thirty-six-week-old male aging spontaneously hypertensive rats were randomly divided into vehicle control (SHR) and PCA (SHR+PCA) groups, while age-matched Wistar–Kyoto rats (WKY) served as the normotensive vehicle control group. The oral PCA (200 mg/kg/day) was administered daily for a total of 12 weeks. When the rats reached the age of 48 weeks, the rat aortas were isolated for the evaluation of vascular reactivity and Western blotting. Also, nitric oxide (NO) production and antioxidant activities were examined among the three groups. The results showed that, when compared with the SHR group, the insulin-induced and IGF-1-induced vasorelaxation were significantly improved in the SHR+PCA group. There was no significant difference in the endothelium-denuded vessels among the three groups. After the pre-incubation of phosphatidylinositol 3-kinase (PI3K) or NO synthase (NOS) inhibitors, the vasorelaxation was abolished and comparable among the three groups. The protein levels of insulin receptors, IGF-1 receptors, phospho-protein kinase B (p-Akt)/Akt, and phospho-endothelial NOS (p-eNOS)/eNOS in aortic tissues were significantly enhanced in the SHR+PCA group when compared with the SHR group. Moreover, significant improvements of nitrate/nitrite concentration and antioxidant activities, including superoxide dismutase, catalase, and total antioxidants, were also found in the SHR+PCA group. In conclusion, the 12 weeks of PCA administration remarkably improved the endothelium-dependent vasorelaxation induced by insulin and IGF-1 in aging hypertension through enhancing the PI3K–NOS–NO pathway. Furthermore, the enhanced antioxidant activities partly contributed to the improved vasorelaxation.

Keywords: polyphenol; high blood pressure; elderly; endothelium; nitric oxide

1. Introduction

Hypertension is recognized as a risk factor for cardiovascular disease (CVD). The prevalence of hypertension has been dramatically increasing worldwide, especially in older adults and the elderly. More than 60% of the population above the age of 65 suffer from hypertension [1]. In older adults with hypertension, more profound pathological processes may exist to induce CVD. Hypertension leads to reversible cardiac and vascular dysfunction, including cardiac hypertrophy, reduced lumen diameter of arteries, increased vascular smooth muscle cell (VSMC) proliferation, and endothelial dysfunction [2–4]. Moreover, in aging heart and vessels, the number of myocardial cells is decreased, cardiac fibrosis is increased, elastic arteries become stiffer, and endothelial function is impaired [5,6]. Since vascular endothelium is critical for homeostasis in the body, its impairment evokes pathological conditions, such as hypertension, diabetes, and CVD (e.g., atherosclerosis, thrombosis) [7]. The impaired bioavailability of nitric oxide (NO) and imbalance of endothelium-derived vasoconstrictive and vasodilatory substances are considered as the key features of endothelial dysfunction. Furthermore, a reduction in activity of antioxidant enzyme, such as superoxide dismutase (SOD), has been suggested to be another mechanism for endothelial dysfunction, which is also associated with cardiac and vascular aging [8–10]. It has been known that insulin and insulin-like growth factor 1 (IGF-1) have important vascular actions that stimulate NO production mainly in the endothelium. They both modulate the endothelium-dependent vasorelaxation by activating phosphatidylinositol 3-kinase (PI3K), protein kinase B (PKB/Akt), and endothelial nitric oxide synthase (eNOS), which results in NO production [11–13]. Previous research has reported that the vascular actions of insulin and IGF-1 are pathologically altered and impaired in cardiovascular disorders, such as hypertension and obesity. Also, the diminished vasorelaxant effects of insulin and IGF-1 have been found in the development of hypertension [14–17]. However, in aging hypertension, the ways insulin and IGF-1 influence the cardiovascular dysfunction remain unclear.

Numerous strategies in prevention and/or treatment for ameliorating high blood pressure have been widely prescribed, such as lifestyle and dietary modifications (e.g., low-sodium intake, and fruit- and vegetable-enriched consumption) [18]. Protocatechuic acid (PCA, 3,4-dihydroxybenzoic acid), a strong antioxidant, is a natural phenolic compound found in many types of food. It has been known for multiple benefits to health, including anti-inflammation, anti-hyperglycemic, anti-hypertensive, and cardiovascular-protective effects [19–21]. A previous study indicated significant preservation of increasing blood pressure and improved antioxidant capacity in dexamethasone-induced hypertensive rats by short-term daily administration of 200 mg/kg PCA [22]. Also, a single dose of intraperitoneal injection of alpinia PCA (5 and 10 mg/kg) for 7 days in aged rats remarkably improved antioxidant activities (i.e., glutathione peroxidase and catalase) and suppressed oxidative stress (malondialdehyde, MDA) [23]. Additionally, administering various doses of PCA decreased blood glucose and hemoglobin A1c ($HbA1_C$) in studies of anti-hyperglycemic effects [24,25]. However, the effectiveness of PCA administration on aging hypertension with regard to the vasorelaxant effects of insulin and IGF-1 and antioxidant activities has not been fully investigated. Therefore, in the present study, we investigated the effects of PCA administration on insulin-induced and IGF-1-induced vasorelaxation and antioxidant activities in aging spontaneously hypertensive rats (SHR).

2. Materials and Methods

2.1. Animals

Eight-week-old male SHR and Wistar–Kyoto rats (WKY) were purchased from the National Laboratory Animal Center (Taipei, Taiwan). All rats were attentively housed in an environment-controlled room at 22–24 °C with a 12-h dark/light cycle (lights on at 06:00 h and off at 18:00 h) and provided standard laboratory chow (Lab Diet 5001; PMI Nutrition International, Brentwood, MO, USA) and water ad libitum. At the age of 36 weeks, the SHR were randomly divided into the vehicle control group (SHR, $n = 8$) and the protocatechuic acid (PCA)-treated group

(SHR+PCA, $n = 8$). The age-matched WKY served as the normotensive vehicle control group (WKY, $n = 8$). The SHR+PCA group was treated with 200 mg/kg body weight of PCA (Sigma Chemical, St. Louis, MO, USA), dissolved in daily water, for a total of 12 weeks [22,24]. The other groups were not treated with PCA in their daily water. The rats in the SHR+PCA group were provided with the PCA-containing water in the afternoon and checked by the assistant every hour to monitor the drinking. After the rats finished drinking the PCA-containing water (2–3 h), they were provided with regular water ad libitum. They drank all of the PCA-containing water every day. All samples were collected at least 24 h after the animals finished the administration of PCA. This study was conducted in conformity under the Guide for the Care and Use of Laboratory Animals of the National Institutes of Health. All experimental procedures were approved by the Institutional Animal Care and Use Committee (IACUC) of the University of Taipei, Taiwan (Ethical approval code: UT104005).

2.2. Resting Blood Pressure and Heart Rate

The heart rate and systolic blood pressure (SBP) were measured noninvasively by the tail-cuff method (BP98A, Softron, Tokyo, Japan) [14]. The hemodynamic data were collected between 9:00 h and 12:00 h, at least 24 h after drinking the PCA.

2.3. Vasoreactivity Experiments

At the end of the experimental period, all rats were fasted overnight and were sacrificed under anesthesia with 2% isoflurane delivered in oxygen (95% O_2 and 5% CO_2). Then, thoracic aortas were carefully isolated. The force displacement transducers (Models FT3E, Grass Instrument, West Warwick, RI, USA) were used to isometrically evaluate the vasorelaxant responses of isolated rings which were submerged in organ chambers containing Krebs–Ringer buffer (118 mM NaCl, 4.8 mM KCl, 2.5 mM $CaCl_2$, 1.2 mM $MgSO_4$, 1.2 mM KH_2PO_4, 24 mM $NaHCO_3$, 0.03 mM Na-EDTA, and 11 mM glucose; pH 7.4) oxygenated with 95% O_2 and 5% CO_2 at 37 °C. After the 60-min equilibration at the optimal passive tension (i.e., 2 g), the drugs were administered. The pre-contraction of aortic rings was induced by phenylephrine (10^{-7} M, Sigma Chemical) before being exposed to various concentrations of insulin (3×10^{-8} to 3×10^{-6} M) and IGF-1 (10^{-9} to 10^{-7} M, PeproTech, NJ, USA) to induce dose-dependent vasorelaxation. The endothelial integrity was confirmed by at least 60% of acetylcholine (10^{-7} M)-induced vasorelaxation in phenylephrine-precontracted vessel rings. The parallel testing of the endothelium-denuded rings was also evaluated among the three groups. The endothelium-denuded rings were indicated by less than 10% of acetylcholine (10^{-7} M)-induced vasorelaxation precontracted with phenylephrine. Moreover, to determine the roles of PI3K and NOS in the insulin- and IGF-1-induced vasorelaxant responses, the selective inhibitors, wortmannin (3×10^{-7} M; an inhibitor of PI3K; Sigma Chemical) and nitro-L-arginine methyl ester (L-NAME) (10^{-6} M; a NOS inhibitor; Sigma Chemical), were pre-incubated for 15 min before the administration of phenylephrine in the endothelium-intact rings. Stock solutions of all drugs were prepared and dissolved in distilled water except for insulin (dissolved in 10^{-2} M HCl). Final dilutions of the drugs were prepared in distilled water immediately before use. None of the vehicles used in final dilutions induced any significant effects on vessel tone [14].

2.4. Blood Collection and Biochemical Analysis

Blood samples were allowed to clot for 30 min at room temperature and then centrifuged at 2000× *g* for 15 min at 4 °C. The serum was collected after the centrifugation and stored at −80 °C for biochemical analysis. Serum nitrate/nitrite concentration was performed using a nitrate/nitrite colorimetric assay kit (Cayman Chemical Company, Ann Arbor, MI, USA). According to the manufacturer's instructions, total nitrate/nitrite concentration was determined by a two-step process. The first step was the conversion of nitrate to nitrite by nitrate reductase. The second step was the addition of Griess Reagents which convert nitrite to a deep purple azo product. The absorbance due to the azo chromophore was measured at 450 nm by a microplate reader (TECAN Infinite

M200PRO, Grödig, Austria). The concentration was expressed in μM in serum samples. Serum MDA concentration, an index of lipid peroxidation marker, was determined using a thiobarbituric acid reactive substances (TBARS) assay kit (Cayman Chemical Company). The TBA reagents prepared according to the manufacturer's protocol was mixed with the serum samples to generate the MDA-TBA adducts under high temperature (90–100 °C) and acidic condition. After completing the reactions, samples were measured colorimetrically at 540 nm by a microplate reader (TECAN Infinite M200PRO). The concentration was expressed in μM in serum samples. Serum SOD activity was determined using a SOD assay kit (Cayman Chemical Company). The assay utilized a tetrazolium salt for the detection of superoxide radicals generated by xanthine oxidase and hypoxanthine. One unit of SOD was defined as the amount of enzyme needed to exhibit 50% dismutation of superoxide radicals. The absorbance was read at 450 nm by a microplate reader (TECAN Infinite M200PRO) and the activity was expressed in U/mL in serum samples. Serum catalase activity was performed using a catalase assay kit (Cayman Chemical Company). The assay relied on the reaction of catalase in the sample with methanol in the presence of hydrogen peroxide (H_2O_2). The absorbance was read at 540 nm by a microplate reader (TECAN Infinite M200PRO) and the activity was expressed in nmol/min/mL in serum samples. Serum total antioxidant capacity was performed using an antioxidant assay kit (Cayman Chemical Company). The assay was based on the ability of antioxidants in the sample to inhibit the oxidation of the 2,2′-azino-di-(3-ethylbenzothiazoline sulphonate) (ABTS) to $ABTS^{\cdot+}$ by metmyoglobin. The capacity of the antioxidants in the sample was compared with that of Trolox, a water-soluble tocopherol analogue, as the standard, and was quantified as millimolar (mM) Trolox equivalents. The absorbance was measured colorimetrically at 750 nm by a microplate reader (TECAN Infinite M200PRO).

2.5. Insulin Resistance Determination

Fasting plasma glucose was determined by the glucose oxidase method using the glucometer (Roche Diagnostics, Indianapolis, IN, USA). According to the manufacturer's instructions, serum insulin was measured using a commercial ELISA kit (Mercodia AB, Uppsala, Sweden). Briefly, adding enzyme conjugate solution incubated with serum sample, the bound conjugate was detected by the reaction with 3,3′-5,5′-tetramethylbenzidine (TMB). The reaction was stopped by the stop solution and the absorbance was measured at 450 nm by a microplate reader (TECAN Infinite M200PRO). The homeostatic model assessment of insulin resistance (HOMA-IR) was calculated by the equation: HOMA-IR = (fasting glucose (mmol/L) × fasting serum insulin (mU/L))/22.5 [26].

2.6. Western Immunoblotting

Western immunoblotting analysis was performed as previously described [14]. Aortic tissue extracts from thoracic aortas were obtained by homogenizing at 4 °C in the tissue protein extraction reagent (T-PER, Thermo Scientific) supplemented with complete protease and phosphatase inhibitors (Sigma Chemical). The supernatant was collected after sequential centrifuge of the homogenates at 10,000 rpm for 10 min. Protein concentration of the aortic tissue extract supernatant was determined by the Bradford method (Bio-Rad Laboratories, Hercules, CA, USA) with bovine serum albumin as a standard. Protein samples (50 μg/lane) were separated by 8% sodium dodecyl sulfate-polyacrylamide gel electrophoresis (SDS-PAGE) with a minigel apparatus (Bio-Rad Laboratories) and subsequently transferred to polyvinylidene difluoride (PVDF) membranes (Millipore, Bedford, MA, USA). The membranes were incubated with blocking buffer (5% nonfat dry milk in tris-buffered saline and Tween 20 (TBST) buffer) for 1 h. Primary antibodies including the anti-insulin receptor, anti-IGF-1 receptor, anti-phospho-Akt, anti-Akt (diluted at a ratio 1:1000; Cell Signaling Technology, Danvers, MA, USA), anti-phospho-eNOS, anti-eNOS (diluted at a ratio 1:1000; BD Transduction Laboratories, Lexington, KY, USA), and actin (diluted at a ratio 1:5000; Millipore) were diluted in antibody-binding buffer overnight at 4 °C. After incubation with the appropriate primary antibody, the peroxidase-conjugated secondary antibodies (1:5000; Millipore) were then incubated at room temperature for 1 h. The immunoblotted proteins were detected by enhanced chemiluminescence by using enhanced chemiluminescence detection reagents in the Gel Doc XR System (Bio-Rad Laboratories).

2.7. Statistical Analysis

All data were presented as means ± standard error (SE). Estimated parameters were compared among the WKY, SHR, and SHR+PCA groups using one-way ANOVA with pre-planned contrast comparison with the control group and then LSD post hoc analysis. Dose responses of vasorelaxation were analyzed by two-way ANOVA with a repeated measures design (using SPSS software v.21). For all statistical tests, $p < 0.05$ was considered to be significant.

3. Results

3.1. General Characteristics

As shown in Table 1, the heart rate and SBP were significantly ($p < 0.05$) increased in the SHR group when compared with the WKY group. After 12 weeks of PCA administration, these indicators were significantly ($p < 0.05$) reduced in the SHR+PCA group compared with the SHR group. In addition, the blood glucose and insulin concentration were significantly ($p < 0.05$) increased in the SHR group when compared with WKY; however, both of them were significantly ($p < 0.05$) decreased in the SHR+PCA group when compared with the SHR. The level of insulin resistance indicated by HOMA-IR was also significantly ($p < 0.05$) augmented in the SHR group, but after the PCA intervention, it was significantly ($p < 0.05$) reduced in the SHR+PCA group. The body weight was similar among the three groups.

Table 1. General characteristics.

Parameters/Groups	WKY	SHR	SHR+PCA
Body weight (g)	395.75 ± 8.47	393.50 ± 5.15	404.50 ± 8.85
Heart rate (bpm)	284.06 ± 3.90	383.19 ± 9.83 $^{\alpha}$	363.38 ± 6.19 $^{\alpha,\beta}$
SBP (mmHg)	121.75 ± 2.15	192.88 ± 2.28 $^{\alpha}$	173.63 ± 0.88 $^{\alpha,\beta}$
Insulin (μg/L)	0.34 ± 0.07	0.66 ± 0.11 $^{\alpha}$	0.37 ± 0.09 $^{\beta}$
Blood glucose (mg/dL)	96.63 ± 2.63	121.25 ± 4.76 $^{\alpha}$	110.13 ± 4.33 $^{\alpha,\beta}$
HOMA-IR	2.02 ± 0.41	4.89 ± 0.82 $^{\alpha}$	2.50 ± 0.54 $^{\beta}$

WKY, Wistar–Kyoto rats; SHR, spontaneously hypertensive rats; PCA, protocatechuic acid; SBP, systolic blood pressure; HOMA-IR, the homeostatic model assessment of insulin resistance. $^{\alpha}$, $p < 0.05$, significant differences from WKY; $^{\beta}$, $p < 0.05$, significant differences from SHR; $n = 8$ in each group.

3.2. Insulin-Induced and IGF-1-Induced Vasorelaxation in Aortas

Figures 1 and 2 revealed the concentration-response curves of insulin-induced and IGF-1-induced vasorelaxation in the isolated aortic rings in the WKY, SHR, and SHR+PCA groups. In endothelial-intact aortic rings, the SHR group had significantly ($p < 0.05$) diminished responses in insulin-induced and IGF-1-induced vasorelaxation when compared with the WKY group. However, these impaired responses were significantly ($p < 0.05$) improved in the SHR+PCA group when compared with the SHR group. As noted, the improvements did not reach the level of vasorelaxation in the WKY group. To determine the endothelium-dependent responses, the parallel investigation of endothelium-denuded of aortic rings showed that no significant difference was found in insulin-induced and IGF-1-induced vasorelaxation among the three groups.

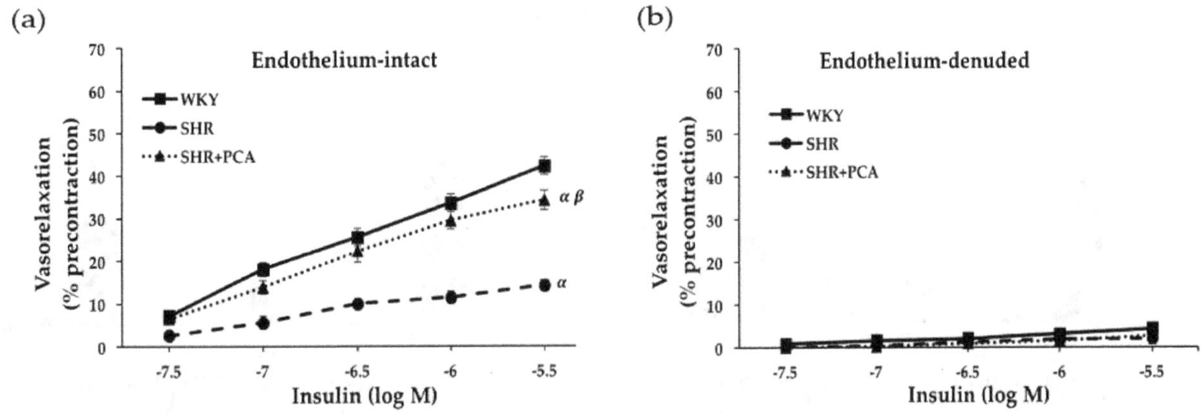

Figure 1. Insulin (3×10^{-8} to 3×10^{-6} M)-induced vasorelaxation at cumulative concentration–response curves in (**a**) endothelium-intact and (**b**) endothelium-denuded aortic rings among the WKY, SHR, and SHR+PCA groups. $^{\alpha}$, $p < 0.05$, significant differences from WKY; $^{\beta}$, $p < 0.05$, significant differences from SHR; $n = 8$ in each group.

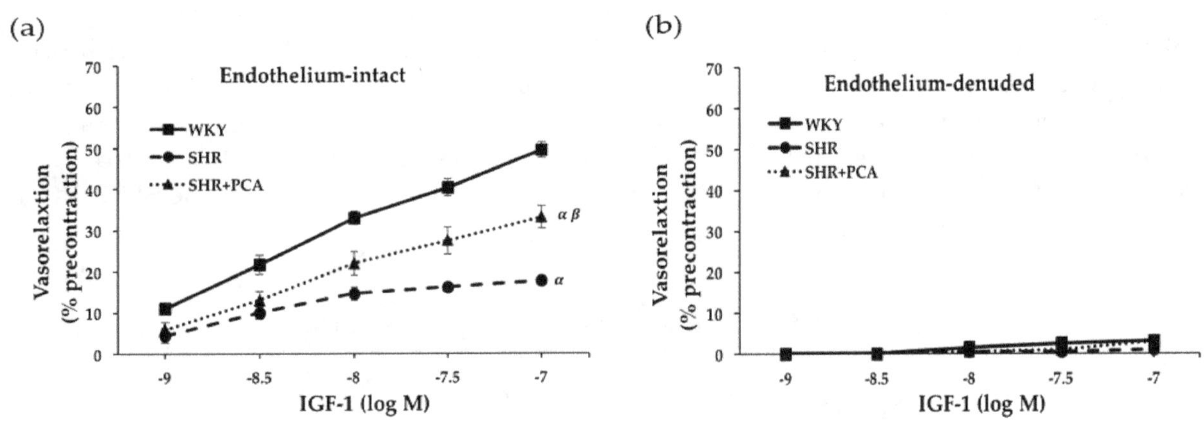

Figure 2. Insulin-like growth factor-1 (IGF-1; 10^{-9} to 10^{-7} M)-induced vasorelaxation at cumulative concentration–response curves in (**a**) endothelium-intact and (**b**) endothelium-denuded aortic rings among the WKY, SHR, and SHR+PCA groups. $^{\alpha}$, $p < 0.05$, significant differences from WKY; $^{\beta}$, $p < 0.05$, significant differences from SHR; $n = 8$ in each group.

3.3. Roles of PI3K and NOS in Insulin-Induced and IGF-1-Induced Vasorelaxation

The selective inhibitors, wortmannin and L-NAME, were pretreated in endothelium-intact aortic rings to verify the roles of PI3K and NOS in insulin-induced and IGF-1-induced vasorelaxation (Figure 3). Before adding wortmannin or L-NAME, the SHR group had significantly ($p < 0.05$) lower insulin-induced and IGF-1-induced vasorelaxation than the WKY group. Nevertheless, the SHR+PCA group had significantly ($p < 0.05$) higher vasorelaxant responses than the SHR group. After the 15-min pre-incubation of wortmanin or L-NAME, the insulin-induced and IGF-1-induced vasorelaxation was significantly ($p < 0.05$) blunted in all groups. Moreover, there was no significant difference in these vasorelaxant responses among the three groups.

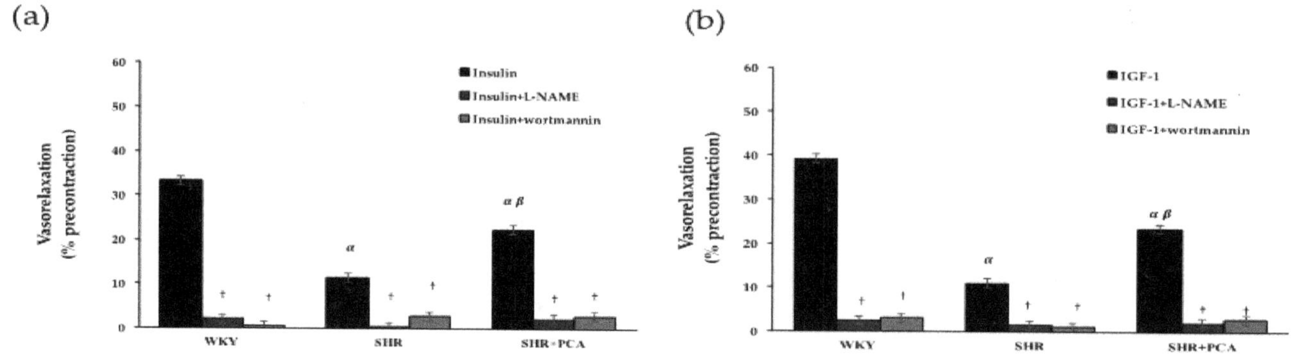

Figure 3. (**a**) Insulin (10^{-6} M)-induced vasorelaxation and (**b**) IGF-1 (3×10^{-8} M)-induced vasorelaxation after the 15-min pre-incubation with wortmannin (3×10^{-7} M) or nitro-L-arginine methyl ester (L-NAME) (10^{-6} M) among the WKY, SHR, and SHR+PCA groups. $^{\alpha}$, $p < 0.05$, significant differences from WKY; $^{\beta}$, $p < 0.05$, significant differences from SHR; †, $p < 0.05$, significant differences from no inhibitors; $n = 8$ in each group.

3.4. Aortic Protein Expression

To determine the effects of PCA administration on aortic protein expression involved in the insulin- and IGF-1-mediated vasorelaxation, the protein levels of insulin receptors, IGF-1 receptors, phospho-Akt (p-Akt), Akt, phospho-eNOS (p-eNOS), and eNOS extracted from thoracic aortas were evaluated by Western blotting (Figure 4 and Supplementary Figure S1). Figure 4 showed that the protein levels of insulin receptors, IGF-1 receptors, p-Akt/Akt, and p-eNOS/eNOS were significantly ($p < 0.05$) diminished in the SHR group ($p < 0.05$) when compared with the WKY group. Netherless, the PCA administration significantly ($p < 0.05$) improved these protein levels in the SHR+PCA group when compared with the SHR group.

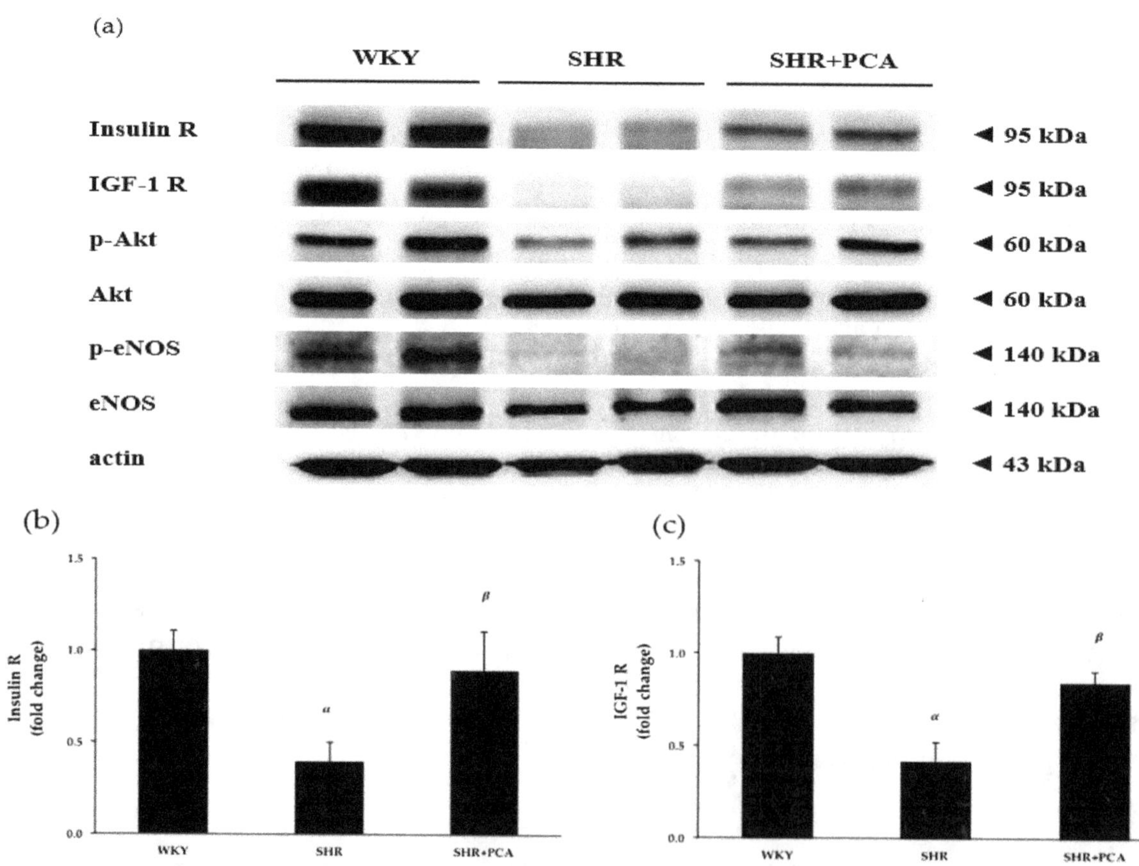

Figure 4. *Cont.*

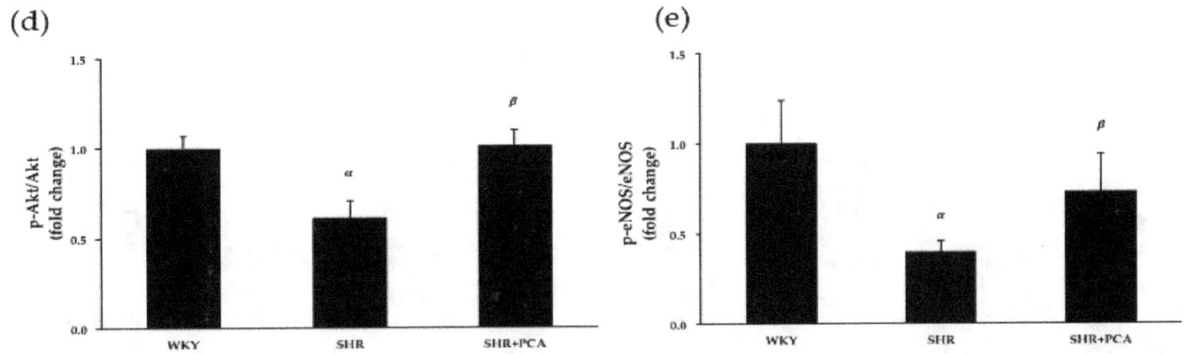

Figure 4. (**a**) Representative immunoblots of insulin receptor (insulin R), insulin-like growth factor-1 receptor (IGF-1 R), phospho-protein kinase B (p-Akt), protein kinase B (Akt), phospho-endothelial nitric oxide synthase (p-eNOS), endothelial nitric oxide synthase (eNOS), and actin extracted from thoracic aortas, and relative protein quantification of (**b**) insulin R, (**c**) IGF-1 R, (**d**) p-Akt/Akt, and (**e**) p-eNOS/eNOS on the basis of actin among the WKY, SHR, and SHR+PCA groups. $^{\alpha}$, $p < 0.05$, significant differences from WKY; $^{\beta}$, $p < 0.05$, significant differences from SHR; $n = 6$ in each group.

3.5. Serum Nitrate/Nitrite Concentration

Figure 5 showed that serum nitrate/nitrite concentration was significantly ($p < 0.05$) reduced in the SHR group when compared with the WKY group. However, after the PCA administration, the nitrate/nitrite concentration was significantly ($p < 0.05$) increased in the SHR+PCA group when compared with the SHR group.

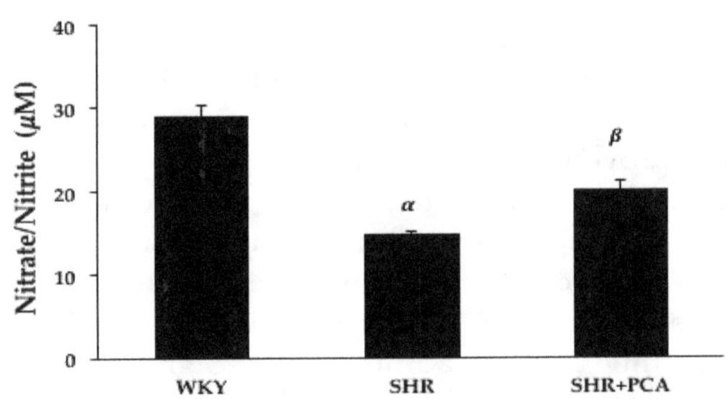

Figure 5. Serum nitrate/nitrite concentration among the WKY, SHR, and SHR+PCA groups. $^{\alpha}$, $p < 0.05$, significant differences from WKY; $^{\beta}$, $p < 0.05$, significant differences from SHR; $n = 8$ in each group.

3.6. Serum MDA and Antioxidant Activities

Serum MDA concentration and antioxidant activities, including SOD, catalase, and total antioxidants, were determined and compared among the three groups. Figure 6 showed that the SHR group had significantly ($p < 0.05$) higher MDA concentration but lower antioxidant activities, including SOD, catalase, and total antioxidants, than the WKY group. On the other hand, the PCA administration significantly ($p < 0.05$) reduced MDA concentration and enhanced these antioxidant activities in the SHR+PCA group when compared with the SHR group.

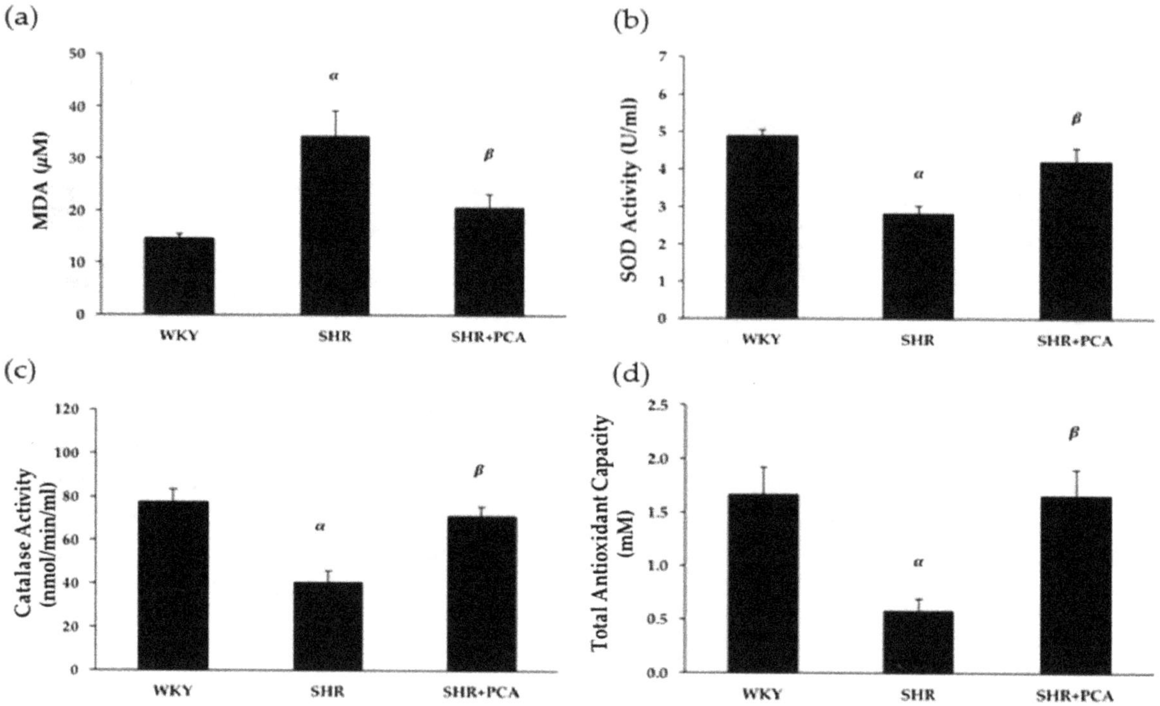

Figure 6. (**a**) Serum malondialdehyde (MDA) concentration, (**b**) superoxide dismutase (SOD) activity, (**c**) catalase activity, and (**d**) total antioxidant capacity among the WKY, SHR, and SHR+PCA groups. $^{\alpha}$, $p < 0.05$, significant differences from WKY; $^{\beta}$, $p < 0.05$, significant differences from SHR; $n = 8$ in each group.

4. Discussion

To the best of our knowledge, the present study was the first to examine the effects of 12 weeks of PCA administration on the vasorelaxation induced by insulin and IGF-1 and antioxidant activities in aging SHR. The main findings of this study were as follows. Firstly, the PCA administration significantly improved the insulin-induced and IGF-1-induced vasorelaxation in aging SHR. However, these improvements did not reach the level of vasorelaxation in the normotensive WKY group. Secondly, in the denuded-endothelium vessels, there were no significant differences in the insulin-induced and IGF-1-induced vasorelaxation among the three groups. Thirdly, the improved vasorelaxation induced by insulin and IGF-1 in aging SHR was mainly mediated by activating the PI3K–NOS–NO signaling. Fourthly, the PCA administration significantly improved the protein levels of insulin receptors, IGF-1 receptors, p-Akt/Akt, and p-eNOS/eNOS in aging SHR. Finally, significant improvements of serum antioxidant activities, including SOD, catalase, and total antioxidants, were also found in aging SHR following the PCA administration, which partly contributed to the improved vasorelaxation.

PCA has been known to evoke multiple health benefits, such as antioxidant, anti-inflammation, anti-hyperglycemia, anti-hypertensive, and cardiovascular-protective effects [19–21]. Previous studies indicated that PCA extracted from the petal of *Hibiscus sabdariffa* also exhibited anti-hypertensive and cardiovascular-protective effects [19,20]. Moreover, oral administration of PCA treatments for 12 weeks significantly improved cardiac function, as shown by increased fractional shortening and left ventricular ejection fraction (LVEF) and decreased low-frequency to high-frequency ratio in streptozotocin (STZ)-induced diabetic rats [25]. Another study has shown that short-term daily supplementation with PCA (50, 100, and 200 mg/kg) dose-dependently reduced SBP and plasma H_2O_2 concentration, and improved antioxidant capacity in dexamethasone-induced hypertensive rats [22]. Consistent with previous studies, our investigation indicated that the 12-weeks PCA administration elicited the decreases in high blood pressure together with restoring vascular function by improving endothelium-dependent vasorelaxation induced by insulin and IGF-1 in aging SHR. Meanwhile,

NO concentration was remarkably improved in aging SHR which received PCA administration. In addition to glucose metabolism, insulin and IGF-1 have vascular protective effects, including the induction of vasorelaxation, inhibition of VSMC proliferation, and anti-inflammation, mainly via stimulating the NO-dependent mechanisms in the endothelium [13]. Several reports have documented that insulin- and IGF-1-mediated vasorelaxant responses are impaired in hypertensive and diabetic animal models, which is associated with the suppressed NO bioavailability [15,27]. Consistently, the present study indicated the impairments of the insulin- and IGF-1-induced vasorelaxant responses and the decreases in NO production in aging SHR compared with the age-matched normotensive WKY. In order to clarify the NO-dependent signaling, the selective inhibitors of PI3K and NOS were administered in the insulin- and IGF-1-induced vasorelaxation. We found that, after the pre-incubation of PI3K or NOS inhibitor, these vasorelaxant differences among the three groups were absent. This suggested that the aging hypertension evoked the decreased activation of PI3K and NOS, partly resulting in the impairments of NO production and insulin- and IGF-1-induced vasorelaxation. In addition, the PCA-induced protective effects on the vasorelaxation were related to the increased activation of PI3K and NOS, resulting in the amelioration of NO production and insulin- and IGF-1-induced vasorelaxation in aging SHR.

Since the upregulation of insulin/IGF-1 receptors and downstream proteins, such as Akt and eNOS, are considered to be involved in the insulin- and IGF-1-induced vasorelaxation, we examined aortic protein expressions among the WKY, SHR, and SHR+PCA groups. We found that aging hypertension significantly decreased aortic protein expressions of insulin and IGF-1 receptors, phospho-Akt/Akt, and phospho-eNOS/eNOS, whereas the PCA administration significantly enhanced expression of these proteins in aging SHR. A previous study, in human visceral adipocytes, indicated that PCA stimulated insulin receptor substrate-1 (IRS-1) tyrosine phosphorylation and the downstream proteins, such as phosphoinositide 3-kinase binding to IRS-1 and Akt phosphorylation. Also, PCA elicited the insulin-sensitizing effects by activating adenosine monophosphate-activated protein kinase [28]. In the present study, we found that the 12-week PCA administration ameliorated the vasorelaxant responses to insulin and IGF-1 in aging SHR through the upregulation of insulin and IGF-1 receptors and downstream Akt/eNOS phosphorylation. In addition to PCA, several phytochemical compounds, such as resveratrol and curcumin, have revealed beneficial effects in reducing cardiovascular risk factors. Resveratrol lowers high blood pressure and improves endothelial function through enhancing eNOS expression and NO production. Moreover, curcumin supplementation ameliorates the impairment in endothelial-dependent dilation with aging by restoring NO bioavailability [29]. However, whether PCA induces the insulin- and IGF-1-sensitizing effects on aortic tissues needs further investigation.

It has been believed that hypertension can cause insulin resistance by altering the delivery of insulin and glucose. Conversely, insulin resistance could cause high blood pressure. In the state of insulin resistance, the insulin-stimulated NO pathway is selectively impaired and the compensatory hyperinsulinemia may activate the mitogen-activated protein kinase (MAPK) pathway, resulting in enhancement of vasoconstriction, pro-inflammation, endothelial dysfunction, increased sodium and water retention, and increases in blood pressure. Insulin resistance and hypertension commonly coexist, especially in older adults. The adverse influences of insulin resistance on blood pressure could be accentuated in an aging population [30]. Furthermore, PCA has been extensively investigated with regards to the anti-hyperglycemia activity and revealed that various doses of administration decreased blood glucose and $HbA1_C$ [24,25]. Consistent with previous studies, we found that fasting blood glucose, insulin concentration, and HOMA were significantly increased in aging SHR. However, after 12 weeks of PCA intervention, these parameters were significantly reduced in aging SHR. This suggested that chronic PCA administration effectively ameliorated the aging hypertension-induced insulin resistance in aging SHR.

Oxidative stress has been considered to promote endothelial dysfunction and lead to vascular damage in hypertension. Moreover, advancing age is associated with the increased oxidative stress and reduced NO bioavailability, mediating the development of endothelial dysfunction and CVD [31–33]. The level of oxidative stress increases as a consequence of greater production of reactive oxygen species (ROS) without a compensatory increase in antioxidant activity. Several sources of increased ROS production include the up-regulation of the oxidant enzyme NADPH oxidase, uncoupling eNOS (due to reduced availability of the cofactor tetrahydrobiopterin), and increased mitochondrial synthesis during oxidative phosphorylation of the electron transport chain. With aging and hypertension, excessive oxidative stress could be the key mechanism mediating impaired NO bioavailability and endothelium-dependent vasorelaxation [32–34]. It is known that PCA administration effectively promotes antioxidant enzymatic activities and inhibits ROS generation [23]. One previous study indicated that 4-week supplementation with PCA reduced serum MDA and hydroperoxide levels, and also improved serum catalase activity, total antioxidant capacity, and glutathione concentration in deoxycorticosterone acetate (DOCA)-salt hypertensive rats [35]. Moreover, evidence has shown that PCA significantly increased the activities of glutathione peroxidase (GPx) and catalase, decreased MDA level, and normalized age–associated alterations in aged rats. This implies that PCA could induce anti-aging effects through upregulating the antioxidant system [23,36,37]. Similarly, our findings showed an increase in oxidative stress (i.e., MDA) and decreases in antioxidant activities, including SOD, catalase, and total antioxidants in aging SHR. Following the 12-week PCA administration, these impairments were significantly ameliorated in aging SHR, which partly contributed to the improved vasorelaxation. A previous study reported that PCA increased the gene expression of GPx and glutathione reductase (GR) in J774A.1 macrophages. The over-expression of glutathione-related enzymes was found by inducing c-Jun N-terminal kinase (JNK)-mediated phosphorylation of nuclear factor erythroid 2 (NF-E2)-related factor 2 (Nrf2). This suggested that PCA improved the endogenous antioxidant potential through the JNK-mediated Nrf2 activation and increased antioxidant enzyme expression [38]. It is plausible to speculate that PCA upregulates the antioxidant enzyme expression which might be responsible for modifying the enzyme activity. In this study, we first demonstrated that PCA had beneficial effects on increasing serum antioxidant activities and reducing MDA level, contributing to improved vasorelaxant responses, in aging hypertensive rats. The potential mechanisms which modify the antioxidant activity and ROS inhibition for these PCA-induced improvements in aging hypertension need to be further clarified.

Reagan-Shaw and coworkers demonstrated the dose translation from animal models to human clinical trials. The estimate of the 200 mg/kg dose in rats yields a human equivalent dose (HED) of 32.4 mg/kg for humans, which is 1944 mg in a 60-kg adult [39]. Moreover, the content of PCA varies considerably depending on the type of food, as seen in *Olea europaea* (olives), *Hibiscus sabdariffa* (roselle), *Eucommia ulmoides* (du-zhong), *Citrus microcarpa* Bunge (calamondin), and *Vitis vinifera* (white wine grapes) [21]. Further studies are recommended to clarify the effective level consumed from the daily diet.

With regard to the limitations of this study, we did not include the placebo/time-control experiments for the insulin-induced vasorelaxation, due to the limited numbers and samples of animals regulated by the IACUC. However, normotensive control (WKY) rats were included in our study, and the results demonstrated a maximal response of insulin-induced vasorelaxation of about 40%, similar to the value shown by Li et al. [40]. Moreover, McCallum and co-workers indicated that incubation with the vehicle control (without insulin) did not affect the phenylephrine-induced vasoconstriction [27]. Therefore, it is plausible to speculate that the vehicle used in final dilution of insulin may not induce significant effects on the vasoreactivity experiments, including vasorelaxation and vasoconstriction. Future work is needed to determine the placebo/time-control effects for the insulin-induced vasorelaxation. Li and co-workers also indicated that insulin produced a dose-dependent vasorelaxation with a maximal response 10–15% in aging-related hypertensive Sprague–Dawley (SD) rats [40], similar to that of the aging SHR in our study. However, the maximum dose of insulin (at 1.5×10^{-6} M) recorded by the Li et al. was much lower than the maximum dose used in our study. The differences of insulin-induced vasorelaxation might be caused by different rat strains and aging effects. The effects of different rat strains and age on the insulin-induced vasorelaxation need to be further investigated.

5. Conclusions

In conclusion, our study demonstrated that 12 weeks of PCA administration remarkably improved the endothelium-dependent vasorelaxation induced by insulin and IGF-1 in aging hypertension through enhancing the PI3K–NOS–NO pathway. Furthermore, it had strong antioxidant effects on aging hypertension, which partly contributed to the amelioration of vascular endothelial function. Based on our findings, PCA might be suggested as an alternative strategy to minimize cardiovascular disorders in the population with aging hypertension.

Author Contributions: Conceptualization, K.M., S.-D.L., and A.-L.Y.; methodology, K.M., Y.-Y.L. and A.-L.Y.; validation, K.M., Y.-Y.L., and A.-L.Y.; formal analysis, K.M., Y.-Y.L., and A.-L.Y.; investigation, K.M., Y.-Y.L., and A.-L.Y.; resources, S.-D.L. and A.-L.Y.; data curation, K.M., Y.-Y.L., and A.-L.Y.; writing—original draft preparation, K.M. and A.-L.Y.; writing—review and editing, K.M., Y.-Y.L., R.C., C.-T.S., S.-D.L., and A.-L.Y.; visualization, K.M., Y.-Y.L., R.C., C.-T.S., and A.-L.Y.; supervision, S.-D.L. and A.-L.Y.; project administration, S.-D.L. and A.-L.Y.; funding acquisition, S.-D.L. and A.-L.Y.

Acknowledgments: We would like to thank Michael Burton of Asia University for proof-reading the manuscript.

References

1. Whelton, P.K.; Carey, R.M.; Aronow, W.S.; Casey, D.E., Jr.; Collins, K.J.; Dennison Himmelfarb, C.; DePalma, S.M.; Gidding, S.; Jamerson, K.A.; Jones, D.W.; et al. 2017 ACC/AHA/AAPA/ABC/ACPM/AGS/APhA/ASH/ASPC/NMA/PCNA Guideline for the Prevention, Detection, Evaluation, and Management of High Blood Pressure in Adults: Executive Summary: A Report of the American College of Cardiology/American Heart Association Task Force on Clinical Practice Guidelines. *Hypertension* **2017**. [CrossRef]
2. Burnier, M.; Wuerzner, G. Pathophysiology of Hypertension. In *Pathophysiology and Pharmacotherapy of Cardiovascular Disease*; Jagadeesh, G., Balakumar, P., Maung-U, K., Eds.; Springer International Publishing: Cham, Switzerland, 2015; pp. 655–683.
3. Hall, J.E.; Granger, J.P.; do Carmo, J.M.; da Silva, A.A.; Dubinion, J.; George, E.; Hamza, S.; Speed, J.; Hall, M.E. Hypertension: Physiology and pathophysiology. *Compr. Physiol.* **2012**, *2*, 2393–2442. [CrossRef] [PubMed]
4. Park, C.G. Hypertension and Vascular Aging. *Korean Circ. J.* **2006**, *36*, 477–481. [CrossRef]
5. Harvey, A.; Montezano, A.C.; Touyz, R.M. Vascular biology of ageing-Implications in hypertension. *J. Mol. Cell. Cardiol.* **2015**, *83*, 112–121. [CrossRef] [PubMed]
6. Papakatsika, S.; Stabouli, S.; Antza, C.; Kotsis, V. Early Vascular Aging: A New Target for Hypertension Treatment. *Curr. Pharm. Des.* **2016**, *22*, 122–126. [CrossRef]
7. Cahill, P.A.; Redmond, E.M. Vascular endothelium—Gatekeeper of vessel health. *Atherosclerosis* **2016**, *248*, 97–109. [CrossRef]
8. Giles, T.D.; Sander, G.E.; Nossaman, B.D.; Kadowitz, P.J. Impaired vasodilation in the pathogenesis of hypertension: Focus on nitric oxide, endothelial-derived hyperpolarizing factors, and prostaglandins. *J. Clin. Hypertens. (Greenwich)* **2012**, *14*, 198–205. [CrossRef]
9. Guerrero, F.; Thioub, S.; Goanvec, C.; Theunissen, S.; Feray, A.; Balestra, C.; Mansourati, J. Effect of tetrahydrobiopterin and exercise training on endothelium-dependent vasorelaxation in SHR. *J. Physiol. Biochem.* **2013**, *69*, 277–287. [CrossRef] [PubMed]
10. Versari, D.; Daghini, E.; Virdis, A.; Ghiadoni, L.; Taddei, S. Endothelium-dependent contractions and endothelial dysfunction in human hypertension. *Br. J. Pharmacol.* **2009**, *157*, 527–536. [CrossRef]
11. Abbas, A.; Grant, P.J.; Kearney, M.T. Role of IGF-1 in glucose regulation and cardiovascular disease. *Expert Rev. Cardiovasc. Ther.* **2008**, *6*, 1135–1149. [CrossRef] [PubMed]
12. Bertrand, L.; Horman, S.; Beauloye, C.; Vanoverschelde, J.L. Insulin signalling in the heart. *Cardiovasc. Res.* **2008**, *79*, 238–248. [CrossRef]

13. Muniyappa, R.; Montagnani, M.; Koh, K.K.; Quon, M.J. Cardiovascular actions of insulin. *Endocr. Rev.* **2007**, *28*, 463–491. [CrossRef]
14. Lin, Y.Y.; Lee, S.D.; Su, C.T.; Cheng, T.L.; Yang, A.L. Long-term treadmill training ameliorates endothelium-dependent vasorelaxation mediated by insulin and insulin-like growth factor-1 in hypertension. *J. Appl. Physiol. (1985)* **2015**, *119*, 663–669. [CrossRef]
15. Vecchione, C.; Colella, S.; Fratta, L.; Gentile, M.T.; Selvetella, G.; Frati, G.; Trimarco, B.; Lembo, G. Impaired insulin-like growth factor I vasorelaxant effects in hypertension. *Hypertension* **2001**, *37*, 1480–1485. [CrossRef]
16. Yang, A.L.; Chao, J.I.; Lee, S.D. Altered insulin-mediated and insulin-like growth factor-1-mediated vasorelaxation in aortas of obese Zucker rats. *Int. J. Obes.* **2007**, *31*, 72–77. [CrossRef] [PubMed]
17. Yang, A.L.; Yeh, C.K.; Su, C.T.; Lo, C.W.; Lin, K.L.; Lee, S.D. Aerobic exercise acutely improves insulin- and insulin-like growth factor-1-mediated vasorelaxation in hypertensive rats. *Exp. Physiol.* **2010**, *95*, 622–629. [CrossRef] [PubMed]
18. Seals, D.R.; Kaplon, R.E.; Gioscia-Ryan, R.A.; LaRocca, T.J. You're only as old as your arteries: Translational strategies for preserving vascular endothelial function with aging. *Physiology* **2014**, *29*, 250–264. [CrossRef] [PubMed]
19. Mojiminiyi, F.B.; Dikko, M.; Muhammad, B.Y.; Ojobor, P.D.; Ajagbonna, O.P.; Okolo, R.U.; Igbokwe, U.V.; Mojiminiyi, U.E.; Fagbemi, M.A.; Bello, S.O.; et al. Antihypertensive effect of an aqueous extract of the calyx of Hibiscus sabdariffa. *Fitoterapia* **2007**, *78*, 292–297. [CrossRef] [PubMed]
20. Sarr, M.; Ngom, S.; Kane, M.O.; Wele, A.; Diop, D.; Sarr, B.; Gueye, L.; Andriantsitohaina, R.; Diallo, A.S. In vitro vasorelaxation mechanisms of bioactive compounds extracted from Hibiscus sabdariffa on rat thoracic aorta. *Nutr. Metab.* **2009**, *6*, 45. [CrossRef]
21. Semaming, Y.; Pannengpetch, P.; Chattipakorn, S.C.; Chattipakorn, N. Pharmacological properties of protocatechuic Acid and its potential roles as complementary medicine. *Evid.-Based Complement. Altern. Med.* **2015**, *2015*, 593902. [CrossRef] [PubMed]
22. Safaeian, L.; Hajhashemi, V.; Haghjoo Javanmard, S.; Sanaye Naderi, H. The Effect of Protocatechuic Acid on Blood Pressure and Oxidative Stress in Glucocorticoid-induced Hypertension in Rat. *Iran J. Pharm. Res.* **2016**, *15*, 83–91. [PubMed]
23. Shi, G.F.; An, L.J.; Jiang, B.; Guan, S.; Bao, Y.M. Alpinia protocatechuic acid protects against oxidative damage in vitro and reduces oxidative stress in vivo. *Neurosci. Lett.* **2006**, *403*, 206–210. [CrossRef]
24. Harini, R.; Pugalendi, K.V. Antihyperglycemic effect of protocatechuic acid on streptozotocin-diabetic rats. *J. Basic Clin. Physiol. Pharmacol.* **2010**, *21*, 79–91. [CrossRef] [PubMed]
25. Semaming, Y.; Kumfu, S.; Pannangpetch, P.; Chattipakorn, S.C.; Chattipakorn, N. Protocatechuic acid exerts a cardioprotective effect in type 1 diabetic rats. *J. Endocrinol.* **2014**, *223*, 13–23. [CrossRef] [PubMed]
26. Liu, R.; Li, H.; Fan, W.; Jin, Q.; Chao, T.; Wu, Y.; Huang, J.; Hao, L.; Yang, X. Leucine Supplementation Differently Modulates Branched-Chain Amino Acid Catabolism, Mitochondrial Function and Metabolic Profiles at the Different Stage of Insulin Resistance in Rats on High-Fat Diet. *Nutrients* **2017**, *9*, 565. [CrossRef]
27. McCallum, R.W.; Hamilton, C.A.; Graham, D.; Jardine, E.; Connell, J.M.; Dominiczak, A.F. Vascular responses to IGF-I and insulin are impaired in aortae of hypertensive rats. *J. Hypertens.* **2005**, *23*, 351–358. [CrossRef]
28. Scazzocchio, B.; Vari, R.; Filesi, C.; Del Gaudio, I.; D'Archivio, M.; Santangelo, C.; Iacovelli, A.; Galvano, F.; Pluchinotta, F.R.; Giovannini, C.; et al. Protocatechuic acid activates key components of insulin signaling pathway mimicking insulin activity. *Mol. Nutr. Food Res.* **2015**, *59*, 1472–1481. [CrossRef] [PubMed]
29. Pagliaro, B.; Santolamazza, C.; Simonelli, F.; Rubattu, S. Phytochemical Compounds and Protection from Cardiovascular Diseases: A State of the Art. *Biomed. Res. Int.* **2015**, *2015*, 918069. [CrossRef]
30. Zhou, M.S.; Wang, A.; Yu, H. Link between insulin resistance and hypertension: What is the evidence from evolutionary biology? *Diabetol. Metab. Syndr.* **2014**, *6*, 12. [CrossRef]
31. Montezano, A.C.; Dulak-Lis, M.; Tsiropoulou, S.; Harvey, A.; Briones, A.M.; Touyz, R.M. Oxidative stress and human hypertension: Vascular mechanisms, biomarkers, and novel therapies. *Can. J. Cardiol.* **2015**, *31*, 631–641. [CrossRef]
32. Seals, D.R.; Jablonski, K.L.; Donato, A.J. Aging and vascular endothelial function in humans. *Clin. Sci. (Lond.)* **2011**, *120*, 357–375. [CrossRef]
33. Guzik, T.J.; Touyz, R.M. Oxidative Stress, Inflammation, and Vascular Aging in Hypertension. *Hypertension* **2017**, *70*, 660–667. [CrossRef] [PubMed]

34. Masodsai, K.; Lin, Y.Y.; Lee, S.D.; Yang, A.L. Exercise and Endothelial Dysfunction in Hypertension. *Adapt. Med.* **2017**, *9*, 1–14. [CrossRef]
35. Safaeian, L.; Emami, R.; Hajhashemi, V.; Haghighatian, Z. Antihypertensive and antioxidant effects of protocatechuic acid in deoxycorticosterone acetate-salt hypertensive rats. *Biomed. Pharmacother.* **2018**, *100*, 147–155. [CrossRef] [PubMed]
36. Kim, Y.S.; Seo, H.W.; Lee, M.H.; Kim, D.K.; Jeon, H.; Cha, D.S. Protocatechuic acid extends lifespan and increases stress resistance in Caenorhabditis elegans. *Arch. Pharm. Res.* **2014**, *37*, 245–252. [CrossRef] [PubMed]
37. Zhang, X.; Shi, G.F.; Liu, X.Z.; An, L.J.; Guan, S. Anti-ageing effects of protocatechuic acid from Alpinia on spleen and liver antioxidative system of senescent mice. *Cell Biochem. Funct.* **2011**, *29*, 342–347. [CrossRef] [PubMed]
38. Varì, R.; D'Archivio, M.; Filesi, C.; Carotenuto, S.; Scazzocchio, B.; Santangelo, C.; Giovannini, C.; Masella, R. Protocatechuic acid induces antioxidant/detoxifying enzyme expression through JNK-mediated Nrf2 activation in murine macrophages. *J. Nutr. Biochem.* **2011**, *22*, 409–417. [CrossRef]
39. Reagan-Shaw, S.; Nihal, M.; Ahmad, N. Dose translation from animal to human studies revisited. *FASEB J.* **2008**, *22*, 659–661. [CrossRef]
40. Li, Q.X.; Xiong, Z.Y.; Hu, B.P.; Tian, Z.J.; Zhang, H.F.; Gou, W.Y.; Wang, H.C.; Gao, F.; Zhang, Q.J. Aging-associated insulin resistance predisposes to hypertension and its reversal by exercise: The role of vascular vasorelaxation to insulin. *Basic Res. Cardiol.* **2009**, *104*, 269–284. [CrossRef]

13

Amino Acids and Hypertension in Adults

Eleonora Poggiogalle [1,*], Mario Fontana [2], Anna Maria Giusti [1], Alessandro Pinto [1], Gino Iannucci [3], Andrea Lenzi [1] and Lorenzo Maria Donini [1]

1. Department of Experimental Medicine-Medical Pathophysiology, Food Science and Endocrinology Section; Sapienza University of Rome, 00185 Rome, Italy
2. Department of Biochemical Sciences "A. Rossi-Fanelli"; Sapienza University of Rome, Piazzale Aldo Moro 5, 00185 Rome, Italy
3. Department of Internal Medicine and Medical Specialties, Sapienza University of Rome, Viale del Policlinico 155, 00165 Rome, Italy

* Correspondence: eleonora.poggiogalle@uniroma1.it

Abstract: Accumulating evidence suggests a potential role of dietary protein among nutritional factors interfering with the regulation of blood pressure. Dietary protein source (plant versus animal protein), and especially, protein composition in terms of amino acids has been postulated to interfere with mechanisms underlying the development of hypertension. Recently, mounting interest has been directed at amino acids in hypertension focusing on habitual dietary intake and their circulating levels regardless of single amino acid dietary supplementation. The aim of the present review was to summarize epidemiological evidence concerning the connection between amino acids and hypertension. Due to the large variability in methodologies used for assessing amino acid levels and heterogeneity in the results obtained, it was not possible to draw robust conclusions. Indeed, some classes of amino acids or individual amino acids showed non-causative association with blood pressure as well as the incidence of hypertension, but the evidence was far from being conclusive. Further research should be prompted for a thorough understanding of amino acid effects and synergistic actions of different amino acid classes on blood pressure regulation.

Keywords: amino acids; blood pressure; humans

---

1. Introduction

According to recent epidemiological projections, the global burden of hypertension is associated with a remarkable increase in poor health outcomes. The global age-standardized prevalence of elevated blood pressure was 24.1% in men and 20.1% in women in 2015 [1]. The overall global prevalence of hypertension is expected to increase by 15–20% by 2025. Based on the Global Burden of Disease report, in 2015 a 1.4 fold increase was detected in mortality and disability-adjusted life years (DALYs) due to the presence of elevated systolic blood pressure since 1990 [2].

The association between hypertension and dietary and lifestyle factors is well established, with excess weight, lack of sufficient physical activity, and high sodium intake acknowledged as the main contributors [3]. Nonetheless, dietary interventions play a pivotal role in the extant treatment strategies for hypertension [4].

Growing interest has been directed to the potential effect of specific nutrients on blood pressure. Association between dietary protein and hypertension has been described, with a high-protein diet exerting beneficial effects on blood pressure [5]; however, the inverse relationship between dietary protein intake and blood pressure described in short-term studies appears to be weakened when considering longer study duration [6]. One potential mechanism for anti-hypertensive effects connected to elevated protein intake may be represented by the replacement of other macronutrients, mainly carbohydrates: if hypotensive effects are attributable to increased protein intake per se or to the concomitant reduction in the proportions of fat and carbohydrate is still unclear [6].

Data regarding the potential effect of the type (plant versus animal source) of dietary protein and blood pressure are not consistent [7]. Evidence from observational studies suggesting a favorable effect on blood pressure due to the vegetable protein intake is not further supported by a meta-analysis including data from forty randomized controlled studies [8], with no differences on blood pressure levels related to dietary protein source. Different protein amino acid compositions, and thus, amino acid intake could be the reason for such discrepant results. It is the case of soy protein, a largely investigated source of vegetable protein, in which some amino acids with antihypertensive properties are abundant (i.e., arginine, and cysteine) [9]. Furthermore, amino acids as part of bioactive peptides derived from food proteins may also be relevant in blood pressure regulation through the inhibition of angiotensin converting enzymes [10]. In recent years, several studies have focused on amino acids and hypertension, with conclusive evidence yet to be established.

The aim of the present review is to summarize epidemiological evidence concerning the connection between amino acids and hypertension.

2. Methods

Relevant peer-reviewed journal articles published in English were identified in the MEDLINE database (the last search was conducted on 31 January 2019); different combinations of the following search terms were used: "amino acids", "hypertension", and "blood pressure". Bibliographic references from eligible articles were reviewed for selection of any additional studies.

Also, the following exclusion criteria were used: any articles concerning secondary hypertension or central hypertension; any paper evaluating inherited disorders of amino acid metabolism; any study regarding hepatic, renal, or musculoskeletal diseases; any article based on amino acid supplementation; any study assessing amino acid derivatives; any study carried out in children and adolescents; and any study conducted in animals. Review articles, letters in response to published articles, editorials, commentaries, and conference abstracts were excluded.

3. Results

A total of seventeen studies were included. Study characteristics, study participants, amino acids investigated, and main outcomes are summarized in Table 1. Ten out of seventeen studies evaluated dietary amino acid intake based on different dietary recall methods (e.g., food-frequency questionnaire, 3 day food diary, 4 day dietary record, 24 h dietary recall, and cross-check dietary history method). In six studies, either plasma or serum amino acid concentrations were assessed, and just one study considered urinary amino acids. In one study, the levels of amino acids in the cerebrospinal fluid were also assessed. Three studies relied on principal component analysis. A marked variability was observed in terms of the number and groups of amino acids investigated, varying from one single amino acid to the calculation of a ratio among different amino acids. Ten out of seventeen studies were cross-sectional, six studies had a prospective design (though in the study by Venho et al. [11], only data at the baseline were considered), and in one study, both the cross-sectional and the prospective analyses were performed [12]. In longitudinal studies, the longest duration of follow-up was 10 years.

Table 1. Study characteristics and main findings.

Authors	Year	Study Participants (n) and Study Design	Ethnicity	Age (Year) *	Amino Acids (Dietary or Biological Fluid Analysis)	Main Findings
Altorf-van der Kuil W et al. [12]	2013	3086 men and women (cross-sectional analysis) + 1810 men and women (prospective analysis, 6 year follow-up)	Dutch	66 ± 7	Glutamic acid, Arginine, cysteine, Lysine, Tyrosine (FFQ)	A higher intake of Tyr (~0.3% of protein) was related to a 2.4 mm Hg lower SBP (p-trend = 0.05) but not to DBP (p = 0.35). The other AA were not significantly associated with BP levels in a cross-sectional analysis. None of the AA were associated with incident hypertension (HR: 0.81–1.18; p-trend> 0.2).
Cheng Y et al. [13]	2018	103 men and women DASH-Sodium trial—considering only the arm on a US diet (cross-sectional study)	US-American	49 ± 10	Urinary AAs	Significant positive associations with SBP for urinary cysteine (p = 0.008), Cit (p = 0.003), and Lys (p = 0.009); significant positive associations with DBP for urinary cystine (p = 0.005) but not the other metabolites.
Hu W et al. [14]	2016	1302 men and women Huai'an Diabetes Prevention Program (cross-sectional study)	Chinese	40–79	Serum BCAAs (Val, Ile, and Leu)	No significant correlation between either single BCAAs or total BCAAs, SBP, and DBP.
Jennings A et al. [15]	2016	1997 female twins Twin-UK cohort (cross-sectional study)	British	41.7 ± 12.1	Dietary BCAA (FFQ)	Higher BCAA intake was also associated with significantly lower SBP (Q5–Q1 = −2.3 mmHg, p-trend 0.01) comparing those in the highest and lowest quintiles of intake. Lower prevalence ratio for hypertension in the highest versus lowest quintile of BCAA intake (p = 0.02).
Ntzouvani A et al. [16]	2017	100 men (cross-sectional study)	Greek	54.6 ± 8.9	Five AA patterns by PCA: Factor 1: BCAAs and AAAs, glutamic and aspartic acid, Ala, Lys, and Met; Factor 2: Gln, Gly, Ser, Asn, Thr, Orn, Lys, His, and Pro; Factor 3: total homocysteine, cystathionine, creatinine, trimethyllysine, methylmalonic acid, Pro and kynurenine; Factor 4: betaine, choline, SDMA, dimethylglycine, and creatinine; Factor 5: Arg, TMAO, Orn and Met. (plasma)	Factor 2 was negatively associated with SBP ($r = -0.296$, $p \leq 0.005$).
Ogawa M et al. [17]	1985	12 normotensive subjects and 12 patients with essential hypertension under nutritional control after at least 10 days of standard hospital diet (cross-sectional study)	Japanese	23–70	Plasma taurine, Ser, Met (sulfur AAs)(plasma and csf)	Plasma taurine, Ser, Met, and Thr were significantly lower in patients with essential hypertension than in normotensive patients. The levels of plasma taurine, Ser, Met, and total sulfur AAs correlated inversely to SBP. No difference was observed in the CSF levels of free AA in normotensive and hypertensive patients.
Oomen CM et al. [18]	2000	806 men The Zutphen Elderly Study (prospective cohort study, 10 year follow-up)	Dutch	64–84	Dietary arginine (cross-check dietary history method)	Non-significant lower SBP of approximately 2 mmHg with a 2.5 g/day higher Arg intake (p = 0.25).
Siomakajlo M et al. [19]	2017	263 men (cross-sectional study)	Polish	36–60	BCAAs, Phe, and AAAs: 2 factors by PCA: Factor 1: BCAAs—Leu, Ile, Val-, and Phe; Factor 2: Tyr and Trp (plasma)	Significant positive associations between Factor 1 and SBP (r = 0.15, 95% CI: 0.01; 0.3), and Factor 1 and DBP (r = 0.17, 95% CI: 0.03; 0.33).
Stamler J et al. [20]	2009	4680 men and women (cross-sectional study)	Chinese, Japanese, British, and US-American	40–59	Glutamic acid (24-h dietary recall)	Glutamic acid intake (as percentage of total protein) higher by 2 SD corresponded to lower DBP (z-score −2.15 to −3.57) and SBP (z-score −2.21 to −3.66).
Stamler J et al. [21]	2013	4680 men and women INTERMAP study (cross-sectional study)	Chinese, Japanese, British, and US-American	40–59	Glycine (24-h dietary recall)	Estimated average BP differences associated with a 2-SD higher Gly intake (0.71 g/24 h) were 2.0–3.0 mm Hg systolic BP (z = 2.97–4.32) stronger in Western than in East Asian participants.

Table 1. *Cont.*

Authors	Year	Study Participants (n) and Study Design	Ethnicity	Age (Year) *	Amino Acids (Dietary or Biological Fluid Analysis)	Main Findings
Teymoori F et al. [22]	2019	4288 men and women (prospective analysis, 3.1 year follow-up)	Iranian	39.7 ± 12.8	Aromatic amino acids (FFQ)	The adjusted OR of hypertension for percentage of AAAs from total protein intake was 1.63 (95% CI, 1.06–2.50; $p = 0.03$) when comparing the highest quartile to the lowest. A positive relationship was observed between the highest versus the lowest quartile Phe intake (OR = 1.66; 95% CI, 1.14–2.47; $p = 0.03$). No significant association of Tyr and Trp intakes with hypertension risk.
Teymoori F et al. [23]	2017	4288 men and women (prospective analysis, 3.1 year follow-up)	Iranian	39.7 ± 12.8	Three AA patterns by PCA: 1st pattern: Branched chain AAs, aromatic AAs, and Pro. 2nd pattern: acidic AAs, and proline. 3rd pattern: sulfuric AAs, and small AAs (Gly and Ala) (FFQ)	The OR for incidence of hypertension of the highest quartile score of the first pattern was 1.83 (95% CI: 1.21–2.77, p for trend = 0.002), compared to the lowest. For the 2nd and 3rd patterns of dietary AA intake, no significant association with incident hypertension was found, although the 3rd pattern did have a slight tendency to reduce the risk of hypertension (OR = 0.81; 95% CI: 0.65–1.16, p for trend = 0.20).
Teymoori F et al. [24]	2018	4288 men and women (prospective analysis, 3.1 years follow-up)	Iranian	39.7 ± 12.8	AA ratios of Leu.Ser/Thr.Trp, Leu/Trp, Leu/Thr, and Ser/Thr (FFQ)	The OR of the highest quartile of dietary Leu.Ser/Thr.Trp intake was 1.48 (95% CI: 1.04–2.09, p for trend: 0.02), compared with the lowest one. The OR of hypertension in the highest, compared with the lowest quartile of the Leu/Thr ratio (2.19 versus 2.02) was 1.46 (1.01–2.12), p for trend = 0.07.
Tuttle KR et al. [25]	2012	92 men and women THIS-DIET study (nested cohort, prospective analysis, 2 year follow-up)	95% White	59 ± 9	Methionine, alanine, threonine, histidine. (3-day food diary)	Met and Ala were positively associated with higher SBP (OR (95% CI): 1.29 (1.14–1.46), $p < 0.001$, and 1.17 (1.05–1.30), $p = 0.005$) and higher DBP (OR (95% CI): 1.21 (1.05–1.39), $p = 0.007$, and 1.22 (1.07–1.38), $p = 0.002$). Thr and His were inversely associated with SBP (OR (95% CI): 0.84 (0.74–0.96), $p = 0.01$, and 0.92 (0.86–1.00), $p = 0.04$) and DBP (His only: OR (95% CI): 0.89 (0.82–0.97), $p = 0.01$)
Venho B et al. [11]	2002	1981 men The Kuopio Ischaemic Heart Disease Risk Factor Study (KIHD) (prospective cohort study, dietary arginine assessment just at baseline)	Finnish	52.3 ± 5.3	Total dietary arginine, animal-derived arginine, plant-derived arginine (4-day dietary record)	The regression coefficients between SBP and the intake of total, animal-derived and plant-derived Arg were 0.01 ($p = 0.674$), <0.01 ($p = 0.931$), and 0.02 ($p = 0.420$), respectively. The regression coefficients between DBP and the intake of total, animal-derived, and plant-derived Arg were <0.01 ($p = 0.746$), 0.01 ($p = 0.831$), and <0.03 ($p = 0.195$), respectively.
Yamaguchi N et al. [26]	2017	8589 men and women (cross-sectional study)	Japanese	>20	19 plasma free amino acids were measured: Ala, Arg, Asn, Cit, Gln, Gly, His, Ile, Leu, Lys, Met, Orn, Phe, Pro, Ser, Thr, Trp, Tyr, and Val	BCAAs and AAAs showed moderately positive correlation with SBP and DBP.
Yang R et al. [27]	2014	272 men and 200 women (cross-sectional study)	Chinese	70.1 ± 6.6	Serum BCAAs (Val, Ile, and Leu) and AAAs (Tyr and Phe)	Positive correlations between total AAAs and DBP ($r = 0.127$), and total BCAAs and DBP ($r = 0.197$) (all $p < 0.05$) as well as Val and SBP ($p < 0.05$). All single AAAs and single BCAA were positively correlated with DBP (all $p < 0.05$).

Legend: BP: blood pressure; CSF: cerebrospinal fluid; SBP: systolic blood pressure; DBP: diastolic blood pressure; DASH: Dietary Approaches to Stop Hypertension; AA: amino acid; AAAs: aromatic amino acids; BCAAs: branched chain amino acids; PCA: principal component analysis; FFQ: food frequency questionnaire; Ala: alanine; Arg: arginine; Asp: asparagine; Cit: citrulline; Gln: glutamine; Gly: glycine; His: histidine; Ile: isoleucine; Leu: leucine; Lys: lysine; Met: methionine; Orn: ornithine; Phe: phenylalanine; Pro: proline; Ser: serine; SDMA: symmetric dimethylarginine; Thr: threonine; TMAO: trimethylamine N-oxide; Trp: tryptophane; Tyr: tyrosine; Val: valine. SD: standard deviation; * Age expressed as mean ± SD, or age range when mean age of total participants was not clearly stated.

4. Discussion

The present review article provides evidence concerning the connections between amino acids and hypertension, focusing on associations between either blood pressure levels or risk of hypertension, and dietary amino acids or amino acid levels in biological fluids.

Only the study by Stamler et al. [20] reported a favorable relationship between dietary glutamic acid and blood pressure, showing that an elevated dietary intake of glutamic acid was associated with lower values of both systolic and diastolic blood pressure. This finding is not in accordance with results from a Dutch study describing no association between dietary glutamic acid either blood pressure levels or incidence of hypertension [12]. Vegetable proteins are especially rich in glutamic acids. Glutamate is included in the glutathione molecule, with potential antioxidant effects improving blood pressure homeostasis [28]. Ethnicity-related differences in dietary sources of glutamic acid may explain those conflicting observations: in the INTERMAP study the association between glutamic acid and reduced blood pressure was ascribed to the elevated presence of glutamic acid in vegetable protein, in line with prior evidence indicating a lowering effect of plant protein on blood pressure [20]. Nonetheless, a more recent meta-analysis by Rebholz et al. [8] did not support a different association of animal versus plant protein with blood pressure.

Regarding tyrosine, results are conflicting: in the Rotterdam study [12], a cross-sectional analysis revealed that a high dietary intake of tyrosine was related to lower systolic blood pressure (though results were statistically just marginally significant when considering quartiles of tyrosine intake, but they become statistically significant when considering tyrosine intake as a continuous variable), but no relationship emerged between dietary tyrosine and diastolic blood pressure. However, no association with the incidence of hypertension was described in findings from prospective analysis after a 6 year follow-up.

Tyrosine effects on hypertension were also evaluated in another study investigating all aromatic amino acids [24] in an Iranian adult study cohort: dietary tyrosine, as well as dietary tryptophan, did not show any association with incident hypertension after a 3.1 year follow-up. Just phenylalanine intake in the highest quartile was associated to significant increased risk of hypertension compared to the lowest quartile. Nonetheless, when considered globally, high total dietary aromatic amino acid intake exhibited a positive significant association with increased risk of incident hypertension [19,22,26,27]. In a Polish observational study assessing plasma amino acid levels, principal component analysis identified phenylalanine in a separated cluster from tyrosine and tryptophan [19]. Tyrosine acts as a precursor for norepinephrine synthesis, therefore, it can modulate norepinephrine levels and affect the sympathetic tone on the vasculature. Findings from animal studies revealed that tyrosine administration in rats lowered blood pressure through central catecholamine action on alpha-receptors [29,30]. However, data from rodents were not confirmed in hypertensive adults undergoing chronic dietary tyrosine supplementation [31]. The majority of phenylalanine is converted to tyrosine, and effects on blood pressure are potentially due to the changes in tyrosine levels. However, phenylalanine *per se* can interfere with tetrahydrobiopterin (BH4) production, a cofactor for aromatic amino acid hydroxylation, involved in the relaxation of the endothelium [32]. In the presence of the high availability of aromatic amino acids, the oxidation of BH4 may result in alterations of its vasoactive properties with detrimental effects on the endothelium [33]. Tryptophan is a precursor for the synthesis of serotonin (5-hydroxytryptamine, 5-HT), a monoaminergic neurotransmitter. Serotonin receptors are present on adrenergic nerves at the level of the sympathetic–vascular junction, potentially explaining the mechanism underlying the influence of 5-HT on the vascular tone [34]. Administration of L-tryptophan induced a reduction in blood pressure in animals [35], and analogous short-term effects were described in hypertensive patients but not in normotensive controls [36]. However, derangements of 5-HT metabolism have been shown in hypertensive patients, and in the long-term, tryptophan effects on blood pressure are unclear. These reasons may explain the lack of association of habitual dietary intake or circulating tryptophan with blood pressure related outcomes [37]. Moreover, tryptophan-containing peptides obtained from enzymatic hydrolysis of food protein have been shown to interfere with the renin–angiotensin axis inhibiting angiotensin-converting enzymes, though further evidence from human studies is needed [38]. Plasma phenylalanine, together with branched chain amino acids (BCAAs) in the same cluster, showed a positive association with both systolic and diastolic blood pressure, whereas no association was found with blood pressure when the other cluster, including the two remaining aromatic amino acids, was taken into account.

Dietary BCAAs clustered with aromatic amino acids (AAAs), and proline based on principal component analysis in a longitudinal study conducted in an Iranian cohort, showed a positive association with incidence of hypertension [23]. Analogous findings of a positive relationship between BCAAs and AAAs emerged in two Asian studies [26,27]. In the TwinUK cohort, dietary BCAAs were associated with decreased risk of hypertension [15], whereas no relationship was observed in a Chinese study considering serum BCAA levels [14]. In one study taking into account the ratio between different dietary amino acids, the leucine–serine/threonine–tryptophan ratio results were significantly positively associated with the risk of hypertension [22].

Branched chain amino acid concentrations in biological fluids (serum/plasma) were positively associated with high blood pressure, though data were discrepant in some studies based on dietary records. Plenty of studies indicated that alterations in BCAA metabolism, leading to the accumulation of BCAAs and their byproducts, are linked to remarkable metabolic derangements such as insulin resistance, the latter being associated with increased risk of hypertension [39,40]. Furthermore, BCAA ingestion was able to reduce brain tryptophan and tyrosine uptake, affecting serotonin and catecholamine synthesis with consequences on central blood pressure regulation [41,42]. Nonetheless, BCAA effects on blood pressure may be counterbalanced in the presence of other nutrients: whey protein is rich in both BCAAs and lactokinins, the latter with inhibiting properties on the angiotensin-converting enzyme; thus, ingestion of whey protein may induce opposite effects on hypertension mediated by BCAAs and lactokinins [43]. Interestingly, AAAs and BCAAs have hydrophobic or bulky residues that can be relevant for the binding of bioactive peptides to the angiotensin-converting enzyme which is crucial in blood pressure control [44].

Concerning dietary glycine, findings from the INTERMAP study were not in line with other studies including glycine in factors obtained by principal component analysis [16,21,23].

In the INTERMAP study [21], dietary intake of glycine (expressed as a percentage of total protein and based on 24 h dietary recall) was positively associated with both systolic and diastolic blood pressure. Conversely, in a Greek study, plasma glycine levels—clustering with glutamine, serine, asparagine, threonine, lysine, histidine, and proline in the principal component analysis—showed a negative relationship with systolic blood pressure [16]. Also, in another study, the principal component analysis pattern encompassing glycine, sulfur amino acids, and alanine, tended to be associated to a diminished risk of hypertension [23]. An inverse correlation was observed between systolic blood pressure and sulfur amino acids in plasma, but not in cerebrospinal fluid, in a small Japanese cohort [17]. Stamler et al. [21] postulated that dietary glycine intake was positively associated with blood pressure, as glycine is abundant in animal-derived protein and meat consumption may be a dietary factor for elevated blood pressure. Conversely, the opposite findings may be supported by the important role played by glycine in reducing oxidative stress, favoring nitric oxide action; moreover, glycine is involved in the synthesis of structural protein, such as elastin; alterations in elastin formation have been connected to impaired elastic properties of vessels, a remarkable aspect in the pathogenesis of hypertension [45].

Dietary alanine showed a positive relation to blood pressure in the INTERMAP study (expressed as percentage of total protein intake) and in a nested cohort within the THIS-DIET study (as daily intake in absolute value) [21,25].

With respect to methionine, results based on dietary records [25] were in disagreement with findings from plasma amino acid levels [17]. Elevated dietary methionine intake was associated with augmented systolic and diastolic blood pressure [25]. Methionine is an essential amino acid; among its metabolic byproducts, homocysteine, when elevated, is well known for its ability to influence endothelial function inducing the production of asymmetrical dimethylarginine (ADMA), which in turn, can inhibit the synthesis of nitric oxide [46]. Thus, methionine effects on blood pressure appear to be indirect and mediated by the increase in homocysteine levels, as shown in studies relying on dietary supplementation with methionine in animals and humans [47,48].

Several amino acids interfere with vascular physiology; among them, arginine is well known to have relevant vasogenic properties [49]. Despite a wealth of studies demonstrating the beneficial effects from dietary supplementation with L-arginine including lowering both systolic and diastolic blood pressure levels [50,51], studies focusing on dietary arginine considering only a usual diet, excluding supraphysiological intake through dietary supplementation, did not support any association between this amino acid and blood pressure [11,18]. In middle-aged men participating in the Kuopio Ischaemic Heart Disease Risk Factor Study (KIHD), no association was found between dietary arginine and blood pressure levels, regardless of the dietary source (either plant-derived or animal-derived arginine) [11]. Similarly, dietary arginine did not associate with blood pressure in a Dutch elderly male population [18].

In the only study assessing urinary amino acids, a positive association was described between urinary cysteine, citrulline, and lysine and systolic blood pressure, and between urinary cysteine and diastolic blood pressure [13]. These data regarding urinary cysteine, as well as the lack of association for dietary cysteine and blood pressure [12] are in contrast with evidence showing antihypertensive effects mediated by cysteine through its free sulfhydryl group. The majority of studies on cysteine were based on supplementation with its stable analogue N-acetyl-cysteine [52]. Cysteine is able to modulate blood pressure by decreasing oxidative stress, increasing nitric oxide bioavailability, and ameliorating insulin sensitivity [52]. In addition, cysteine is part of the tripeptide glutathione with glutamic acid and glycine. Glutathione is in turn well known for its antioxidant ability with additional beneficial consequences on blood pressure regulation [52].

5. Conclusions

Due to the large variability in methodologies used for assessing amino acid levels and heterogeneity in results obtained, it was not possible to draw robust conclusions. In fact, the use of any type of dietary records was affected by under- or overreporting [53,54]. Data based on direct measurements in plasma and other biological fluids are more reliable, though they can be affected by derangements in metabolic cascades leading to alterations in amino acid metabolic byproducts.

Further research should be prompted for a thorough understanding of the synergistic actions of different amino acid classes on blood pressure regulation. In addition, the interplay between gut microbiota and amino acid metabolism in hypertension [55] deserves future investigation.

Author Contributions: Conceptualization, E.P. and M.F.; methodology, L.M.D., A.M.G., A.P.; investigation, E.P., M.F., G.I.; writing—original draft preparation, E.P., A.M.G.; writing—review and editing, E.P., M.F., A.L.; supervision, L.M.D., A.L., G.I.

References

1. NCD Risk Factor Collaboration (NCD-RisC). Worldwide trends in blood pressure from 1975 to 2015: A pooled analysis of 1479 population-based measurement studies with 19·1 million participants. *Lancet* **2017**, *389*, 37–55. [CrossRef]
2. Forouzanfar, M.H.; Liu, P.; Roth, G.A.; Ng, M.; Biryukov, S.; Marczak, L.; Alexander, L.; Estep, K.; Abate, K.H.; Akinyemiju, T.F.; et al. Global Burden of Hypertension and Systolic Blood Pressure of at Least 110 to 115 mm Hg, 1990–2015. *JAMA* **2017**, *317*, 165–182. [CrossRef] [PubMed]
3. Geleijnse, J.M.; Kok, F.J.; Grobbee, D.E. Impact of dietary and lifestyle factors on the prevalence of hypertension in Western populations. *Eur. J. Public Health* **2004**, *14*, 235–239. [CrossRef] [PubMed]

4. Williams, B.; Mancia, G.; Spiering, W.; Agabiti Rosei, E.; Azizi, M.; Burnier, M.; Clement, D.L.; Coca, A.; De Simone, G.; Dominiczak, A.; et al. 2018 ESC/ESH Guidelines for the management of arterial hypertension. *Eur. Heart J.* **2018**, *39*, 3021–3104. [CrossRef] [PubMed]
5. Appel, L.J.; Sacks, F.M.; Carey, V.J.; Obarzanek, E.; Swain, J.F.; Miller, E.R., 3rd; Conlin, P.R.; Erlinger, T.P.; Rosner, B.A.; Laranjo, N.M.; et al. Effects of protein, monounsaturated fat, and carbohydrate intake on blood pressure and serum lipids: Results of the OmniHeart randomized trial. *JAMA* **2005**, *294*, 2455–2464. [CrossRef] [PubMed]
6. Teunissen-Beekman, K.F.; van Baak, M.A. The role of dietary protein in blood pressure regulation. *Curr. Opin. Lipidol.* **2013**, *24*, 65–70. [CrossRef]
7. Altorf-van der Kuil, W.; Engberink, M.F.; Brink, E.J.; van Baak, M.A.; Bakker, S.J.; Navis, G.; van't Veer, P.; Geleijnse, J.M. Dietary protein and blood pressure: A systematic review. *PLoS ONE* **2010**, *5*, e12102. [CrossRef]
8. Rebholz, C.M.; Friedman, E.E.; Powers, L.J.; Arroyave, W.D.; He, J.; Kelly, T.N. Dietary protein intake and blood pressure: A meta-analysis of randomized controlled trials. *Am. J. Epidemiol.* **2012**, *176*, S27–S43. [CrossRef]
9. Vasdev, S.; Stuckless, J. Antihypertensive effects of dietary protein and its mechanism. *Int. J. Angiol.* **2010**, *19*, e7–e20. [CrossRef]
10. Aluko, R.E. Antihypertensive peptides from food proteins. *Annu. Rev. Food Sci. Technol.* **2015**, *6*, 235–262. [CrossRef]
11. Venho, B.; Voutilainen, S.; Valkonen, V.P.; Virtanen, J.; Lakka, T.A.; Rissanen, T.H.; Ovaskainen, M.L.; Laitinen, M.; Salonen, J.T. Arginine intake, blood pressure, and the incidence of acute coronary events in men: The Kuopio Ischaemic Heart Disease Risk Factor Study. *Am. J. Clin. Nutr.* **2002**, *76*, 359–364. [CrossRef] [PubMed]
12. Altorf-van der Kuil, W.; Engberink, M.F.; De Neve, M.; van Rooij, F.J.; Hofman, A.; van't Veer, P.; Witteman, J.C.; Franco, O.H.; Geleijnse, J.M. Dietary amino acids and the risk of hypertension in a Dutch older population: The Rotterdam Study. *Am. J. Clin. Nutr.* **2013**, *97*, 403–410. [CrossRef] [PubMed]
13. Cheng, Y.; Song, H.; Pan, X.; Xue, H.; Wan, Y.; Wang, T.; Tian, Z.; Hou, E.; Lanza, I.R.; Liu, P.; et al. Urinary Metabolites Associated with Blood Pressure on a Low- or High-Sodium Diet. *Theranostics* **2018**, *8*, 1468–1480. [CrossRef] [PubMed]
14. Hu, W.; Sun, L.; Gong, Y.; Zhou, Y.; Yang, P.; Ye, Z.; Fu, J.; Huang, A.; Fu, Z.; Yu, W.; et al. Relationship between Branched-Chain Amino Acids, Metabolic Syndrome, and Cardiovascular Risk Profile in a Chinese Population: A Cross-Sectional Study. *Int. J. Endocrinol.* **2016**, *2016*, 8173905. [CrossRef] [PubMed]
15. Jennings, A.; MacGregor, A.; Pallister, T.; Spector, T.; Cassidy, A. Associations between branched chain amino acid intake and biomarkers of adiposity and cardiometabolic health independent of genetic factors: A twin study. *Int. J. Cardiol.* **2016**, *223*, 992–998. [CrossRef] [PubMed]
16. Ntzouvani, A.; Nomikos, T.; Panagiotakos, D.; Fragopoulou, E.; Pitsavos, C.; McCann, A.; Ueland, P.M.; Antonopoulou, S. Amino acid profile and metabolic syndrome in a male Mediterranean population: A cross-sectional study. *Nutr. Metab. Cardiovasc. Dis.* **2017**, *27*, 1021–1030. [CrossRef] [PubMed]
17. Ogawa, M.; Takahara, A.; Ishijima, M.; Tazaki, S. Decrease of plasma sulfur amino acids in essential hypertension. *Jpn. Circ. J.* **1985**, *49*, 1217–1224. [CrossRef]
18. Oomen, C.M.; van Erk, M.J.; Feskens, E.J.; Kok, F.J.; Kromhout, D. Arginine intake and risk of coronary heart disease mortality in elderly men. *Arterioscler. Thromb. Vasc. Biol.* **2000**, *20*, 2134–2139. [CrossRef]
19. Siomkajło, M.; Rybka, J.; Mierzchała-Pasierb, M.; Gamian, A.; Stankiewicz-Olczyk, J.; Bolanowski, M.; Daroszewski, J. Specific plasma amino acid disturbances associated with metabolic syndrome. *Endocrine* **2017**, *58*, 553–562. [CrossRef]
20. Stamler, J.; Brown, I.J.; Daviglus, M.L.; Chan, Q.; Kesteloot, H.; Ueshima, H.; Zhao, L.; Elliott, P. INTERMAP Research Group. Glutamic acid, the main dietary amino acid, and blood pressure: The INTERMAP Study (International Collaborative Study of Macronutrients, Micronutrients and Blood Pressure). *Circulation* **2009**, *120*, 221–228. [CrossRef]
21. Stamler, J.; Brown, I.J.; Daviglus, M.L.; Chan, Q.; Miura, K.; Okuda, N.; Ueshima, H.; Zhao, L.; Elliott, P. Dietary glycine and blood pressure: The International Study on Macro/Micronutrients and Blood Pressure. *Am. J. Clin. Nutr.* **2013**, *98*, 136–145. [CrossRef] [PubMed]
22. Teymoori, F.; Asghari, G.; Farhadnejad, H.; Mirmiran, P.; Azizi, F. Do dietary amino acid ratios predict risk of incident hypertension among adults? *Int. J. Food Sci. Nutr.* **2019**, *70*, 387–395. [CrossRef] [PubMed]

23. Teymoori, F.; Asghari, G.; Mirmiran, P.; Azizi, F. Dietary amino acids and incidence of hypertension: A principle component analysis approach. *Sci. Rep.* **2017**, *7*, 16838. [CrossRef] [PubMed]
24. Teymoori, F.; Asghari, G.; Mirmiran, P.; Azizi, F. High dietary intake of aromatic amino acids increases risk of hypertension. *J. Am. Soc. Hypertens.* **2018**, *12*, 25–33. [CrossRef] [PubMed]
25. Tuttle, K.R.; Milton, J.E.; Packard, D.P.; Shuler, L.A.; Short, R.A. Dietary amino acids and blood pressure: A cohort study of patients with cardiovascular disease. *Am. J. Kidney Dis.* **2012**, *59*, 803–809. [CrossRef] [PubMed]
26. Yamaguchi, N.; Mahbub, M.H.; Takahashi, H.; Hase, R.; Ishimaru, Y.; Sunagawa, H.; Amano, H.; Kobayashi-Miura, M.; Kanda, H.; Fujita, Y.; et al. Plasma free amino acid profiles evaluate risk of metabolic syndrome, diabetes, dyslipidemia, and hypertension in a large Asian population. *Environ. Health Prev. Med.* **2017**, *22*, 35. [CrossRef] [PubMed]
27. Yang, R.; Dong, J.; Zhao, H.; Li, H.; Guo, H.; Wang, S.; Zhang, C.; Wang, S.; Wang, M.; Yu, S.; et al. Association of branched-chain amino acids with carotid intima-media thickness and coronary artery disease risk factors. *PLoS ONE* **2014**, *9*, e99598. [CrossRef]
28. Vasdev, S.; Gill, V.D.; Singal, P.K. Modulation of oxidative stress-induced changes in hypertension and atherosclerosis by antioxidants. *Exp. Clin. Cardiol.* **2006**, *11*, 206–216.
29. Sved, A.F.; Fernstrom, J.D.; Wurtman, R.J. Tyrosine administration reduces blood pressure and enhances brain norepinephrine release in spontaneously hypertensive rats. *Proc. Natl. Acad. Sci. USA* **1979**, *76*, 3511–3514. [CrossRef]
30. Yamori, Y.; Fujiwara, M.; Horie, R.; Lovenberg, W. The hypotensive effect of centrally administered tyrosine. *Eur. J. Pharmacol.* **1980**, *68*, 201–204. [CrossRef]
31. Sole, M.J.; Benedict, C.R.; Myers, M.G.; Leenen, F.H.; Anderson, G.H. Chronic dietary tyrosine supplements do not affect mild essential hypertension. *Hypertension* **1985**, *7*, 593–596. [CrossRef] [PubMed]
32. Mitchell, B.M.; Dorrance, A.M.; Webb, R.C. Phenylalanine improves dilation and blood pressure in GTP cyclohydrolase inhibition-induced hypertensive rats. *J. Cardiovasc. Pharmacol.* **2004**, *43*, 758–763. [CrossRef]
33. Ichinose, H.; Nomura, T.; Sumi-Ichinose, C. Metabolism of tetrahydrobiopterin: Its relevance in monoaminergic neurons and neurological disorders. *Chem. Rec.* **2008**, *8*, 378–385. [CrossRef] [PubMed]
34. Watts, S.W.; Morrison, S.F.; Davis, R.P.; Barman, S.M. Serotonin and blood pressure regulation. *Pharmacol. Rev.* **2012**, *64*, 359–388. [CrossRef] [PubMed]
35. Ardiansyah Shirakawa, H.; Inagawa, Y.; Koseki, T.; Komai, M. Regulation of blood pressure and glucose metabolism induced by L-tryptophan in stroke-prone spontaneously hypertensive rats. *Nutr. Metab.* **2011**, *8*, 45. [CrossRef]
36. Feltkamp, H.; Meurer, K.A.; Godehardt, E. Tryptophan-induced lowering of blood pressure and changes of serotonin uptake by platelets in patients with essential hypertension. *Klin. Wochenschr.* **1984**, *62*, 1115–1119. [CrossRef] [PubMed]
37. Kamal, L.A.; Le Quan-Bui, K.H.; Meyer, P. Decreased uptake of 3H-serotonin and endogenous content of serotonin in blood platelets in hypertensive patients. *Hypertension* **1984**, *6*, 568–573. [CrossRef]
38. Khedr, S.; Deussen, A.; Kopaliani, I.; Zatschler, B.; Martin, M. Effects of tryptophan-containing peptides on angiotensin-converting enzyme activity and vessel tone ex vivo and in vivo. *Eur. J. Nutr.* **2018**, *57*, 907–915. [CrossRef]
39. Batch, B.C.; Shah, S.H.; Newgard, C.B.; Turer, C.B.; Haynes, C.; Bain, J.R.; Muehlbauer, M.; Patel, M.J.; Stevens, R.D.; Appel, L.J.; et al. Branched chain amino acids are novel biomarkers for discrimination of metabolic wellness. *Metabolism* **2013**, *62*, 961–969. [CrossRef]
40. Soleimani, M. Insulin resistance and hypertension: New insights. *Kidney Int.* **2015**, *87*, 497–499. [CrossRef]
41. Fernstrom, J.D. Large neutral amino acids: Dietary effects on brain neurochemistry and function. *Amino Acids* **2013**, *45*, 419–430. [CrossRef] [PubMed]
42. Choi, S.; DiSilvio, B.; Fernstrom, M.H.; Fernstrom, J.D. Effect of chronic protein ingestion on tyrosine and tryptophan levels and catecholamine and serotonin synthesis in rat brain. *Nutr. Neurosci.* **2011**, *14*, 260–267. [CrossRef] [PubMed]
43. Pal, S.; Ellis, V. Acute effects of whey protein isolate on blood pressure, vascular function and inflammatory markers in overweight postmenopausal women. *Br. J. Nutr.* **2011**, *105*, 1512–1519. [CrossRef] [PubMed]
44. Martin, M.; Deussen, A. Effects of natural peptides from food proteins on angiotensin converting enzyme activity and hypertension. *Crit. Rev. Food Sci. Nutr.* **2019**, *59*, 1264–1283. [CrossRef] [PubMed]

45. El Hafidi, M.; Pérez, I.; Baños, G. Is glycine effective against elevated blood pressure? *Curr. Opin. Clin. Nutr. Metab. Care* **2006**, *9*, 26–31. [CrossRef] [PubMed]
46. Böger, R.H.; Lentz, S.R.; Bode-Böger, S.M.; Knapp, H.R.; Haynes, W.G. Elevation of asymmetrical dimethylarginine may mediate endothelial dysfunction during experimental hyperhomocyst(e)inaemia in humans. *Clin. Sci.* **2001**, *100*, 161–167. [CrossRef] [PubMed]
47. Robin, S.; Maupoil, V.; Groubatch, F.; Laurant, P.; Jacqueson, A.; Berthelot, A. Effect of a methionine-supplemented diet on the blood pressure of Wistar-Kyoto and spontaneously hypertensive rats. *Br. J. Nutr.* **2003**, *89*, 539–548. [CrossRef] [PubMed]
48. Ditscheid, B.; Fünfstück, R.; Busch, M.; Schubert, R.; Gerth, J.; Jahreis, G. Effect of L-methionine supplementation on plasma homocysteine and other free amino acids: A placebo-controlled double-blind cross-over study. *Eur. J. Clin. Nutr.* **2005**, *59*, 768–775. [CrossRef] [PubMed]
49. Moncada, S.; Higgs, A. The L-arginine-nitric oxide pathway. *N. Engl. J. Med.* **1993**, *329*, 2002–2012.
50. Dong, J.Y.; Qin, L.Q.; Zhang, Z.; Zhao, Y.; Wang, J.; Arigoni, F.; Zhang, W. Effect of oral L-arginine supplementation on blood pressure: A meta-analysis of randomized, double-blind, placebo-controlled trials. *Am. Heart J.* **2011**, *162*, 959–965. [CrossRef]
51. Menzel, D.; Haller, H.; Wilhelm, M.; Robenek, H. L-arginine and B vitamins improve endothelial function in subjects with mild to moderate blood pressure elevation. *Eur. J. Nutr.* **2018**, *57*, 557–568. [CrossRef] [PubMed]
52. Vasdev, S.; Singal, P.; Gill, V. The antihypertensive effect of cysteine. *Int. J. Angiol.* **2009**, *18*, 7–21. [CrossRef] [PubMed]
53. Westerterp, K.R.; Goris, A.H. Validity of the assessment of dietary intake: Problems of misreporting. *Curr. Opin. Clin. Nutr. Metab. Care* **2002**, *5*, 489–493. [CrossRef] [PubMed]
54. Castro-Quezada, I.; Ruano-Rodríguez, C.; Ribas-Barba, L.; Serra-Majem, L. Misreporting in nutritional surveys: Methodological implications. *Nutr. Hosp.* **2015**, *31*, 119–127. [PubMed]
55. Richards, E.M.; Pepine, C.J.; Raizada, M.K.; Kim, S. The Gut, Its Microbiome, and Hypertension. *Curr. Hypertens. Rep.* **2017**, *19*, 36. [CrossRef] [PubMed]

14

Hypertension Associated with Fructose and High Salt: Renal and Sympathetic Mechanisms

Dragana Komnenov [1,2], Peter E. Levanovich [1] and Noreen F. Rossi [1,2,3,*]

1 Department of Physiology, Wayne State University, 4160 John R Street #908, Detroit, MI 48201, USA; dkomneno@med.wayne.edu (D.K.); plevanov@med.wayne.edu (P.E.L.)
2 Department of Internal Medicine, Wayne State University, 4160 John R Street #908, Detroit, MI 48201, USA
3 John D. Dingell VA Medical Center, 4646 John R Street, Detroit, MI 48201, USA
* Correspondence: nrossi@wayne.edu

Abstract: Hypertension is a leading cause of cardiovascular and chronic renal disease. Despite multiple important strides that have been made in our understanding of the etiology of hypertension, the mechanisms remain complex due to multiple factors, including the environment, heredity and diet. This review focuses on dietary contributions, providing evidence for the involvement of elevated fructose and salt consumption that parallels the increased incidence of hypertension worldwide. High fructose loads potentiate salt reabsorption by the kidney, leading to elevation in blood pressure. Several transporters, such as NHE3 and PAT1 are modulated in this milieu and play a crucial role in salt-sensitivity. High fructose ingestion also modulates the renin-angiotensin-aldosterone system. Recent attention has been shifted towards the contribution of the sympathetic nervous system, as clinical trials demonstrated significant reductions in blood pressure following renal sympathetic nerve ablation. New preclinical data demonstrates the activation of the renal sympathetic nerves in fructose-induced salt-sensitive hypertension, and reductions of blood pressure after renal nerve ablation. This review further demonstrates the interplay between sodium handling by the kidney, the renin-angiotensin-aldosterone system, and activation of the renal sympathetic nerves as important mechanisms in fructose and salt-induced hypertension.

Keywords: fructose; hypertension; renin-angiotensin-aldosterone system; renal transporters; sodium; renal sympathetic nerve activity

1. Introduction

Hypertension is a multifactorial condition rather than a single disease entity whose onset can be brought about through a variety of factors originating from environmental, dietary, or hereditary factors. The complex interplay of these components has frustrated our understanding of hypertension, despite decades of research spent attempting to identify its causes and develop viable treatments. Even today, less than 20% of all hypertensive cases have a known etiology (referred to as secondary hypertension) with the basis for the remaining majority of cases being unknown (referred to as primary or essential hypertension) [1,2]. Studies of the U.S. population have found that 29% of adults are hypertensive, and this number is only expected to increase dramatically in the near future [3]. Unfortunately, elevated blood pressure is becoming increasingly prevalent in people under the age of 40 years [4]. Despite the fact that the proportion of individuals with controlled blood pressure (systolic < 140 mmHg; diastolic < 90 mmHg) in the U.S. has increased from 28.4% to 43.5%, in low and middle-income countries it has actually decreased to 7.7% [5,6]. Indeed, even mild increases in either systolic or diastolic pressure (<10 mmHg) are accompanied by increases in mortality rates [7]. The increased prevalence of hypertension has coincided with an equally sharp increase in the incidence of chronic kidney disease that has been attributed, at least in part, to substantial changes in dietary intake and sedentary lifestyle [4,8]. Hence, there has been an increased effort to develop new models of hypertension that better reflect the environmental and dietary behaviors of modern society. Several models of diet-induced hypertension exist that are well established, namely those high in fat or sodium [9,10]. Models of metabolic syndrome induce a constellation of medical conditions accompanying insulin resistance such as obesity, hyperglycemia, hypertension and dyslipidemia [11]. Given the widespread use of fructose as a sweetener in food products, several recent reviews have discussed the impact of fructose ingestion on obesity and hypertension within the metabolic syndrome [12,13] and the hormones involved [14]. The present review focuses on recent interest in the consequences of even mild fructose consumption independent of full-blown metabolic syndrome with particular attention to the role of the kidney and the sympathetic nervous system on blood pressure.

Study selection: We searched PubMed (https://www.ncbi.nlm.nih.gov/pubmed/), the Cochrane Registry (http://www.cochranelibrary.com/about/central-landing-page.html), and the Web of Science Core Collection (https://www.library.ethz.ch/en/Resources/Databases/Web-of-Science-Core-Collection) from January 1975 to January 2019. The following search terms were used: fructose and blood pressure or hypertension; fructose and sodium; fructose and kidney; fructose and sympathetic nervous system. Then the search terms were refined with the addition of sodium to the search. Human and animal studies were included. This resulted in 428 articles whose abstracts were screened for relevancy to our topic of renal and sympathetic mechanisms involved in blood pressure control in the presence of fructose and high salt diets.

2. Fructose Consumption, Hypertension and Mortality

Total fructose consumption includes that which is found in high fructose corn syrup (HFCS) and sucrose. Generation of HFCS began in the late 1950s when it was discovered that glucose, hydrolyzed from corn starch extracts, could be partially converted to fructose through enzymatic isomerization [15]. Over time, this process was industrialized and led to the development of the corn-derived sweetener, HFCS, which can be synthesized with varying ratios of fructose to glucose content. Ease of synthesis, comparable flavor, and low cost of this ingredient have contributed to its widespread use as a sweetener [16]. Between 1970 and 2006, fructose consumption drastically increased, amounting to approximately 50% of all per capita added sugar consumption. This increase is accounted for solely by an exponential increase in free fructose consumption in the form of HFCS. During this time, caloric intake from total sugar (HFCS, sucrose, and other natural sugars) and fats increased significantly contributing to a 41% increase in total carbohydrate intake, of which fructose consumption provided a primary source [17].

HFCS appeals to nearly every demographic leading to its widespread use in food products. Statistical analysis of data collected in the National Health and Nutrition Examination Survey (NHANES I-III) determined that HFCS is most heavily consumed in the form soft drinks, and this trend is consistent throughout all age groups and sexes. Although a recent meta-analysis of three prospective studies fails to show incident hypertension associated with fructose, these studies relied on self-reports of physician-diagnosed hypertension and did not include concurrent sodium intake [18]. In contrast, another meta-analysis (n = 240,508) that includes data from the Coronary Artery Risk Development in Young Adults (CARDIA) cohort (n = 240,508) [19] and quoted by the recent American Heart Association update on stroke reports a 12% greater risk of hypertension with consumption of sugar sweetened beverages when controlled for sex, age, race, BMI and smoking behaviors [20]. Compared with the increased risk associated with more traditional factors such as alcohol consumption (61%), smoking (21%), and red meat intake (35%) and sedentary life style (48%) [21–24] or the non-traditional risk of stress (5–12%) [25], the risk associated with fructose intake may appear small but is nonetheless real. Whether the risk of hypertension associated with fructose is modified by combination with higher sodium intake has not yet been evaluated in humans, but the role of combined intake in preclinical studies is discussed below.

Adolescents and young adults are the highest consumers overall, and people in lower income population sectors are more likely to consume HFCS than those in more affluent demographic groups [13]. The rise in fructose consumption over the past several decades has been accompanied by an increase in obesity in the United States, and these rates parallel those of hypertension in a nearly linear relationship between body mass index and blood pressure [26,27]. Although several human studies have shown that high fructose consumption contributes to weight gain and blood pressure elevation, there is still controversy over the extent to which HFCS consumption is correlated with the historical obesity and hypertension trends [28]. Factors such as overall increase in national carbohydrate consumption make it challenging to discern increased fructose intake as a primary etiologic source for these disease states [17]. Nevertheless, the ingestion of fructose induces several physiologic responses that favor weight gain and increased blood pressure.

The most recent NHANES III survey found that as of 2004, the average daily intake of fructose (49 g) in the U.S. equated to 9.1% of total energy intake [17]. Interestingly, commercially available soft drinks using HFCS have up to 140 calories from added sugars per 12 fluid ounce container. Given the most commonly used HFCS composition of 55% fructose and 45% glucose, this amounts to approximately 25 g or 100 calories from fructose alone. This quantity from one drink alone nearly surpasses the American Heart Association recommendation of only 150 and 100 calories from added sugars per day for men and women, respectively [29]. Animal studies designed to model this trend in human dietary intake have used various dietary fructose compositions—many of which exceed 60% of total daily caloric intake [30–32]. Increased fructose ingestion in either humans or animal studies have demonstrated significant hemodynamic changes even after limited periods of time [28,33,34]. Interestingly, the majority of animal studies were unaccompanied by significant increases in body weight, suggesting that factors apart from obesity may contribute to the hypertensive phenotype [30,31]. Chronic animal models using more moderate fructose intake that is consistent with heavy human consumption (15–20% of daily caloric intake) demonstrate cardiovascular and metabolic changes similar to human subjects, although the timeline by which these occur may be skewed [35,36]. The role of endothelial dysfunction has been reviewed in detail [37,38]. Mechanisms involved in the early phases of sodium absorption by the intestine have been studied to a greater extent [39]; however, renal sodium reabsorption [40], the renal renin-angiotensin-aldosterone (RAS) system [41], and sympathetic nervous system [32,42] have received more limited attention.

3. Fructose Influences Sodium Handling and Blood Pressure

3.1. *Fructose Influences Gastrointestinal Sodium Absorption*

Sodium homeostasis is a critical component of blood pressure regulation and has been linked to various cardiovascular and renal complications, including hypertension [43–46]. Glucose intake is coupled to Na^+ transport via the luminal sodium-glucose-linked transporter 1 (SGLT1). Intracellular glucose concentration is largely maintained through the glucose transporter 2 (GLUT2) isoform along the basolateral membrane. Chronically, fructose and glucose (but not other sugars) lead to an increase in GLUT2 protein expression along the basolateral membrane [47]. Similar to GLUT5, GLUT2 has a much lower affinity for glucose than other isoforms and therefore functions primarily as a fructose transporter [48]. Fructose transport is facilitated by a downhill concentration gradient between the intestinal lumen and intracellular space [39,49,50]. On the other hand, sodium absorption occurs throughout the small intestine via a variety of transport systems. SLC26A6 (human), also known as the putative anion transporter 1 (PAT1), is a multifunctional apical chloride/base exchanger that increases with fructose feeding in both the jejunum [39,51] and kidney [52]. The function of PAT1 is coupled with that of the intestinal Na/H exchanger 3 (NHE3) so that Na^+ is reabsorbed with Cl^- in an electroneutral manner [53,54]. The presence of fructose amplifies NHE3 function, thereby enhancing absorption of Na^+ and secretion of H^+ [39,40,42]. PAT1 also co-localizes with GLUT5 (Slca5), a member of the glucose transporter family, with low affinity for glucose and high affinity for fructose (Figure 1). GLUT5 is the dominant fructose transporter in the jejunum.

Despite the changes in both sodium and sugar transporters, the impact of fructose on overall gastrointestinal absorption and the resulting fecal excretion of sodium has been given scant investigative attention. An increase in dietary sodium does not increase absolute fecal sodium excretion in Sprague Dawley rats independent of whether the high sodium chow is delivered with glucose or fructose in the drinking water or with water alone. Thus, gastrointestinal sodium absorption increases as dietary intake of sodium increases regardless of the presence or type of sugars in the diet (Figure 1). The task for excretion of the greater total body sodium content relies on the kidney. Notably, urinary sodium excretion is significantly diminished in fructose-fed rats resulting in a positive sodium balance [41]. The renal mechanisms that are understood to date are detailed below.

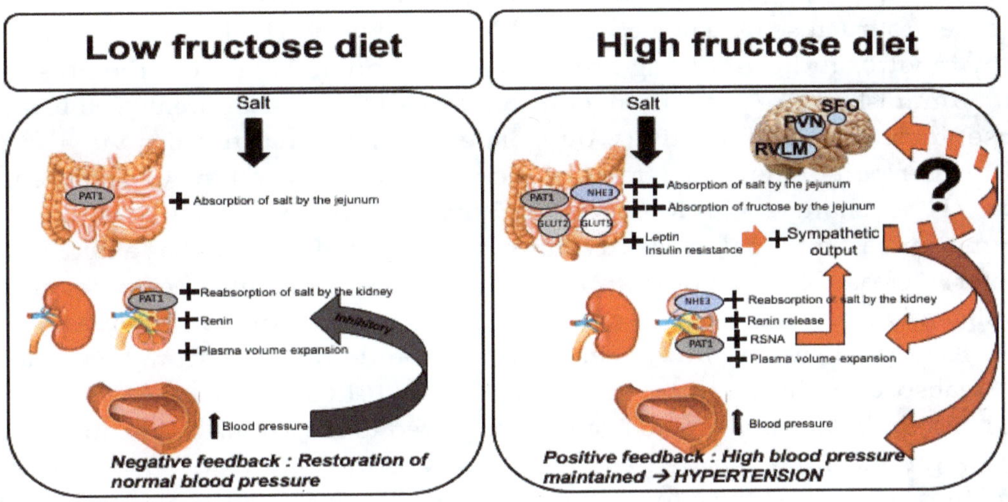

Figure 1. Mechanisms of fructose-induced salt-sensitive hypertension. Left panel: In the absence of high dietary fructose, absorption of salt in the small intestine (jejunum) and proximal tubule of the kidney is accomplished by PAT1. Increased sodium load leads to plasma volume expansion which activates RAS, resulting in elevation of blood pressure. Either increased plasma renin activity or increased blood pressure alone are capable of initiating the negative feedback mechanism to dampen NaCl reabsorption and decrease RAS activation, resulting in restoration of blood pressure back to normal. Right panel: When dietary fructose intake is high in conjunction with high salt, intestinal fructose absorption with Glut 5 and Glut 2 and sodium is absorption via PAT1 and NHE3 in increase. Proximal tubular sodium reabsorption is increased by both PAT1 and NHE3. Elevated fructose load leads to increased levels of circulating leptin and insulin, resulting in insulin resistance. These hormones lead to increased sympathetic outputs. In addition to activation of RAS and Na^+ reabsorption, increased RSNA also participates in elevating blood pressure, ultimately resulting in the loss of the negative feedback mechanism. Increased afferent inputs to the central barosensitive regions may also contribute to hypertension by creating a feedforward situation via efferent sympathetic nerves. PAT1, putative anion transporter 1; NHE3, sodium/hydrogen exchanger 3; Glut 5 and Glut 2, glucose transporters 5 and 2, respectively; RAS, renin-angiotensin-aldosterone system; RSNA, renal sympathetic nerve activity; SFO, subfornical organ; PVN, paraventricular nucleus; RVLM, rostral ventrolateral medulla.

3.2. *Fructose Influences Renal Sodium Reabsorption and RAS*

The bulk of Na^+ reabsorption in the mammalian kidney occurs in the proximal tubule, which is responsible for reabsorption of 60–70% of all Na^+ and fluid filtered by the glomerulus [55]. Similar to the intestine, GLUT2, GLUT5, NHE3, and several isoforms from the SGLT family facilitate the reabsorption of Na^+. Proximal tubule Na^+ reabsorption is reliant on secondary active transport by co-transporters such as NHE3 and SGLT isoforms, particularly SGLT2 [56]. Fine tuning of ionic concentrations and gradients is critical to blood pressure homeostasis. Perturbation such as augmented proximal tubule Na^+ reabsorption results in increased fluid reabsorption, leading to a net positive sodium balance predisposing to hypertension (Figure 1). This mechanism has been linked to hypertension in spontaneously hypertensive rats [57] and Dahl salt-sensitive rats [58]. In carefully executed balance studies, Gordish et al. [41] showed that rats given 20% fructose in their drinking water and placed on high salt diet displayed significantly greater cumulative Na^+ balance compared with rats given only water or 20% glucose in their drinking water. These findings strongly supported a role for fructose-feeding on renal Na^+ balance. Notably, except for elevated triglyceride levels in the fructose-fed high salt group, there were no differences in fasting plasma glucose and body weights between fructose-high salt-fed rats and glucose or water controls either with standard or high salt intake [41].

In the proximal tubule, the majority of Na^+ and all bicarbonate ($HCO3^-$) reabsorption occurs via Na^+/H^+ exchange, via NHE3 [59]. Acute in vivo microperfusion studies of proximal tubules from Wistar rats exposed to fructose revealed enhanced NHE3 activity. The increase in NHE3 activity was corroborated by in vitro studies showing greater Na^+ dependent H^+ flux in the presence of fructose associated with diminished PKA activity in cultured LLC-PK1 cells, a porcine cell line [60]. Fructose, but not glucose, increased NHE3 activity by isolated rat proximal tubules via a PKC-dependent pathway and further potentiated the effects of picomolar concentrations of angiotensin II (Ang II) to increase Na^+/H^+ exchange. Na/K-ATPase activity did not change [40]. Moderate amounts of fructose consumption (approximately 40% of daily caloric intake provided as a 20% fructose solution in drinking water) increased tail cuff blood pressure in rats. Proximal tubule expression levels of NHE3 increased significantly in the fructose-fed compared to that of control rats, whereas $\alpha 1$ subunit of the basolateral Na/K-ATPase did not. Moreover, proximal tubules isolated from these rats also showed enhanced Na^+ reabsorption that was potentiated by Ang II [61,62].

The proximal tubule thus appears to become sensitized to Ang II via a PKC mechanism, to which the addition of high Na^+ intake leads to substantial reabsorption rates. Further, this sensitization extends beyond the proximal tubule into the thick ascending limb and other Na^+ transport mechanisms in the distal nephron although studies have reported some conflicting results. An early study with 65% dietary fructose failed to observe a change in overall $Na^+/K^+/2Cl^-$ co-transporter 2 (NKCC2) abundance in the kidney [63]. In vitro and in vivo studies have shown similar effects on NKCC2 expression and activity. Acute in vitro administration of fructose to the thick ascending limb increases NKCC2 activity by increasing protein expression and not phosphorylation along the apical membrane [64]. Chronic in vivo studies using furosemide, an NKCC2 antagonist, to measure acute diuretic and natriuretic responses following NKCC2 blockade found that high fructose-induced hypertension led to significant increases in urine output as well as in urinary potassium, chloride, and sodium concentration. This was reflected by significant increases in NKCC2 mRNA and protein expression [65]. Together, these alterations in transporter expression and activity throughout the nephron facilitate plasma volume expansion which is responsible, at least in part, for the observed hypertension.

The importance of sensitization to Ang II also cannot be understated. Several preclinical studies have shown that even moderate consumption of fructose and Na^+ can have considerable adverse effects on blood pressure [41,42,61,66]. With the profound increases in Na^+ retention observed in the various models of fructose-induced hypertension with expected extracellular volume expansion, it would be anticipated that plasma renin activity (PRA) would be suppressed. Further investigation by others reported blunted suppression of PRA in Sprague Dawley rats given 20% fructose for one week, followed by one week of fructose plus 4% NaCl diet [41,66]. In contrast, extending the high salt intake period to three weeks, Soncrant et al. confirmed the elevation in blood pressure using telemetric monitoring and were able to demonstrate inhibition of PRA and plasma Ang II in fructose-fed rats [42]. Thus, it appears that PRA which is typically inhibited by either high blood pressure or expanded extracellular volume requires a longer period of exposure to either of these inhibitory influences in the context of high fructose intake. In other words, a much greater expansion of extracellular volume and, therefore a longer period of positive cumulative Na^+ balance, may be required to inhibit renin secretion with concomitant fructose-feeding.

It is also possible that intrarenal RAS contributes to hypertension and increased Na^+ reabsorption with fructose feeding. Early studies indicated that renal tissue renin expression was suppressed in fructose-fed mice [39] yet increased in rats fed 20% fructose for 12 weeks [65]. Renal tissue Ang II levels were not statistically different from control glucose-fed rats on high salt diet for three weeks despite higher blood pressure [42]. Notably, renal angiotensin AT1 receptor mRNA was increased in adipose tissue but not kidney after three weeks of high fructose ingestion [67]. When fructose was given in greater amounts (60 to 66% in the drinking water) and for longer periods of time (8 to 16 weeks), both Ang I and Ang II as well as AT1 receptor protein expression was increased in kidney tissue [68,69]. Alternatively, the third influence on renin secretion involves sympathetic inputs to the macula densa. Indeed, switching from standard diet (0.4% NaCl) to a high salt (4% NaCl) diet, in fructose-fed rats, increased renal sympathetic nerve activity by ~50% [42]. Denervation of the kidneys bilaterally using cryo-techniques further decreased the already suppressed PRA suggesting sympathetic inputs to the kidney were responsible for the enhanced renin secretion. Notably, tissue Ang II content was not altered by any of the diets compared with controls [42].

In addition to the experimental dietary manipulations, some of the variability in these studies likely stems from methodology used such as the technique for blood pressure assessment (tail cuff vs. telemetry), the time when fructose is initiated relative to the high salt diet, the length of exposure to each component of the diet, and the collection of blood or tissue for measurements of renin, plasma Ang II or their tissue levels. Regardless of the impact of these factors, the findings that a diet enriched for fructose sensitizes the nephron to Ang II such that even minimal activation of the RAS can have profound sodium reabsorption effects.

3.3. Fructose Influences the Renal Sympathetic Nervous System

The scientific interest in sympathetic innervation of the kidney has increased recently after the demonstration of marked reductions in blood pressure in individuals with resistant hypertension after denervation using the catheter-based approach [70,71]. Renal sympathetic nerve activity (RSNA) is significantly increased in many forms of experimental hypertension (reviewed by Osborn and Foss [72]), underlying the vital role of RSNA in blood pressure regulation. The mechanisms of increased RSNA in the pathogenesis of hypertension include increased tubular sodium reabsorption and water retention, decreased renal blood flow and glomerular filtration rate, and increased renin secretion from the juxtaglomerular cells which activates RAS [73]. Since moderately high dietary fructose and salt cause hypertension via similar mechanisms, it has been hypothesized that sympathetic activity increases in this dietary milieu. In fact, ingestion of fructose has been shown to result in changes in secretion of hormones that regulate energy balance [74], a shift associated with increased sympathetic nervous system activity [75]. The hormone leptin which promotes satiety is released from adipose tissue cells to maintain energy balance by promoting satiety. In contrast, ghrelin opposes this action and promotes hunger. Ingestion of fructose leads to simultaneously increased secretion of ghrelin and decreased secretion of leptin; however, after chronic ingestion of excess dietary fructose (over one to four weeks), fasting plasma concentrations of leptin are significantly higher [76]. The mechanistic basis for elevated leptin levels likely stems from fructose-induced fatty acid re-esterification and synthesis of VLDL-triglycerides. This pathway causes a shift towards the fat-storing mode, prompting the adipose cells to respond by elevating leptin production. Simultaneously, augmentation of RSNA occurs initiating the onslaught of hypertension-promoting effects.

Multiple studies have shown that uncontrolled increases in RSNA contribute to both the onset and maintenance of hypertension in both humans and in animal models [72,77], suggesting that coupled with the metabolic changes and energy balance shifts, fructose-induced salt-sensitive hypertension also likely leads to increased RSNA. When rats fed 20% fructose were switched to the high salt diet for one week, they developed hypertension, accompanied by net positive sodium balance, but persistently high PRA [41]. The inability of net positive sodium retention and elevated mean arterial pressure to reduce PRA suggests that increased RSNA is acting upon the juxtaglomerular apparatus to secrete renin and activate RAS. In fact, a preclinical study demonstrated a direct involvement of increased RSNA in fructose-induced salt-sensitive hypertension in conscious rats chronically instrumented with nerve telemetry devices [42]. High salt intake in rats on 20% fructose, but not glucose, resulted in a 41% increase in RSNA after 1 week. Further confirmation of the role of RSNA was provided by demonstrating a decrease in blood pressure after bilateral renal denervation using the cryo-technique. Although the rats did not display the full complement of metabolic syndrome, insulin sensitivity was also reduced in the hypertensive fructose-fed rats. This restoration of RSNA to baseline following cryoablation was accompanied by decreased blood pressure and improved insulin sensitivity [42].

The attenuation of PRA suppression in fructose and high salt-fed rats is mitigated when the rats ingest a high salt diet for at least three weeks. Therefore, it appears that the initial mechanism of fructose-induced salt-sensitive hypertension involves persistently elevated PRA that eventually subsides after two to three weeks of high salt feeding. During this period augmentation of RSNA is initiated, which serves as a feed-forward mechanism that takes over when PRA returns to baseline in order to maintain elevated arterial pressure (Figure 1).

Concurrently, an indirect mechanism involving reactive oxygen species generation may be partially responsible for blunted suppression of PRA initially, followed by increases in RSNA. High fructose and salt feeding in rats leads to increased oxidative stress as measured by 8-isoprostane excretion, and supplementation with the superoxide dismutase mimetic, Tempol, attenuates both the increase in mean arterial pressure and reactive oxygen species generation [66]. Furthermore, oxygen radicals can activate the sympathetic sites that are involved in the pathogenesis of hypertension [78]. Thus, moderately high fructose and salt feeding in rats causes hypertension in at least two phases. Firstly, an increase in blood pressure results from the direct action of renin, which eventually returns to baseline as a result of the negative feedback mechanism evoked by the net positive, albeit greater, cumulative sodium balance and increase in blood pressure. Additionally, generation of reactive oxygen species contributes to high PRA. Secondly, after two to three weeks of high salt feeding, PRA decreases and hypertension is maintained via increased RSNA. Oxygen radicals further contribute to sympathoexcitation, providing a collateral mechanism to maintain increased blood pressure.

4. Conclusions

High fructose and salt intakes are contributing to the increased incidence and prevalence of hypertension in the U.S. and globally. Even prior to the development of full blown metabolic syndrome, fructose-induced enhancement of renal Na^+ reabsorption with greater positive net cumulative Na^+ balance can lead to elevations of blood pressure. The inhibition of PRA is also blunted despite higher blood pressure and extracellular volume and is driven by enhanced renal sympathetic nerve inputs. Activation of circulating RAS, therefore, further augments blood pressure. After longer periods of fructose and high salt ingestion, intrarenal RAS is also increased which may further drive tubular Na^+ reabsorption. The combined inputs from afferent nerves, reactive oxygen species and increased metabolic hormones such as leptin work centrally to stimulate sympathetic outputs and further increase blood pressure (Figure 1). Thus, combined fructose and high salt diets may lead to hypertension and increased cardiovascular risks even short term and in individuals without the full metabolic syndrome.

Author Contributions: P.E.L.—writing, review and editing; D.K.—conceptualization, writing, review and editing; N.F.R.—conceptualization, writing, review and editing, supervision and funding acquisition. D.K. and P.E.L. contributed equally to this manuscript.

Abbreviations

Ang II	angiotensin II
AT1	angiotensin receptor type 1
CARDIA	Coronary Artery Risk Development in Young Adults

GLUT	glucose transporter
HFCS	high fructose corn syrup
NHANES	National Health and Nutrition Examination Survey
NHE	sodium hydrogen exchanger
NKCC2	sodium potassium chloride transporter
PAT1	putative anion transporter 1
PKA	protein kinase A
PKC	protein kinase C
PRA	plasma renin activity
PVN	paraventricular nucleus
RAS	renin angiotensin system
RSNA	renal sympathetic nerve activity
RVLM	rostral ventrolateral medulla
SFO	subfornical organ.

References

1. Carretero, O.A.; Oparil, S. Essential hypertension. Part I: Definition and etiology. *Circulation* **2000**, *101*, 329–335. [CrossRef] [PubMed]
2. Messerli, F.H.; Williams, B.; Ritz, E. Essential hypertension. *Lancet* **2007**, *370*, 591–603. [CrossRef]
3. Egan, B.M.; Zhao, Y.; Axon, R.N. US trends in prevalence, awareness, treatment, and control of hypertension, 1988–2008. *JAMA* **2010**, *303*, 2043–2050. [CrossRef] [PubMed]
4. Yano, Y.; Reis, J.P.; Colangelo, L.A.; Shimbo, D.; Viera, A.J.; Allen, N.B.; Gidding, S.S.; Bress, A.P.; Greenland, P.; Muntner, P.; et al. Association of Blood Pressure Classification in Young Adults Using the 2017 American College of Cardiology/American Heart Association Blood Pressure Guideline with Cardiovascular Events Later in Life. *JAMA* **2018**, *320*, 1774–1782. [CrossRef] [PubMed]
5. Dorans, K.S.; Mills, K.T.; Liu, Y.; He, J. Trends in Prevalence and Control of Hypertension According to the 2017 American College of Cardiology/American Heart Association (ACC/AHA) Guideline. *J. Am. Heart Assoc.* **2018**, *7*. [CrossRef] [PubMed]
6. Mills, K.T.; Bundy, J.D.; Kelly, T.N.; Reed, J.E.; Kearney, P.M.; Reynolds, K.; Chen, J.; He, J. Global Disparities of Hypertension Prevalence and Control: A Systematic Analysis of Population-Based Studies From 90 Countries. *Circulation* **2016**, *134*, 441–450. [CrossRef] [PubMed]
7. Taylor, B.C.; Wilt, T.J.; Welch, H.G. Impact of diastolic and systolic blood pressure on mortality: Implications for the definition of "normal". *J. Gen. Intern. Med.* **2011**, *26*, 685–690. [CrossRef] [PubMed]
8. Bowe, B.; Xie, Y.; Li, T.; Mokdad, A.H.; Xian, H.; Yan, Y.; Maddukuri, G.; Al-Aly, Z. Changes in the US Burden of Chronic Kidney Disease From 2002 to 2016: An Analysis of the Global Burden of Disease Study. *JAMA Netw. Open* **2018**, *1*, e184412. [CrossRef] [PubMed]
9. Lerman, L.O.; Chade, A.R.; Sica, V.; Napoli, C. Animal models of hypertension: An overview. *J. Lab. Clin. Med.* **2005**, *146*, 160–173. [CrossRef] [PubMed]
10. Warden, C.H.; Fisler, J.S. Comparisons of diets used in animal models of high-fat feeding. *Cell Metab.* **2008**, *7*, 277. [CrossRef] [PubMed]
11. Alberti, K.G.; Eckel, R.H.; Grundy, S.M.; Zimmet, P.Z.; Cleeman, J.I.; Donato, K.A.; Fruchart, J.C.; James, W.P.; Loria, C.M.; Smith, S.C., Jr.; et al. Harmonizing the metabolic syndrome: A joint interim statement of the International Diabetes Federation Task Force on Epidemiology and Prevention; National Heart, Lung, and Blood Institute; American Heart Association; World Heart Federation; International Atherosclerosis Society; and International Association for the Study of Obesity. *Circulation* **2009**, *120*, 1640–1645. [CrossRef] [PubMed]
12. Bray, G.A.; Nielsen, S.J.; Popkin, B.M. Consumption of high-fructose corn syrup in beverages may play a role in the epidemic of obesity. *Am. J. Clin. Nutr.* **2004**, *79*, 537–543. [CrossRef] [PubMed]
13. Tappy, L.; Le, K.A. Metabolic effects of fructose and the worldwide increase in obesity. *Physiol. Rev.* **2010**, *90*, 23–46. [CrossRef] [PubMed]

14. Zhang, D.M.; Jiao, R.Q.; Kong, L.D. High Dietary Fructose: Direct or Indirect Dangerous Factors Disturbing Tissue and Organ Functions. *Nutrients* **2017**, *9*, 335. [CrossRef] [PubMed]
15. Marshall, R.O.; Kooi, E.R. Enzymatic conversion of D-glucose to D-fructose. *Science* **1957**, *125*, 648–649. [CrossRef] [PubMed]
16. Hanover, L.M.; White, J.S. Manufacturing, composition, and applications of fructose. *Am. J. Clin. Nutr.* **1993**, *58*, 724S–732S. [CrossRef] [PubMed]
17. Marriott, B.P.; Cole, N.; Lee, E. National estimates of dietary fructose intake increased from 1977 to 2004 in the United States. *J. Nutr.* **2009**, *139*, 1228S–1235S. [CrossRef] [PubMed]
18. Jayalath, V.H.; Sievenpiper, J.L.; de Souza, R.J.; Ha, V.; Mirrahimi, A.; Santaren, I.D.; Blanco Mejia, S.; Di Buono, M.; Jenkins, A.L.; Leiter, L.A.; et al. Total fructose intake and risk of hypertension: A systematic review and meta-analysis of prospective cohorts. *J. Am. Coll. Nutr.* **2014**, *33*, 328–339. [CrossRef] [PubMed]
19. Jayalath, V.H.; de Souza, R.J.; Ha, V.; Mirrahimi, A.; Blanco-Mejia, S.; Di Buono, M.; Jenkins, A.L.; Leiter, L.A.; Wolever, T.M.; Beyene, J.; et al. Sugar-sweetened beverage consumption and incident hypertension: A systematic review and meta-analysis of prospective cohorts. *Am. J. Clin. Nutr.* **2015**, *102*, 914–921. [CrossRef] [PubMed]
20. Benjamin, E.J.; Virani, S.S.; Callaway, C.W.; Chamberlain, A.M.; Chang, A.R.; Cheng, S.; Chiuve, S.E.; Cushman, M.; Delling, F.N.; Deo, R.; et al. Heart Disease and Stroke Statistics-2018 Update: A Report From the American Heart Association. *Circulation* **2018**, *137*, e67–e492. [CrossRef] [PubMed]
21. Beunza, J.J.; Martinez-Gonzalez, M.A.; Ebrahim, S.; Bes-Rastrollo, M.; Nunez, J.; Martinez, J.A.; Alonso, A. Sedentary behaviors and the risk of incident hypertension: The SUN Cohort. *Am. J. Hypertens.* **2007**, *20*, 1156–1162. [CrossRef] [PubMed]
22. Bowman, T.S.; Gaziano, J.M.; Buring, J.E.; Sesso, H.D. A prospective study of cigarette smoking and risk of incident hypertension in women. *J. Am. Coll. Cardiol.* **2007**, *50*, 2085–2092. [CrossRef] [PubMed]
23. Forman, J.P.; Stampfer, M.J.; Curhan, G.C. Diet and lifestyle risk factors associated with incident hypertension in women. *JAMA* **2009**, *302*, 401–411. [CrossRef] [PubMed]
24. Wang, L.; Manson, J.E.; Buring, J.E.; Sesso, H.D. Meat intake and the risk of hypertension in middle-aged and older women. *J. Hypertens.* **2008**, *26*, 215–222. [CrossRef] [PubMed]
25. Ford, C.D.; Sims, M.; Higginbotham, J.C.; Crowther, M.R.; Wyatt, S.B.; Musani, S.K.; Payne, T.J.; Fox, E.R.; Parton, J.M. Psychosocial Factors Are Associated with Blood Pressure Progression among African Americans in the Jackson Heart Study. *Am. J. Hypertens.* **2016**, *29*, 913–924. [CrossRef] [PubMed]
26. Hall, J.E. The kidney, hypertension, and obesity. *Hypertension* **2003**, *41*, 625–633. [CrossRef] [PubMed]
27. Jones, D.W.; Kim, J.S.; Andrew, M.E.; Kim, S.J.; Hong, Y.P. Body mass index and blood pressure in Korean men and women: The Korean National Blood Pressure Survey. *J. Hypertens.* **1994**, *12*, 1433–1437. [CrossRef] [PubMed]
28. Le, M.T.; Frye, R.F.; Rivard, C.J.; Cheng, J.; McFann, K.K.; Segal, M.S.; Johnson, R.J.; Johnson, J.A. Effects of high-fructose corn syrup and sucrose on the pharmacokinetics of fructose and acute metabolic and hemodynamic responses in healthy subjects. *Metabolism* **2012**, *61*, 641–651. [CrossRef] [PubMed]
29. Johnson, R.J.; Perez-Pozo, S.E.; Sautin, Y.Y.; Manitius, J.; Sanchez-Lozada, L.G.; Feig, D.I.; Shafiu, M.; Segal, M.; Glassock, R.J.; Shimada, M.; et al. Hypothesis: Could excessive fructose intake and uric acid cause type 2 diabetes? *Endocr. Rev.* **2009**, *30*, 96–116. [CrossRef] [PubMed]
30. Hwang, I.S.; Ho, H.; Hoffman, B.B.; Reaven, G.M. Fructose-induced insulin resistance and hypertension in rats. *Hypertension* **1987**, *10*, 512–516. [CrossRef] [PubMed]
31. Martinez, F.J.; Rizza, R.A.; Romero, J.C. High-fructose feeding elicits insulin resistance, hyperinsulinism, and hypertension in normal mongrel dogs. *Hypertension* **1994**, *23*, 456–463. [CrossRef] [PubMed]
32. Tran, L.T.; Yuen, V.G.; McNeill, J.H. The fructose-fed rat: A review on the mechanisms of fructose-induced insulin resistance and hypertension. *Mol. Cell. Biochem.* **2009**, *332*, 145–159. [CrossRef] [PubMed]
33. Brown, C.M.; Dulloo, A.G.; Yepuri, G.; Montani, J.P. Fructose ingestion acutely elevates blood pressure in healthy young humans. *Am. J. Physiol. Regul. Integr. Comp. Physiol.* **2008**, *294*, R730–R737. [CrossRef] [PubMed]
34. Perez-Pozo, S.E.; Schold, J.; Nakagawa, T.; Sanchez-Lozada, L.G.; Johnson, R.J.; Lillo, J.L. Excessive fructose intake induces the features of metabolic syndrome in healthy adult men: Role of uric acid in the hypertensive response. *Int. J. Obes. (Lond.)* **2010**, *34*, 454–461. [CrossRef] [PubMed]

35. Dai, S.; Mcneill, J.H. Fructose-Induced Hypertension in Rats Is Concentration-Dependent and Duration-Dependent. *J. Pharmacol. Toxicol. Methods* **1995**, *33*, 101–107. [CrossRef]
36. Glushakova, O.; Kosugi, T.; Roncal, C.; Mu, W.; Heinig, M.; Cirillo, P.; Sanchez-Lozada, L.G.; Johnson, R.J.; Nakagawa, T. Fructose induces the inflammatory molecule ICAM-1 in endothelial cells. *J. Am. Soc. Nephrol.* **2008**, *19*, 1712–1720. [CrossRef] [PubMed]
37. Aroor, A.R.; Demarco, V.G.; Jia, G.; Sun, Z.; Nistala, R.; Meininger, G.A.; Sowers, J.R. The role of tissue Renin-Angiotensin-aldosterone system in the development of endothelial dysfunction and arterial stiffness. *Front. Endocrinol. (Lausanne)* **2013**, *4*, 161. [CrossRef] [PubMed]
38. Katakam, P.V.; Ujhelyi, M.R.; Hoenig, M.E.; Miller, A.W. Endothelial dysfunction precedes hypertension in diet-induced insulin resistance. *Am. J. Physiol.* **1998**, *275*, R788–R792. [CrossRef] [PubMed]
39. Singh, A.K.; Amlal, H.; Haas, P.J.; Dringenberg, U.; Fussell, S.; Barone, S.L.; Engelhardt, R.; Zuo, J.; Seidler, U.; Soleimani, M. Fructose-induced hypertension: Essential role of chloride and fructose absorbing transporters PAT1 and Glut5. *Kidney Int.* **2008**, *74*, 438–447. [CrossRef] [PubMed]
40. Cabral, P.D.; Hong, N.J.; Hye Khan, M.A.; Ortiz, P.A.; Beierwaltes, W.H.; Imig, J.D.; Garvin, J.L. Fructose stimulates Na/H exchange activity and sensitizes the proximal tubule to angiotensin II. *Hypertension* **2014**, *63*, e68–e73. [CrossRef] [PubMed]
41. Gordish, K.L.; Kassem, K.M.; Ortiz, P.A.; Beierwaltes, W.H. Moderate (20%) fructose-enriched diet stimulates salt-sensitive hypertension with increased salt retention and decreased renal nitric oxide. *Physiol. Rep.* **2017**, *5*. [CrossRef] [PubMed]
42. Soncrant, T.; Komnenov, D.; Beierwaltes, W.H.; Chen, H.; Wu, M.; Rossi, N.F. Bilateral renal cryodenervation decreases arterial pressure and improves insulin sensitivity in fructose-fed Sprague-Dawley rats. *Am. J. Physiol. Regul. Integr. Comp. Physiol.* **2018**, *315*, R529–R538. [CrossRef] [PubMed]
43. De Wardener, H.E.; He, F.J.; MacGregor, G.A. Plasma sodium and hypertension. *Kidney Int.* **2004**, *66*, 2454–2466. [CrossRef] [PubMed]
44. Haddy, F.J. Role of dietary salt in hypertension. *Life Sci.* **2006**, *79*, 1585–1592. [CrossRef] [PubMed]
45. Karppanen, H.; Mervaala, E. Sodium intake and hypertension. *Prog. Cardiovasc. Dis.* **2006**, *49*, 59–75. [CrossRef] [PubMed]
46. Meneton, P.; Jeunemaitre, X.; de Wardener, H.E.; MacGregor, G.A. Links between dietary salt intake, renal salt handling, blood pressure, and cardiovascular diseases. *Physiol. Rev.* **2005**, *85*, 679–715. [CrossRef] [PubMed]
47. Cheeseman, C.I.; Harley, B. Adaptation of glucose transport across rat enterocyte basolateral membrane in response to altered dietary carbohydrate intake. *J. Physiol.* **1991**, *437*, 563–575. [CrossRef] [PubMed]
48. Gould, G.W.; Thomas, H.M.; Jess, T.J.; Bell, G.I. Expression of human glucose transporters in Xenopus oocytes: Kinetic characterization and substrate specificities of the erythrocyte, liver, and brain isoforms. *Biochemistry* **1991**, *30*, 5139–5145. [CrossRef] [PubMed]
49. Kane, S.; Seatter, M.J.; Gould, G.W. Functional studies of human GLUT5: Effect of pH on substrate selection and an analysis of substrate interactions. *Biochem. Biophys. Res. Commun.* **1997**, *238*, 503–505. [CrossRef] [PubMed]
50. Leturque, A.; Brot-Laroche, E.; Le Gall, M.; Stolarczyk, E.; Tobin, V. The role of GLUT2 in dietary sugar handling. *J. Physiol. Biochem.* **2005**, *61*, 529–537. [CrossRef] [PubMed]
51. Wang, Z.; Petrovic, S.; Mann, E.; Soleimani, M. Identification of an apical Cl(-)/HCO3(-) exchanger in the small intestine. *Am. J. Physiol. Gastrointest. Liver Physiol.* **2002**, *282*, G573–G579. [CrossRef] [PubMed]
52. Soleimani, M.; Alborzi, P. The role of salt in the pathogenesis of fructose-induced hypertension. *Int. J. Nephrol.* **2011**, *2011*, 392708. [CrossRef] [PubMed]
53. Dudeja, P.K.; Rao, D.D.; Syed, I.; Joshi, V.; Dahdal, R.Y.; Gardner, C.; Risk, M.C.; Schmidt, L.; Bavishi, D.; Kim, K.E.; et al. Intestinal distribution of human Na^+/H^+ exchanger isoforms NHE-1, NHE-2, and NHE-3 mRNA. *Am. J. Physiol.* **1996**, *271*, G483–G493. [CrossRef] [PubMed]
54. Seidler, U.; Rottinghaus, I.; Hillesheim, J.; Chen, M.; Riederer, B.; Krabbenhoft, A.; Engelhardt, R.; Wiemann, M.; Wang, Z.; Barone, S.; et al. Sodium and chloride absorptive defects in the small intestine in Slc26a6 null mice. *Pflugers Arch.* **2008**, *455*, 757–766. [CrossRef] [PubMed]
55. Dantzler, W.H. *Comparative Physiology of the Vertebrate Kidney*; Springer: Berlin, Germany; New York, NY, USA, 1989; p. x, 198p.
56. Boron, W.F.; Boulpaep, E.L. *Medical Physiology: A Cellular and Molecular Approach*, Updated 2nd ed.; Saunders/Elsevier: Philadelphia, PA, USA, 2012; p. xiii. 1337p.

57. Aldred, K.L.; Harris, P.J.; Eitle, E. Increased proximal tubule NHE-3 and H+-ATPase activities in spontaneously hypertensive rats. *J. Hypertens.* **2000**, *18*, 623–628. [CrossRef] [PubMed]
58. Tank, J.E.; Moe, O.W.; Henrich, W.L. Abnormal regulation of proximal tubule renin mRNA in the Dahl/Rapp salt-sensitive rat. *Kidney Int.* **1998**, *54*, 1608–1616. [CrossRef] [PubMed]
59. Alpern, R.J.; Cogan, M.G.; Rector, F.C., Jr. Effect of luminal bicarbonate concentration on proximal acidification in the rat. *Am. J. Physiol.* **1982**, *243*, F53–F59. [CrossRef] [PubMed]
60. Queiroz-Leite, G.D.; Crajoinas, R.O.; Neri, E.A.; Bezerra, C.N.; Girardi, A.C.; Reboucas, N.A.; Malnic, G. Fructose acutely stimulates NHE3 activity in kidney proximal tubule. *Kidney Blood Press. Res.* **2012**, *36*, 320–334. [CrossRef] [PubMed]
61. Gonzalez-Vicente, A.; Cabral, P.D.; Hong, N.J.; Asirwatham, J.; Yang, N.; Berthiaume, J.M.; Dominici, F.P.; Garvin, J.L. Dietary Fructose Enhances the Ability of Low Concentrations of Angiotensin II to Stimulate Proximal Tubule Na(+) Reabsorption. *Nutrients* **2017**, *9*, 885. [CrossRef] [PubMed]
62. Gonzalez-Vicente, A.; Hong, N.J.; Yang, N.; Cabral, P.D.; Berthiaume, J.M.; Dominici, F.P.; Garvin, J.L. Dietary Fructose Increases the Sensitivity of Proximal Tubules to Angiotensin II in Rats Fed High-Salt Diets. *Nutrients* **2018**, *10*, 1244. [CrossRef] [PubMed]
63. Song, J.; Hu, X.; Shi, M.; Knepper, M.A.; Ecelbarger, C.A. Effects of dietary fat, NaCl, and fructose on renal sodium and water transporter abundances and systemic blood pressure. *Am. J. Physiol. Ren. Physiol.* **2004**, *287*, F1204–F1212. [CrossRef] [PubMed]
64. Ares, G.R.; Kassem, K.M.; Ortiz, P.A. Fructose acutely stimulates NKCC2 activity in rat thick ascending limbs (TALs) by increasing surface NKCC2 expression. *Am. J. Physiol. Ren. Physiol.* **2018**. [CrossRef]
65. Xu, C.; Lu, A.; Lu, X.; Zhang, L.; Fang, H.; Zhou, L.; Yang, T. Activation of Renal (Pro)Renin Receptor Contributes to High Fructose-Induced Salt Sensitivity. *Hypertension* **2017**, *69*, 339–348. [CrossRef] [PubMed]
66. Zenner, Z.P.; Gordish, K.L.; Beierwaltes, W.H. Free radical scavenging reverses fructose-induced salt-sensitive hypertension. *Integr. Blood Press. Control* **2018**, *11*, 1–9. [CrossRef] [PubMed]
67. Giacchetti, G.; Sechi, L.A.; Griffin, C.A.; Don, B.R.; Mantero, F.; Schambelan, M. The tissue renin-angiotensin system in rats with fructose-induced hypertension: Overexpression of type 1 angiotensin II receptor in adipose tissue. *J. Hypertens.* **2000**, *18*, 695–702. [CrossRef] [PubMed]
68. Dhar, I.; Dhar, A.; Wu, L.; Desai, K.M. Increased methylglyoxal formation with upregulation of renin angiotensin system in fructose fed Sprague Dawley rats. *PLoS ONE* **2013**, *8*, e74212. [CrossRef] [PubMed]
69. Yokota, R.; Ronchi, F.A.; Fernandes, F.B.; Jara, Z.P.; Rosa, R.M.; Leite, A.P.O.; Fiorino, P.; Farah, V.; do Nascimento, N.R.F.; Fonteles, M.C.; et al. Intra-Renal Angiotensin Levels Are Increased in High-Fructose Fed Rats in the Extracorporeal Renal Perfusion Model. *Front. Physiol.* **2018**, *9*, 1433. [CrossRef] [PubMed]
70. Esler, M.D.; Bohm, M.; Sievert, H.; Rump, C.L.; Schmieder, R.E.; Krum, H.; Mahfoud, F.; Schlaich, M.P. Catheter-based renal denervation for treatment of patients with treatment-resistant hypertension: 36 month results from the SYMPLICITY HTN-2 randomized clinical trial. *Eur. Heart J.* **2014**, *35*, 1752–1759. [CrossRef] [PubMed]
71. Krum, H.; Schlaich, M.P.; Sobotka, P.A.; Bohm, M.; Mahfoud, F.; Rocha-Singh, K.; Katholi, R.; Esler, M.D. Percutaneous renal denervation in patients with treatment-resistant hypertension: Final 3-year report of the Symplicity HTN-1 study. *Lancet* **2014**, *383*, 622–629. [CrossRef]
72. Osborn, J.W.; Foss, J.D. Renal Nerves and Long-Term Control of Arterial Pressure. *Compr Physiol* **2017**, *7*, 263–320. [CrossRef] [PubMed]
73. DiBona, G.F. Physiology in perspective: The Wisdom of the Body. Neural control of the kidney. *Am. J. Physiol. Regul. Integr. Comp. Physiol.* **2005**, *289*, R633–R641. [CrossRef] [PubMed]
74. Teff, K.L.; Elliott, S.S.; Tschop, M.; Kieffer, T.J.; Rader, D.; Heiman, M.; Townsend, R.R.; Keim, N.L.; D'Alessio, D.; Havel, P.J. Dietary fructose reduces circulating insulin and leptin, attenuates postprandial suppression of ghrelin, and increases triglycerides in women. *J. Clin. Endocrinol. Metab.* **2004**, *89*, 2963–2972. [CrossRef] [PubMed]
75. Zeng, W.; Pirzgalska, R.M.; Pereira, M.M.; Kubasova, N.; Barateiro, A.; Seixas, E.; Lu, Y.H.; Kozlova, A.; Voss, H.; Martins, G.G.; et al. Sympathetic neuro-adipose connections mediate leptin-driven lipolysis. *Cell* **2015**, *163*, 84–94. [CrossRef] [PubMed]
76. Tappy, L.; Le, K.A. Does fructose consumption contribute to non-alcoholic fatty liver disease? *Clin. Res. Hepatol. Gastroenterol.* **2012** *36*, 554–560. [CrossRef] [PubMed]

77. DiBona, G.F.; Kopp, U.C. Neural control of renal function. *Physiol. Rev.* **1997**, *77*, 75–197. [CrossRef] [PubMed]
78. Campese, V.M.; Ye, S.; Zhong, H.; Yanamadala, V.; Ye, Z.; Chiu, J. Reactive oxygen species stimulate central and peripheral sympathetic nervous system activity. *Am. J. Physiol. Heart Circ. Physiol.* **2004**, *287*, H695–H703. [CrossRef] [PubMed]

15

Weight Loss and Hypertension in Obese Subjects

Francesco Fantin *, Anna Giani, Elena Zoico, Andrea P. Rossi, Gloria Mazzali and Mauro Zamboni

Department of Medicine, Section of Geriatrics, University of Verona Healthy Aging Center, Verona, Piazzale Stefani 1, 37126 Verona, Italy

* Correspondence: francesco.fantin@univr.it

Abstract: Arterial hypertension is strongly related to overweight and obesity. In obese subjects, several mechanisms may lead to hypertension such as insulin and leptin resistance, perivascular adipose tissue dysfunction, renal impairment, renin-angiotensin-aldosterone-system activation and sympathetic nervous system activity. Weight loss (WL) seems to have positive effects on blood pressure (BP). The aim of this review was to explain the mechanisms linking obesity and hypertension and to evaluate the main studies assessing the effect of WL on BP. We analysed studies published in the last 10 years (13 studies either interventional or observational) showing the effect of WL on BP. Different WL strategies were taken into account—diet and lifestyle modification, pharmacological intervention and bariatric surgery. Although a positive effect of WL could be identified in each study, the main difference seems to be the magnitude and the durability of BP reduction over time. Nevertheless, further follow-up data are needed: there is still a lack of evidence about long term effects of WL on hypertension. Hence, given the significant results obtained in several recent studies, weight management should always be pursued in obese patients with hypertension.

Keywords: hypertension; weight loss; obesity

1. Introduction

Arterial hypertension is considered one of the most important cardiovascular (CV) risk factors and its connection to overweight and obesity has been extensively proved [1,2]. The prevalence of hypertension among obese patients may range from 60% to 77%, increasing with body–mass index (BMI), in all age groups [3] and it is significantly higher compared to the 34% found in normal weight subjects [3]. These percentages are relevant even when compared to high blood pressure (BP) prevalence in the general population: in 2015, the global age-standardized prevalence was 24.1% (21.4–27.1) in men and 20.1% (17.8–22.5) in women [4]. As shown from the Framingham Heart Study [5], weight gain is responsible for a large percentage of hypertension and it is associated with higher risk of having high BP, even when occurring late in life [6].

The latest definition of hypertension, provided by European Guidelines, is focused on the level of BP (considering office BP, as measured during medical evaluation) at which the benefits of treatment offset its risk, as documented by clinical trials [7]. BP ranges are also defined: the last classification identifies three grades of hypertension (beginning from grade 1, with systolic BP 140–159 mmHg and diastolic BP 90–99 mmHg, followed by grade 2, with SBP 160–179 mmHg and DBP 100–109 mmHg and grade 3, with SBP $\geq$ 180 mmHg and DBP $\geq$ 110 mmHg) and isolated systolic hypertension (SBP $\geq$ 140 and DBP lower than 90 mmHg) [7]. Regardless of the grade, treatment, either with lifestyle interventions or drugs [7], is indicated.

Both obesity and hypertension are considered CV risk factors, therefore their combined management is of utmost importance [8]. It has been shown that moderate weight loss (WL) has a BP lowering effect in both hypertensive and non-hypertensive patients [9]. Furthermore, the magnitude of WL correlates with better results in terms of CV risk reduction [10]. In obese patients with metabolic syndrome, a moderate WL improves renal function [11] and may lead to a 15% reduction of all-cause mortality [12].

Both the latest American and European hypertension guidelines underline the effect of lifestyle modification [7,13] as the first step to be considered in all patients with hypertension and of course in overweight and obese patients. According to the European Society of Cardiology, weight reduction and WL maintenance are mandatory lifestyle changes [7]. American Heart Association highlights that among obese patients, reducing body weight (BW) can lower the risk of developing hypertension to the level of those patients who have never been obese [13]. Moreover, American obesity guidelines report a dose-response effect of the magnitude of WL on BP reduction [14]. Given the strong connection between obesity, overweight and BP and the strong evidence of the possible benefits that can be obtained through weight reduction, the underlying mechanisms and WL strategies should be further explained.

2. Mechanisms Linking Obesity to Hypertension

The pathophysiology of hypertension in obese subjects should be considered as a complex phenomenon. The cardiovascular system is affected by structural, functional and hemodynamical changes [15] which can directly increase hypertension risk. The consequences of these changes will not be discussed in the following paragraphs, since they are beyond the purpose of this review. Our attention is focused on the role of different kinds of adipose tissue. The role of Renin Angiotensin Aldosterone System (RAAS) and sympathetic nervous system activation is also considered.

2.1. Visceral Adipose Tissue

Fat distribution has been shown to be strongly related to cardiovascular morbidity and mortality [16], independent of the other classical CV risk factors. The distribution of adipose tissue is one of the factors which links obesity to hypertension, along with age of onset of obesity, its duration and degree and weight variation across lifespan [17] (Figure 1). Visceral adiposity, in fact, plays a central role in BP increase, through a greater release of free fatty acid (FFA) in systemic circulation and a consequent increase in insulin resistance and hyperinsulinemia (Figure 1). These changes are firmly related to augmented arterial stiffness and a decrease in vasodilation [17]. Although insulin is a vasodilator hormone, insulin resistance can reduce insulin vasodilation capacity, thereby reducing the nitric oxide (NO) production by endothelial cells [18,19]. Also, the increased levels of insulin are responsible for lumbar SNA promotion, through brain receptor pattern activation, which is directly involved in BP increase [20]. Hyperinsulinemia is found to precede the onset of hypertension in high risk patients and this corroborates the hypothesis of the effect of insulin resistance on BP increase [17].

Furthermore, a strong association has been reported between visceral adipose tissue and greater serum levels of cytokine, such as leptin, interleukin-6, plasminogen activator inhibitor-1, all of which are related both to endothelial dysfunction and hypertension [21–23]. The inflammation pattern promoted by cytokines release is involved in an inflammation-dependent aortic stiffening [24] and it can also lead to left ventricular stiffness and mass increase [24]. This hypothesis is well described in the clinical model of metabolic syndrome [24]. Moreover, all the components of metabolic syndrome are shown to be related to augmented carotid-femoral pulse wave velocity [25,26], whereas the same relation cannot be described with the cardio-ankle vascular index [25].

Even if classical effects of leptin include food intake reduction and increasing energy expenditure due to leptin's central action on the hypothalamus, leptin receptors are also located in the vessels and mainly in the aorta [27], as well as in tunica media and adventitia of arteries and inside atherosclerotic plaques [28]. Through these receptors, leptin may promote vascular smooth muscle cell proliferation and migration, contributing to arterial stiffness [29]. Leptin has been shown also to promote angiogenesis and to activate immune system (both monocytes and T-cell); it is also involved in atherogenesis onset, by increased platelet aggregation and Radical Oxygen Species (ROS) production [30]. As demonstrated in experimental studies in human cells models, leptin also induces endothelial oxidative stress and reactive oxygen species formation [31,32], mechanisms known to increase the risk to develop hypertension. The increased level of leptin is often associated with hypoadiponectinemia [33]: visceral fat, in particular, has also been shown to be negatively associated with adiponectin levels, whose protective effect on arteries is known [34].

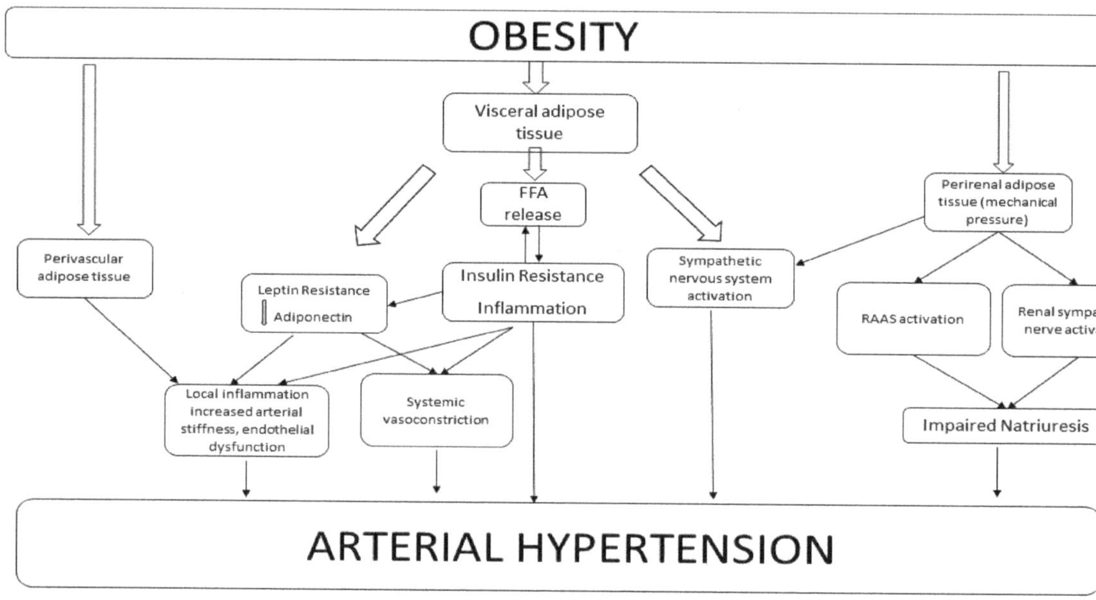

Figure 1. Mechanisms Linking Obesity to Hypertension.

2.2. *Perivascular Adipose Tissue*

Perivascular adipose tissue (PVAT) represents adipose tissue (AT) that surrounds blood vessels. Its main function is to provide mechanical support to vessels and even regulate vascular homeostasis. In experimental models of angiotensin II-induced hypertension and deoxycorticosterone acetate (DOCA)-salt hypertension, complement cascade activation is described [35]. In particular, the effector C5a is recognized to promote macrophage infiltration of PVAT, which is responsible for further inflammatory activation [35].

It has been widely shown that PVAT releases biologically active adipokines, with paracrine effects on the vessels [36] (e.g., leptin, adiponectin, omentin, visfatin, resistin, apelin), cytokines/chemokines (e.g., interleukin-6, IL-6; tumour necrosis factor-α, TNF-α; monocyte chemoattractant protein-1, MCP-1), NO, prostacyclin, angiotensin-1 to 7 Angiotensin II and reactive oxygen species (ROS) [37–41]. Obesity leads to a dysfunction of PVAT which releases elevated levels of pro-inflammatory factors adipokines such as leptin, cytokines and chemokines directly to the vascular wall, contributing to endothelial dysfunction and inflammation [39].

All these molecules act with different effects on vascular tone regulation. PVAT-derived relaxing factors (adiponectin, NO, H2S prostacylcin) promote vasodilation and on the other hand PVAT-derived contractile factors, such as leptin, Ang II and ROS induce vasoconstriction. In obese subjects PVAT dysfunction results in augmented production of contractile factors, inducing increased arterial vasoconstriction and greater vascular tone [39,42]. PVAT anticontractile activity is shown to be reduced in hypertensive patients [41].

Moreover, it has been shown that the expression of factors involved in immune cell infiltration and even vascular smooth muscle cells (VSMC) proliferation, are increased in obese subjects, which leads to a general state of inflammation of PVAT and thickening of the arterial wall and probably contributes to an increased risk of hypertension. It has been observed that during the progression of hypertension, immune cells accumulate mainly in perivascular fat tissue surrounding both large and resistance vessels such as the aorta and mesenteric arteries. In particular, one study showed that in non-obesity-induced hypertension inflammation is highly pronounced in PVAT, whereas in non-perivascular visceral fat, immune cell infiltration is less pronounced [42–44].

2.3. Renal Adipose Tissue

In obese subjects, renal-pressure natriuresis may be impaired through mechanical compression of the kidneys by fat in and around the kidneys [1,45,46]. Increased sodium reabsorption caused by adipose renal tissue mechanical compression could indirectly contribute to renal vasodilation, glomerular hyperfiltration and stimulate increased renin secretion in obese subjects. Moreover, ectopic fat accumulation in and around kidneys seems to have "lipotoxic" effects on kidneys through increased oxidative stress, mitochondrial dysfunction and endoplasmic reticulum stress [47].

Furthermore, natriuresis can be also affected by the activation of the renin-angiotensin-aldosterone system and increased sympathetic nervous system activity, especially by the renal sympathetic nerve activity. (Figure 1). A neural pathway has been hypothesized between renal fat and sympathetic activation [48]. A study by Shi et al. showed an increase in renal sympathetic outflow following enhanced afferent signals from adipose tissue, leading to increased arterial BP in rats. The authors called this reflex the "adipose afferent reflex" (AAR) [49].

Moreover, it has been demonstrated that intra-adipose administration of capsaicin, bradykinin, adenosine or leptin can activate the afferent nerves and consequent AAR [50–52], showing a greater enhancement in hypertensive rats compared to normotensive ones. These data seem to show that AAR might be a contributing factor in the pathogenesis of obesity-related hypertension. Altered activities of the adipose-innervating sensory neurons could regulate the cardiovascular system via neural reflex and enhanced hypertension. Nevertheless, more studies are needed to confirm the role of perirenal AAR activation in hypertension pathogenesis, since the anatomical distribution and function of the primary afferent neurons innervating perirenal fat still remains unclear.

2.4. Renin Angiotensin Aldosterone System

An important role explaining the increased risk of hypertension in obese patients is surely played by the activation of the renin angiotensin aldosterone system (RAAS) [53–55]. In obese subjects, increased renal adipose tissue activates the RAAS through mechanical compression in the kidney. Also, the RAAS can be activated by the increased Sympathetic Nervous System (SNS) activity of obese subjects. (Figure 1). Interestingly, it has been hypothesized that angiotensinogen, produced even by adipocytes, may play a role in determining increased BP in obesity [20,53], even if there is a lack of studies showing a direct effect of angiotensinogen or angiotensin II on BP regulation in obesity. Furthermore, there is evidence that adipocytes can synthesize aldosterone and it may be involved in a paracrine control of vascular function [20].

2.5. Sympathetic Nervous System Activation

Several studies showed an increased sympathetic activity in obese subjects, as assessed by direct recordings of muscle sympathetic nerve activity (MSNA) [56–60]. Grassi et al. showed that both heart rate and MSNA baroreflex changes were attenuated in hypertensive obese subjects compared to normotensive subjects. They concluded that the association between obesity and hypertension triggers sympathetic activation together with baroreflex cardiovascular control, which could contribute to the increased incidence of hypertension in obese subjects. Finally, increased levels of leptin, together with the increased levels of pro-inflammatory cytokines, activate the SNS, leading to a BP increase in obese subjects.

Figure 1 describes the complex network which links obesity to arterial hypertension. The effect of different kinds of adipose tissue is shown—PVAT directly promotes local inflammation and contributes to endothelial dysfunction. Visceral AT can induce leptin and insulin resistance, which increase both systemic vasoconstriction and endothelial dysfunction. Moreover, visceral adipose tissue can directly activate the sympathetic nervous system. Perirenal adipose tissue, through mechanical compression, is involved in the RAAS activation and in renal sympathetic system activity. All these pathways, widely interrelated among each other, lead to increased arterial BP in obese subjects.

3. Weight Loss and Blood Pressure

Several studies showed that WL may reduce BP: we analysed the studies looking at the effect of WL on BP in the last 10 years; we found 13 studies (either interventional or observational) that showed an association between WL and BP decrease (Table 1). Different WL strategies were taken into account: diet and lifestyle modification, pharmacological intervention and bariatric surgery. Although a positive effect of WL could be identified in each study, the main difference seems to be the magnitude and the durability of BP reduction over time. Some of these results were also corroborated by the evidence of 8 reviews published in the last ten years.

Interestingly, all the studies providing specific WL strategies in obese hypertensive patients showed a significant improvement either in BP decrease and or in body weight reduction. On the contrary, an observational study led by Ho et al., on 2906 obese subjects who developed incident hypertension and achieved BP control within 12 months after diagnosis, showed that the majority of patients did not achieve a significant WL [8]. Therefore, combined management should be pursued.

Table 1. This table summarizes selected studies from the last 10 years, showing a positive effect of weight loss (WL) on blood pressure (BP), achieved by diet and lifestyle modifications, pharmacological intervention and bariatric surgery. The table includes only studies with available data regarding number of participants, WL strategies, quantifiable mean WL and mean BP decrease, median follow-up time. * mean values referred to patients who achieved the major waist circumference reduction.

Author, Year	**Number of Participants**	**WL Intervention**	**Mean WL ΔBW (Kg) ΔBMI (kg/m²)**		**Mean BP Reduction (mmHg)**	**Median Follow up**
			Diet and Lifestyle modification			
Blumenthal, 2010 (*ENCORE study*)	144	DASH diet alone	−0.3		11.2 (SBP) 7.5 (DBP)	4 months
		DASH diet plus weight management	−8.7		16.1 (SBP) 9.9 (DBP)	
Rocha-Goldberg, 2010	17	behavioral intervention	1.5 ± 3.2 lb		10.4 ± 10.6 (SBP)	6 weeks
Rothberg, 2017	344	behavioral intervention		−6 ± 3	8 (SBP) *	6 months
	170	behavioral intervention		−5 ± 4	8 (SBP) *	2 years
Straznicky, 2011	59	dietary and moderate-intensity aerobic exercise	−7.1 ± 0.6 (dietary)	−2.4 ± 0.2 (dietary)	10±2 (SBP)	12 weeks
			−8.4 ± 1.0 (dietary + exercise)	−2.8± 0.3 (dietary + exercise)		
Wing, 2011 (*look AHEAD study*)	5154	intensive lifestyle intervention or diabetes support and education	−4.8 ± 7.6		2.40 (DBP) 4.76 (SBP)	1 year

Table 1. *Cont.*

Author, Year	Number of Participants	WL Intervention	Mean WL ΔBW (Kg) ΔBMI (kg/m^2)	Mean BP Reduction (mmHg)	Median Follow up
Pharmacological intervention					
Marso, 2016	9340	Pharmacologic (liraglutide vs placebo)	2.3 kg *higher in Liraglutide group*	1.2 (SBP) *lower in Liraglutide group*	36 weeks
Wijkman, 2019	124	Pharmacologic (liraglutide vs placebo)	>3%	9.2 (SBP)	24 weeks
Bariatric Surgery					
Ghanim, 2018	15	Surgery (RYGB)	−11.7	11 (SBP)	6 months
Hallersund, 2013 (*SOS study*)	2473 (277 gastric bypass, 1064 purely restricted proedures, 1132 control)	Surgery (GBP, VBG/B)	−10.1 (GBP group)	−5.1 (SBP) −5.6 (DBP) (GBP group)	10 years
Seravalle, 2014	20 (10 surgery + 10 control)	Surgery (vertical sleeve gastrectomy)	−9.1 ± 1.4	10.2 ± 4.5 (SBP)	6 months
			−10.8 ± 1.6	13.9 ± 5.0 (SBP)	1 year

3.1. Diet and Lifestyle Modification

According to published guidelines [7,13], diet and lifestyle modifications aimed at BW reduction are the first step in treating hypertension (COR I, LOE A) [13]. Weight reduction may reduce blood pressure and delay the need of pharmacological antihypertensive therapy [7] and it is also recommended in order to control other associated metabolic risk factors [7]. Straznicky et al. evaluated whether energy restriction could reduce BP in a group of 59 patients affected by obesity. Subjects were treated with dietary intervention or dietary intervention with moderate-intensity aerobic exercise or no treatment, for a period of 12 weeks. In both groups, BW reduction was associated with a significant systolic BP decrease and sympathetic neural activity downregulation [11].

Rothberg et al. enrolled obese patients in a 2-year, intensive, behavioural, weight management program [61] and showed that waist circumference (WC) reduction was related to metabolic syndrome component improvement. After subdividing the study population according to the amount of WC reduction, they observed higher systolic BP reduction in subjects with greater WC decrease, both at the 6-month and 2-year follow-up.

The Look AHEAD study [10,62], an intensive behavioural lifestyle intervention, evaluated the effect of BW loss on CV mortality and morbidity, in a study sample of 5154 patients with type 2 diabetes and overweight or obesity. Patients were randomized to diabetes support and education or to an intensive lifestyle intervention. The average WL was different in the two groups and the magnitude of WL was positively related to improvements in both BP and cardiovascular risk. Subjects who lost 5% to 10% of their initial BW were more likely to show a greater improvement in BP. Moreover, at 1 year, both systolic and diastolic BP declined in those patients who underwent an intensive lifestyle intervention, as compared to those who received only diabetes support and education. Only systolic BP maintained a decreased trend throughout the following progression of the study [62].

Behavioural intervention was also studied in another selected sub-population and its feasibility has been proved—in Hispanics/Latinos, for example, Rocha Goldberg et al. showed the effectiveness of educational lifestyle intervention on BW and BP control [63]; WL was observed along with a decrease in systolic BP. The ENCORE study, a large randomized controlled trial, was conducted on 144 obese or overweight hypertensive patients: subjects were randomized to a low-calorie Dietary Approach to Stop Hypertension (DASH diet) or DASH diet alone or usual diet. After four months, the subgroup assigned to DASH diet combined with a weight management program achieved both WL and a greater and significant reduction of BP [13,64,65].

3.2. Pharmacological Intervention

Wijkman et al. recently conducted a double-blind, placebo-controlled parallel group trial in overweight and obese patients with type 2 diabetes, randomized to receive liraglutide or placebo for 24 weeks. Compared to the placebo group, subjects who received liraglutide presented greater reduction of both BW and BP, 33% had a BP decrease of more than 5 mmHg (versus only 15% in the placebo group, ($p < 0.01$), 35% lost more than 3% in BW (vs just 3% of patients with placebo, $p < 0.0001$) and 22% of patients decreased both WL and BP versus 2% of patients in the placebo group [66]. Furthermore, the SCALE Obesity and Prediabetes trial provided evidence that overweight or obese patients, randomized to liraglutide for a period of three years, had a significant decrease in BMI, WC, systolic and diastolic BP as compared with placebo ($p < 0.001$ for all) [67]. In a multicentre, double-blind, placebo-controlled trial, Marso et al. confirmed these findings—the liraglutide group had a greater decrease in WL, as well in systolic but not in diastolic BP, than in the control group [68].

Beside the WL, other mechanisms explaining the effect of Liraglutide on BP has been hypothesized. Liraglutide treatment has been shown to increase natriuresis through a raise of natriuretic peptides [69]. Another study found increased levels of cyclic guanyl monophosphate (cGMP) and cyclic adenyl monophosphate (cAMP) which are two vasodilators and reduced plasma concentrations of angiotensinogen, renin and angiotensin after GLP-1 receptors therapy [70]. Moreover, as GLP 1 receptors are expressed in endothelial cells [71], it has been hypothesized that GLP-1 receptor agonists may improve endothelial dysfunction contributing to lower BP levels.

A review by Siebenhofer et al., of nine randomized controlled trials conducted for at least 24 weeks in hypertensive adult patients, comparing different weight reducing drugs (orlistat, sibutramine or phentermine/topiramate) to placebo, showed that treatment with orlistat is associated with WL and a significant drop in BP [72]. Sibutramine, instead, was responsible for diastolic BP increase. Phentermine/topiramate was associated to BP lowering but only one study was considered [69]. The Joint statement of the European Association for the Study of Obesity and the European Society of Hypertension confirms the positive effect of orlistat: compared to placebo, it improved both WL (more 2.7 kg) and diastolic BP, which resulted 2.2 mmHg lower [73].

3.3. Bariatric Surgery

In obese patients of any age, bariatric surgery has been shown to provide, together with WL, consistent improvement in systolic BP [74]. A very high number of patients treated by laparoscopic adjustable gastric banding discontinued anti-hypertensive medication or needed a lower medication dose [74,75]. Furthermore, six months after vertical sleeve gastrectomy, Seravalle et al. observed a significant reduction both in systolic BP and in sympathetic nerve conduction; interestingly, BP decline was also found to be persistent together with sympathetic inhibition 12 months after the surgical intervention [76].

As compared to lifestyle intervention, a surgical approach seems to give much more persistent and durable results [77]. In a large prospective controlled study, the Swedish Obese Subjects (SOS) study, patients were assigned to medical therapy or to different surgical procedures. A total of 4047 obese subjects were initially recruited. Surgically treated patients were matched to control subjects, who underwent a lifestyle intervention or even no treatment [78]. After a median follow-up of ten years, gastric bypass was associated with significant WL, WL maintenance and greater BP decrease, as compared both to non-surgical controls and to purely restrictive procedures such as vertical banded gastroplasty or gastric banding [79].

Nevertheless, a wide Cochrane meta-analysis by Colquitt and colleagues compared different surgical procedures, such as laparoscopic gastric bypass and laparoscopic duodenojejunal bypass with sleeve gastrectomy: however, no statistically significant differences were observed in terms of hypertension remission [80] among the different surgical procedures. In a systematic review of RCTs of bariatric surgery, Chang et al. described a 75% remission of hypertension (95% CI 62–86%) [81] independent of the type of procedure.

Considering the end organ effects of hypertension in obese patients, improvements are described after bariatric surgery. In a large review which considered CV risk factors and CV imaging in patients undergoing bariatric surgery, Vest et al. reported an echocardiographic reduction of left ventricular mass and an improvement in diastolic function, measured by E/A ratio [82]. A reduction in proteinuria, renal function decline and end stage renal disease [83] have been also observed in a recent review of observational studies by Cohen.

In a recent study by Ghanim et al., diabetic obese patients have been evaluated before and six months after Roux-en-Y gastric bypass. At the follow-up analysis, together with a significant decrease in BW and BP, a significant reduction was found in circulating vasoconstrictors (neprilysin, renin, angiotensinogen, angiotensin II and endothelin 1), whereas the vasodilator atrial natriuretic peptide (ANP) was increased [84]. Taken together, these studies show that bariatric surgery may partially explain the mechanisms of the long-term benefits of gastric bypass on BP.

4. Possible Mechanisms Involved in BP Reduction after Weight Loss

The explanation of the BP lowering effect of WL interventions may be identified in adipose tissue decrease. These changes may reverse the complex network of mechanisms linking obesity and hypertension (Figure 1). Visceral adipose tissue reduction, which is directly related to waist circumference reduction [61,67], may attenuate the inflammation pathway and arterial and ventricular stiffening may improve [24]. Moreover, it is well known that a visceral AT decrease, even due to a decrease of FFA release, is related to insulin resistance improvement (as also shown by the positive effect of WL, on diabetes management [10,62,66]) and a lower level of insulin may reduce systemic vasoconstriction that is partially responsible for arterial hypertension. Leptin [30] and adiponectin [34] pathways are also improved.

Since PVAT dysfunction is strongly related to obesity, it is possible to hypothesize that WL may improve PVAT functioning, by reducing the vasoconstriction effect. A reduction in vasoconstriction has been shown also after bariatric surgery [85], along with an improvement of RAAS functioning too. Weight loss may reduce renal adipose tissue as well and benefits may be found in natriuresis and sympathetic activation [45,46,49] and BP levels should consequentially lower. Unfortunately, only a few laboratory-based studies on the effect of weight loss on hypertension in the past decade have been published and new future studies are necessary to confirm possible mechanisms linking WL to the improvement of obesity-related hypertension

5. Conclusions

Lifestyle intervention, including weight loss, should be considered the first step in all patients with hypertension, especially if overweight and obese. All together studies aimed to show that WL induced by dietary intervention alone or associated with physical exercise or even with drugs or bariatric surgery, demonstrates a beneficial effect of WL on BP. However, the effect on BP seems to depend on the amount of WL.

Some considerations must be made. Most lifestyle intervention and pharmacological studies regarding WL and BP have been conducted on relatively small number of participants and have different follow-up lengths too. Only one study had 2 years' follow-up [61], whereas the others had a maximum a 1-year follow-up. The only interventional study showing a long follow-up (10 years) with a persistent WL and BP reduction was the SOS study [79] but it regarded the surgical approach.

Thus, studies with a longer follow-up in wider populations are needed to support these findings and to explain better the mechanisms related to the improvement of BP in obese subjects losing weight.

References

1. Hall, J.E.; Do Carmo, J.M.; Da Silva, A.A.; Wang, Z.; Hall, M.E. Obesity-Induced Hypertension: Interaction of Neurohumoral and Renal Mechanisms. *Circ. Res.* **2015**, *116*, 991–1006. [CrossRef] [PubMed]
2. Seravalle, G.; Grassi, G. Obesity and hypertension. *Pharmacol. Res.* **2017**, *122*, 1–7. [CrossRef] [PubMed]
3. Bramlage, P.; Pittrow, D.; Wittchen, H.U.; Kirch, W.; Boehler, S.; Lehnert, H.; Hoefler, M.; Unger, T.; Sharma, A.M. Hypertension in overweight and obese primary care patients is highly prevalent and poorly controlled. *Am. J. Hypertens.* **2004**, *17*, 904–910. [CrossRef] [PubMed]
4. Zhou, B.; Bentham, J.; Di Cesare, M.; Bixby, H.; Danaei, G.; Cowan, M.J.; Paciorek, C.J.; Singh, G.; Hajifathalian, K.; Bennett, J.E.; et al. Worldwide trends in blood pressure from 1975 to 2015: A pooled analysis of 1479 population-based measurement studies with 19·1 million participants. *Lancet* **2017**, *389*, 37–55. [CrossRef]
5. Kannel, W.B. Framingham study insights into hypertensive risk of cardiovascular disease. *Hypertens. Res.* **1995**, *18*, 181–196. [CrossRef] [PubMed]
6. Shihab, H.M.; Meoni, L.A.; Chu, A.Y.; Wang, N.Y.; Ford, D.E.; Liang, K.Y.; Gallo, J.J.; Klag, M.J. Body mass index and risk of incident hypertension over the life course: The Johns Hopkins Precursors Study. *Circulation* **2012**, *126*, 2983–2989. [CrossRef] [PubMed]
7. Williams, B.; Mancia, G.; Spiering, W.; Rosei, E.A.; Azizi, M.; Burnier, M.; Clement, D.L.; Coca, A.; De Simone, G.; Dominiczak, A.; et al. 2018 ESC/ESH Guidelines for the management of arterial hypertension. *Eur. Heart J.* **2018**, *39*, 3021–3104. [CrossRef]
8. Ho, A.K.; Bartels, C.M.; Thorpe, C.T.; Pandhi, N.; Smith, M.A.; Johnson, H.M. Achieving Weight Loss and Hypertension Control among Obese Adults: A US Multidisciplinary Group Practice Observational Study. *Am. J. Hypertens.* **2016**, *29*, 984–991. [CrossRef]
9. Mertens, I.L.; Van Gaal, L.F. Overweight, obesity, and blood pressure: The effects of modest weight reduction. *Obes. Res.* **2000**, *8*, 270–278. [CrossRef]
10. Wing, R.R.; Lang, W.; Wadden, T.A.; Safford, M.; Knowler, W.C.; Bertoni, A.G.; Hill, J.O.; Brancati, F.L.; Peters, A.; Wagenknecht, L. Benefits of modest weight loss in improving cardiovascular risk factors in overweight and obese individuals with type 2 diabetes. *Diabetes Care* **2011**, *34*, 1481–1486. [CrossRef]
11. Straznicky, N.E.; Lambert, E.A.; Nestel, P.J.; McGrane, M.T.; Dawood, T.; Schlaich, M.P.; Masuo, K.; Eikelis, N.; De Courten, B.; Mariani, J.A.; et al. Sympathetic neural adaptation to hypocaloric diet with or without exercise training in obese metabolic syndrome subjects. *Diabetes* **2010**, *59*, 71–79. [CrossRef] [PubMed]
12. Kritchevsky, S.B.; Beavers, K.M.; Miller, M.E.; Shea, M.K.; Houston, D.K.; Kitzman, D.W.; Nicklas, B.J. Intentional weight loss and all-cause mortality: A meta-analysis of randomized clinical trials. *PLoS ONE* **2015**, *10*, e0121993. [CrossRef] [PubMed]
13. Whelton, P.K.; Carey, R.M.; Aronow, W.S.; Ovbiagele, B.; Casey, D.E., Jr.; Smith, S.C., Jr.; Collins, K.J.; Spencer, C.C.; Himmelfarb, C.D.; Stafford, R.S.; et al. 2017 Guideline for the Prevention, Detection, Evaluation, and Management of High Blood Pressure in Adults: A Report of the American College of Cardiology/American Heart Association, Task Force on Clinical Practice Guidelines. *J. Am. Coll. Cardiol.* **2017**, *71*, 85–87.
14. Jensen, M.D.; Ryan, D.H.; Apovian, C.M.; Ard, J.D.; Comuzzie, A.G.; Donato, K.A.; Hu, F.B.; Hubbard, V.S.; Jakicic, J.M.; Kushner, R.F.; et al. 2013 AHA/ACC/TOS guideline for the management of overweight and obesity in adults: A report of the American college of cardiology/American heart association task force on practice guidelines and the obesity society. *J. Am. Coll. Cardiol.* **2014**, *63 Pt 25*, 2985–3023. [CrossRef]
15. Lavie, C.J.; Milani, R.V.; Ventura, H.O. Obesity and Cardiovascular Disease. Risk Factor, Paradox, and Impact of Weight Loss. *J. Am. Coll. Cardiol.* **2009**, *53*, 1925–1932. [CrossRef] [PubMed]
16. Fantuzzi, G.; Mazzone, T. Adipose tissue and atherosclerosis: Exploring the connection. *Arterioscler. Thromb. Vasc. Biol.* **2007** *27*, 996–1003. [CrossRef] [PubMed]
17. Bosello, O.; Zamboni, M. Visceral obesity and metabolic syndrome. *Obes. Rev.* **2000**, *1*, 47–56. [CrossRef]
18. Caballero, A.E. Endothelial dysfunction in obesity and insulin resistance: A road to diabetes and heart disease. *Obes. Res.* **2003**, *11*, 1278–1289. [CrossRef]

19. Kuboki, K.; Jiang, Z.Y.; Takahara, N.; Ha, S.W.; Igarashi, M.; Yamauchi, T.; Feener, E.P.; Herbert, T.P.; Rhodes, C.J.; King, G.L. Regulation of endothelial constitutive nitric oxide synthase gene expression in endothelial cells and in vivo—A specific vascular action of insulin. *Circulation* **2000**, *101*, 676–681. [CrossRef]
20. Rahmouni, K. Obesity-associated hypertension: Recent progress in deciphering the pathogenesis. *Hypertension* **2014**, *64*, 215–221. [CrossRef]
21. Zachariah, J.P.; Hwang, S.; Hamburg, N.M.; Benjamin, E.J.; Larson, M.G.; Levy, D.; Vita, J.A.; Sullivan, L.M.; Mitchell, G.F.; Vasan, R.S. Circulating Adipokines and Vascular Function: Cross-Sectional Associations in a Community-Based Cohort. *Hypertension* **2016**, *67*, 294–300. [CrossRef]
22. Kofler, S.; Nickel, T.; Weis, M. Role of cytokines in cardiovascular diseases: A focus on endothelial responses to inflammation. *Clin. Sci.* **2005**, *108*, 205–213. [CrossRef]
23. Singhal, A.; Farooqi, S.; Cole, T.J.; O'Rahilly, S.; Fewtrell, M.; Kattenhorn, M.; Lucas, A.; Deanfield, J. Influence of leptin on arterial distensibility: A novel link between obesity and cardiovascular disease? *Circulation* **2002**, *106*, 1919–1924. [CrossRef]
24. Zanoli, L.; Di Pino, A.; Terranova, V.; Di Marca, S.; Pisano, M.; Di Quattro, R.; Ferrara, V.; Scicali, R.; Rabuazzo, A.M.; Fatuzzo, P.; et al. Inflammation and ventricular-vascular coupling in hypertensive patients with metabolic syndrome. *Nutr. Metab. Cardiovasc. Dis.* **2018**, *28*, 1222–1229. [CrossRef]
25. Topouchian, J.; Labat, C.; Gautier, S.; Bäck, M.; Achimastos, A.; Blacher, J.; Cwynar, M.; De La Sierra, A.; Pall, D.; Fantin, F.; et al. Effects of metabolic syndrome on arterial function in different age groups: The Advanced Approach to Arterial Stiffness study. *J. Hypertens.* **2018**, *36*, 824–833. [CrossRef]
26. Fantin, F.; Di Francesco, V.; Rossi, A.; Giuliano, K.; Marino, F.; Cazzadori, M.; Gozzoli, M.P.; Vivian, M.E.; Bosello, O.; Rajkumar, C.; et al. Abdominal obesity and subclinical vascular damage in the elderly. *J. Hypertens.* **2010**, *28*, 333–339. [CrossRef]
27. Purdham, D.M.; Zou, M.-X.; Rajapurohitam, V.; Karmazyn, M. Rat heart is a site of leptin production and action. *Am. J. Physiol. Circ. Physiol.* **2004**, *287*, H2877–H2884. [CrossRef]
28. Parhami, F.; Tintut, Y.; Ballard, A.; Fogelman, A.M.; Demer, L.L. Leptin enhances the calcification of vascular cells artery wall as a target of leptin. *Circ. Res.* **2001**, *88*, 954–960. [CrossRef]
29. Oda, A.; Taniguchi, T.; Yokoyama, M. Leptin stimulates rat aortic smooth muscle cell proliferation and migration. *Kobe J. Med. Sci.* **2001**, *47*, 141–150. [CrossRef]
30. Werner, N.; Nickenig, G. From Fat Fighter to risk factor: The zizag trek of leptin. *Arterioscler. Thromb. Vasc. Biol.* **2004**, *24*, 7–9. [CrossRef]
31. Bouloumie, A.; Marumo, T.; Lafontan, M.; Busse, R. Leptin induces oxidative stress in human endothelial cells. *FASEB J.* **1999**, *13*, 1231–1238. [CrossRef]
32. Yamagishi, S.I.; Edelstein, D.; Du, X.L.; Kaneda, Y.; Guzmán, M.; Brownlee, M. Leptin Induces Mitochondrial Superoxide Production and Monocyte Chemoattractant Protein-1 Expression in Aortic Endothelial Cells by Increasing Fatty Acid Oxidation via Protein Kinase. *J. Biol. Chem.* **2001**, *276*, 25096–25100. [CrossRef]
33. Catharina, A.S.; Modolo, R.; Ritter, A.; Sabbatini, A.; Correa, N.; Brunelli, V.; Fraccaro, N.; Almeida, A.; Lopes, H.; Moreno, H.; et al. [PP.05.34] metabolic syndrome-related features in controlled and resistant hypertensive subjects. *J. Hypertens.* **2017**, *35*, e128. [CrossRef]
34. Mahmud, A.; Feely, J. Adiponectin and arterial stiffness. *Am. J. Hypertens.* **2005**, *18 Pt 1*, 1543–1548. [CrossRef]
35. Ruan, C.C.; Gao, P.J. Role of Complement-Related Inflammation and Vascular Dysfunction in Hypertension. *Hypertension* **2019**, *73*, 965–971. [CrossRef]
36. Lohn, M.; Dubrovska, G.; Lauterbach, B.; Luft, F.C.; Gollasch, M.; Sharma, A.M. Periadventitial fat releases a vascular relaxing factor. *FASEB J.* **2002**, *16*, 1057–1063. [CrossRef]
37. Szasz, T.; Webb, R.C. Perivascular adipose tissue: More than just structural support. *Clin. Sci.* **2011**, *122*, 1–12. [CrossRef]
38. Almabrouk, T.A.M.; Ewart, M.A.; Salt, I.P.; Kennedy, S. Perivascular fat, AMP-activated protein kinase and vascular diseases. *Br. J. Pharmacol.* **2014**, *171*, 595–617. [CrossRef]
39. Fernández-Alfonso, M.S.; Gil-Ortega, M.; García-Prieto, C.F.; Aranguez, I.; Ruiz-Gayo, M.; Somoza, B. Mechanisms of perivascular adipose tissue dysfunction in obesity. *Int. J. Endocrinol.* **2013**, *2013*, 402053. [CrossRef]
40. Xia, N.; Li, H. The role of perivascular adipose tissue in obesity-induced vascular dysfunction. *Br. J. Pharmacol.* **2017**, *174*, 3425–3442. [CrossRef]
41. Szasz, T.; Bomfim, G.F.; Webb, R.C. The influence of perivascular adipose tissue on vascular homeostasis. *Vasc. Health Risk Manag.* **2013**, *9*, 105–116. [CrossRef]

42. Van Dam, A.D.; Boon, M.R.; Berbée, J.F.P.; Rensen, P.C.N.; van Harmelen, V. Targeting white, brown and perivascular adipose tissue in atherosclerosis development. *Eur. J. Pharmacol.* **2017**, *816*, 82–92. [CrossRef]
43. Mikolajczyk, T.P.; Nosalski, R.; Szczepaniak, P.; Budzyn, K.; Osmenda, G.; Skiba, D.; Sagan, A.; Wu, J.; Vinh, A.; Marvar, P.J.; et al. Role of chemokine RANTES in the regulation of perivascular inflammation, T-cell accumulation, and vascular dysfunction in hypertension. *FASEB J.* **2016**, *30*, 1987–1999. [CrossRef]
44. Guzik, T.J.; Hoch, N.E.; Brown, K.A.; McCann, L.A.; Rahman, A.; Dikalov, S.; Goronzy, J.; Weyand, C.; Harrison, D.G. Role of the T cell in the genesis of angiotensin II–induced hypertension and vascular dysfunction. *J. Exp. Med.* **2007**, *204*, 2449–2460. [CrossRef]
45. Nosalski, R.; Guzik, T.J. Perivascular adipose tissue inflammation in vascular disease. *Br. J. Pharmacol.* **2017**, *174*, 3496–3513. [CrossRef]
46. Chandra, A.; Neeland, I.J.; Berry, J.D.; Ayers, C.R.; Rohatgi, A.; Das, S.R.; Khera, A.; McGuire, D.K.; De Lemos, J.A.; Turer, A.T. The relationship of body mass and fat distribution with incident hypertension: Observations from the dallas heart study. *J. Am. Coll. Cardiol.* **2014**, *64*, 997–1002. [CrossRef]
47. Chughtai, H.L.; Morgan, T.M.; Rocco, M.; Stacey, B.; Brinkley, T.E.; Ding, J.; Nicklas, B.; Hamilton, C.; Hundley, W.G. Renal sinus fat and poor blood pressure control in middle-aged and elderly individuals at risk for cardiovascular events. *Hypertension* **2010**, *56*, 901–906. [CrossRef]
48. Bobulescu, I.A.; Lotan, Y.; Zhang, J.; Rosenthal, T.R.; Rogers, J.T.; Adams-Huet, B.; Sakhaee, K.; Moe, O.W. Triglycerides in the human kidney cortex: Relationship with body size. *PLoS ONE* **2014**, *9*, e101285. [CrossRef]
49. Liu, B.X.; Sun, W.; Kong, X.Q. Perirenal Fat: A Unique Fat Pad and Potential Target for Cardiovascular Disease. *Angiology* **2018**, *9*, 3319718799967. [CrossRef]
50. Shi, Z.; Chen, W.W.; Xiong, X.Q.; Han, Y.; Zhou, Y.B.; Zhang, F.; Gao, X.Y.; Zhu, G.Q. Sympathetic activation by chemical stimulation of white adipose tissues in rats. *J. Appl. Physiol.* **2012**, *112*, 1008–1014. [CrossRef]
51. Niijima, A. Reflex effects from leptin sensors in the white adipose tissue of the epididymis to the efferent activity of the sympathetic and vagus nerve in the rat. *Neurosci. Lett.* **1999**, *262*, 125–128. [CrossRef]
52. Smith, J.A.M.; Amagasu, S.M.; Eglen, R.M.; Hunter, J.C.; Bley, K.R. Characterization of prostanoid receptor-evoked responses in rat sensory neurones. *Br. J. Pharmacol.* **1998**, *124*, 513. [CrossRef]
53. Xiong, X.Q.; Chen, W.W.; Zhu, G.Q. Adipose afferent reflex: Sympathetic activation and obesity hypertension. *Acta Physiol.* **2014**, *210*, 468–478. [CrossRef]
54. Thatcher, S.; Yiannikouris, F.; Gupte, M.; Cassis, L. The adipose renin-angiotensin system: Role in cardiovascular disease. *Mol. Cell. Endocrinol.* **2009**, *302*, 111–117. [CrossRef]
55. Jia, G.; Aroor, A.R.; Sowers, J.R. The role ofmineralocorticoid receptor signaling in the cross-talk between adipose tissue and the vascular wall. *Cardiovasc. Res.* **2017**, *113*, 1055–1063. [CrossRef]
56. Schütten, M.T.J.; Houben, A.J.H.M.; de Leeuw, P.W.; Stehouwer, C.D.A. The Link Between Adipose Tissue Renin-Angiotensin-Aldosterone System Signaling and Obesity-Associated Hypertension. *Physiology* **2017**, *32*, 197–209. [CrossRef]
57. Grassi, G.; Mark, A.; Esler, M. The Sympathetic Nervous System Alterations in Human Hypertension. *Circ. Res.* **2015**, *116*, 976–990. [CrossRef]
58. Grassi, G.; Seravalle, G.; Brambilla, G.; Buzzi, S.; Volpe, M.; Cesana, F.; Dell'Oro, R.; Mancia, G. Regional differences in sympathetic activation in lean and obese normotensive individuals with obstructive sleep apnoea. *J. Hypertens.* **2014**, *32*, 383–388. [CrossRef]
59. Grassi, G.; Pisano, A.; Bolignano, D.; Seravalle, G.; D'Arrigo, G.; Quarti-Trevano, F.; Mallamaci, F.; Zoccali, C.; Mancia, G. Sympathetic nerve traffic activation in essential hypertension and its correlates systematic reviews and meta-analyses. *Hypertension* **2018**, *72*, 483–491. [CrossRef]
60. Fonkoue, I.T.; Le, N.A.; Kankam, M.L.; DaCosta, D.; Jones, T.N.; Marvar, P.J.; Park, J. Sympathoexcitation and impaired arterial baroreflex sensitivity are linked to vascular inflammation in individuals with elevated resting blood pressure. *Physiol. Rep.* **2019**, *7*, e14057. [CrossRef]
61. Richard, R.N. Obesity-Related Hypertension. *Ochsner J.* **2009**, *9*, 133–136.
62. Rothberg, A.E.; McEwen, L.N.; Kraftson, A.T.; Ajluni, N.; Fowler, C.E.; Nay, C.K.; Miller, N.M.; Burant, C.F.; Herman, W.H. Impact of weight loss on waist circumference and the components of the metabolic syndrome. *BMJ Open Diabetes Res. Care* **2017**, *5*, e000341. [CrossRef]
63. Johnston, C.A.; Moreno, J.P.; Foreyt, J.P. Cardiovascular Effects of Intensive Lifestyle Intervention in Type 2 Diabetes. *Curr. Atheroscler. Rep.* **2014**, *16*, 457. [CrossRef]

64. Rocha-Goldberg, M.D.P.; Corsino, L.; Batch, B.; Voils, C.I.; Thorpe, C.T.; Bosworth, H.B.; Svetkey, L.P. Hypertension improvement project (HIP) Latino: Results of a pilot study of lifestyle intervention for lowering blood pressure in Latino adults. *Ethn. Health* **2010**, *15*, 269–282. [CrossRef]
65. Sacks, F.M.; Campos, H. Dietary Therapy in Hypertension. *N. Engl. J. Med.* **2010**, *362*, 2102–2112. [CrossRef]
66. Blumenthal, J.A.; Babyak, M.A.; Hinderliter, A.; Watkins, L.L.; Craighead, L.; Lin, P.H.; Caccia, C.; Johnson, J.; Waugh, R.; Sherwood, A. Effects of the DASH diet alone and in combination with exercise and weight loss on blood pressure and cardiovascular biomarkers in men and women with high blood pressure: The ENCORE study. *Arch. Intern. Med.* **2010**, *170*, 126–135. [CrossRef]
67. Wijkman, M.O.; Dena, M.; Dahlqvist, S.; Sofizadeh, S.; Hirsch, I.; Tuomilehto, J.; Mårtensson, J.; Torffvit, O.; Imberg, H.; Saeed, A.; et al. Predictors and correlates of systolic blood pressure reduction with liraglutide treatment in patients with type 2 diabetes. *J. Clin. Hypertens.* **2019**, *21*, 105–115. [CrossRef]
68. Mehta, A.; Marso, S.P.; Neeland, I.J. Liraglutide for weight management: A critical review of the evidence. *Obes. Sci. Pract.* **2016**, *3*, 3–14. [CrossRef]
69. Marso, S.P.; Daniels, G.H.; Brown-Frandsen, K.; Kristensen, P.; Mann, J.F.; Nauck, M.A.; Nissen, S.E.; Pocock, S.; Poulter, N.R.; Ravn, L.S.; et al. Liraglutide and Cardiovascular Outcomes in Type 2 Diabetes HHS Public Access. *N. Engl. J. Med.* **2016**, *375*, 311–322. [CrossRef]
70. Gutzwiller, J.P.; Tschopp, S.; Bock, A.; Zehnder, C.E.; Huber, A.R.; Kreyenbuehl, M.; Gutmann, H.; Drewe, J.; Henzen, C.; Goeke, B.; et al. Glucagon-like peptide 1 induces natriuresis in healthy subjects and in insulin-resistant obese men. *J. Clin. Endocrinol. Metab.* **2004**, *89*, 3055–3061. [CrossRef]
71. Li, C.J.; Yu, Q.; Yu, P.; Yu, T.L.; Zhang, Q.M.; Lu, S.; Yu, D.M. Changes in liraglutide-induced body composition are related to modifications in plasma cardiac natriuretic peptides levels in obese type 2 diabetic patients. *Cardiovasc. Diabetol.* **2014**, *13*, 36. [CrossRef]
72. Ussher, J.R.; Drucker, D.J. Cardiovascular actions of incretin-based therapies. *Circ. Res.* **2014**, *114*, 1788–1803. [CrossRef]
73. Siebenhofer, A.; Jeitler, K.; Horvath, K.; Berghold, A.; Posch, N.; Meschik, J.; Semlitsch, T. Long-term effects of weight-reducing drugs in people with hypertension. *Cochrane Database Syst. Rev.* **2016**, *3*, CD007654. [CrossRef]
74. Jordan, J.; Yumuk, V.; Schlaich, M.; Nilsson, P.M.; Zahorska-Markiewicz, B.; Grassi, G.; Schmieder, R.E.; Engeli, S.; Finer, N. Joint statement of the European Association for the Study of Obesity and the European Society of Hypertension: Obesity and difficult to treat arterial hypertension. *J. Hypertens.* **2012**, *30*, 1047–1055. [CrossRef]
75. Frezza, E.E.; Wei, C.; Wachtel, M.S. Is surgery the next answer to treat obesity-related hypertension? *J. Clin. Hypertens.* **2009**, *11*, 284–288. [CrossRef]
76. Schiavon, C.A.; Bersch-Ferreira, A.C.; Santucci, E.V.; Oliveira, J.D.; Torreglosa, C.R.; Bueno, P.T.; Frayha, J.C.; Santos, R.N.; Damiani, L.P.; Noujaim, P.M.; et al. Effects of bariatric surgery in obese patients with hypertension the GATEWAY randomized trial (gastric bypass to treat obese patients with steady hypertension). *Circulation* **2018**, *137*, 1132–1142. [CrossRef]
77. Seravalle, G.; Colombo, M.; Perego, P.; Giardini, V.; Volpe, M.; Dell'Oro, R.; Mancia, G.; Grassi, G. Long-term sympathoinhibitory effects of surgically induced weight loss in severe obese patients. *Hypertension* **2014**, *64*, 431–437. [CrossRef]
78. Cohen, J.B.; Cohen, D.L. Cardiovascular and Renal Effects of Weight Reduction in Obesity and the Metabolic Syndrome. *Curr. Hypertens. Rep.* **2015**, *17*, 34. [CrossRef]
79. Sjöström, L. Review of the key results from the Swedish Obese Subjects (SOS) trial—A prospective controlled intervention study of bariatric surgery. *J. Intern. Med.* **2013**, *273*, 219–234. [CrossRef]
80. Hallersund, P.; Sjöström, L.; Olbers, T.; Lönroth, H.; Jacobson, P.; Wallenius, V.; Näslund, I.; Carlsson, L.M.; Fändriks, L. Gastric Bypass Surgery Is Followed by Lowered Blood Pressure and Increased Diuresis —Long Term Results from the Swedish Obese Subjects (SOS) Study. *PLoS ONE* **2012**, *7*, e49696. [CrossRef]
81. Colquitt, J.L.; Pickett, K.; Loveman, E.; Frampton, G.K. Surgery for weight loss in adults. *Cochrane Database Syst. Rev.* **2014**, *8*, CD003641. [CrossRef]
82. Chang, S.H.; Stoll, C.R.T.; Song, J.; Varela, J.E.; Eagon, C.J.; Colditz, G.A. The effectiveness and risks of bariatric surgery an updated systematic review and meta-analysis, 2003–2012. *JAMA Surg.* **2014**, *149*, 275–287. [CrossRef]

83. Vest, A.R.; Heneghan, H.M.; Agarwal, S.; Schauer, P.R.; Young, J.B. Bariatric surgery and cardiovascular outcomes: A systematic review. *Heart* **2012**, *98*, 1763–1777. [CrossRef]
84. Cohen, J.B. Hypertension in Obesity and the Impact of Weight Loss. *Curr. Cardiol. Rep.* **2017**, *19*, 98. [CrossRef]
85. Ghanim, H.; Monte, S.; Caruana, J.; Green, K.; Abuaysheh, S.; Dandona, P. Decreases in neprilysin and vasoconstrictors and increases in vasodilators following bariatric surgery. *Diabetes Obes. Metab.* **2018**, *20*, 2029–2033. [CrossRef]

16

Cod Residual Protein Prevented Blood Pressure Increase in Zucker fa/fa Rats, Possibly by Inhibiting Activities of Angiotensin-Converting Enzyme and Renin

Iselin Vildmyren [1,2], Aslaug Drotningsvik [1,3], Åge Oterhals [4], Ola Ween [5], Alfred Halstensen [2,6] and Oddrun Anita Gudbrandsen [1,*]

1 Dietary Protein Research Group, Department of Clinical Medicine, University of Bergen, 5021 Bergen, Norway; iselin.vildmyren@uib.no (I.V.); aslaug.drotningsvik@uib.no (A.D.)
2 K. Halstensen AS, P.O. Box 103, 5399 Bekkjarvik, Norway; alfred.halstensen@uib.no
3 TripleNine Vedde AS, 6030 Langevåg, Norway
4 Nofima AS, P.B. 1425 Oasen, 5844 Bergen, Norway; Aage.Oterhals@Nofima.no
5 Møreforsking Ålesund AS, P.O. Box 5075, 6021 Ålesund, Norway; ola.ween@moreforsk.no
6 Department of Clinical Science, University of Bergen, 5021 Bergen, Norway
* Correspondence: nkjgu@uib.no

Abstract: Hypertension is the leading risk factor for cardiovascular disease, and prevention of high blood pressure through diet and lifestyle should be a preferred approach. High intake of fish is associated with lower blood pressure, possibly mediated through the proteins since peptides with angiotensin-converting enzyme (ACE) inhibiting capacities have been identified in fish skin, backbone, and fillet. The effects of cod meals made from residual materials and fillet on blood pressure were investigated in obese Zucker fa/fa rats which spontaneously develop high blood pressure. Rats were fed diets containing water-soluble (stickwater) or water-insoluble (presscake) fractions of protein-rich meals from cod residual materials (head, gut, backbone with muscle residuals, skin, trimmings) or fillet. Rats were fed diets containing 25% of total protein from cod meal and 75% of protein from casein, or casein as the sole protein source (control group) for four weeks. Results show that a diet containing residual presscake meal with high gut content prevented blood pressure increase, and this cod residual meal also showed the strongest in vitro inhibitions of ACE and renin activities. In conclusion, a diet containing water-insoluble proteins (presscake meal) with high gut content prevented increase in blood pressure in obese Zucker fa/fa rats.

Keywords: fish protein; fish meal; cod; rest raw material; hypertension

---

1. Introduction

The prevalence of hypertension is increasing worldwide, and is estimated to affect 1.56 billion adults by the year of 2025 [1]. Hypertension is the leading risk factor for cardiovascular disease [2], and the goal of prevention of hypertension is to avoid premature cardiovascular disease [3] since hypertension increases the risk of atherosclerosis, stroke, myocardial infarction, heart failure, peripheral vascular disease, disability, and damage to major organs such as heart and kidneys [4,5]. Hypertension can be prevented through dietary changes such as reduced sodium intake; maintaining an adequate intake of potassium; and consuming a diet low in saturated and total fat and rich in fruits, vegetables, whole-grain and low-fat dairy products [6]. Prevention of hypertension through the diet should be a preferred approach and more knowledge on effects of various nutrients on blood pressure is warranted.

Blood pressure is controlled by several mechanisms, of which the renin-angiotensin system may be the best known. Angiotensinogen is cleaved by renin to the biologically inactive angiotensin I, which is further converted to the vasoconstrictor angiotensin II by the angiotensin-converting enzyme (ACE). The cleavage of angiotensinogen to angiotensin I by renin is considered to be the rate determining step in the generation of angiotensin II [7]. ACE also catalyzes the degradation of the vasodilator bradykinin to inactive peptides, thus providing a second way of regulating blood pressure through manipulation of ACE activity [7], and a wide range of synthetic drugs targeting ACE-inhibition has been developed and are commonly used by hypertensive patients all over the world. Other factors that may influence blood pressure include arginine which is a precursor for the formation of the vasodilator nitric oxide [8], and dietary sodium which acts as a vasoconstrictor through its control of blood volume by increasing arterial constriction and peripheral vascular resistance [9] and effects on renin [10].

High intake of fish is reported to be associated with lower blood pressure in both clinical [11–15] and rat [16,17] studies, whereas some studies show no association between fish consumption and blood pressure [18–20]. A possible blood pressure lowering effect of fish may be mediated through the proteins in fish, as peptides with ACE-inhibiting capacities in vitro have been identified in fish fillet, skin, and backbone [21–24]. In addition, studies in spontaneously hypertensive rats have shown anti-hypertensive effects of ACE-inhibitory peptides identified in marine sources [25–27], however little is known of the potential effects of fish proteins on renin activity. Large amounts of protein-rich fish residual materials such as head, gut, bones, trimmings, and other cut-offs are produced by the world's fisheries and aquaculture industries, but very little is used for human consumption [28]. Therefore, fish proteins from both fillet and residual materials as food component are of interest for regulation of blood pressure and thus for prevention of cardiovascular disease and should be investigated in vivo.

The obese Zucker fa/fa rat presents a range of abnormalities similar to those seen in humans with obesity—including insulin resistance, dyslipidemia, mild glucose intolerance, and hypertension—and is a popular rat model for studies of metabolic complications and possible treatments of obesity [29]. The Zucker rat is a valuable experimental model for hypertension as this rat develops an age-related increase in blood pressure, which is also the case for humans [30], and in Zucker fa/fa rats this development starts already before the age of 10 weeks [31,32]. The most used rat model for studies on development and treatment of hypertension is the spontaneously hypertensive rat, although this rat is representative for only a rare subtype of human hypertension; primary hypertension that is inherited in a Mendelian fashion [33]. The Zucker fa/fa rat could therefore be a more relevant model where hypertension co-exists with obesity and other metabolic disturbances in a real-life setting [31].

The aim of the present study was to investigate the effects of diets containing protein-rich meals from a selection of water-soluble and water-insoluble cod residuals or cod fillet on the development of high blood pressure in obese Zucker fa/fa rats which spontaneously develops high blood pressure, compared with Zucker fa/fa rats fed a control diet devoid of fish. Circulating nitrite + nitrate (as a measure of nitric oxide) and renin were measured to elucidate possible mechanisms involved in blood pressure regulation that were affected by the cod meals, and the in vitro potential of the dietary proteins to inhibit ACE and renin activities were investigated. Our hypothesis was that cod meal prepared from residual materials and fillet would prevent or delay the development of high blood pressure in obese Zucker fa/fa rats, possibly through inhibition of the renin-angiotensin system.

2. Materials and Methods

2.1. Ethical Approval

The animal experiment was approved in accordance with the Norwegian regulation on animal experimentation (approval no 11603). The protocol was approved by the Norwegian State Board of Biological Experiments with Living Animals.

2.2. Design

Thirty-eight male Zucker fa/fa rats (Crl:ZUC(Orl)-Lepr fa, from Charles River Laboratories, Calco, Italy) were randomly assigned to six experimental groups with six rats in each of the groups receiving cod meal, with eight rats in the control group. Groups had comparable mean body weight at baseline. The rats were housed in pairs in individually ventilated cages (IVC type 4, blue line from Tecniplast, Buguggiate, VA, Italy) with plastic housing, under standard conditions with a temperature of 21 ± 1 °C, and a light-dark cycle of 12 h. The intervention period started after at least one week of acclimatization under these conditions, i.e., when the rats were 9–11 weeks old and weighing 339 ± 14 g.

The intervention period was four weeks, and rats had ad libitum access to feed and tap water. Freshly thawed feed was provided daily. Systolic and diastolic blood pressures of conscious rats were measured at baseline (Day 0), on Day 14 and three days before endpoint (i.e., on Day 25). Rats were prewarmed in a heating cabinet at 32 °C for 30 min before blood pressure was measured 10 times using the tail-cuff method (CODA™ Non-Invasive Blood Pressure System, Kent Scientific Corporation, Litchfield, CT, USA). Mean arterial pressure (MAP) was calculated as (diastolic blood pressure + 1/3 (systolic blood pressure − diastolic blood pressure)).

Rats were housed individually for 24 h in metabolic cages without fasting in advance to evaluate feed and water intake, and urine volume. To allow for the rats to recover after housing in the metabolic cages before measurements of end-point blood pressure on Day 25, the rats were housed in metabolic cages on Day 17.

At the end of the feeding period (after four weeks of intervention), after a 12 h fast with access to tap water, the rats were euthanized while under anaesthesia with isoflurane (Isoba vet, Intervet, Schering-Plough Animal Health, Boxmeer, The Netherlands) mixed with oxygen. Blood was drawn directly from the heart and was collected in BD Vacutainer SST II Advance gel tubes (Becton, Dickinson, and Company, Franklin Lakes, NJ, USA) for isolation of serum. Serum samples were stored at minus 80 °C until analysis. Staff handling the rats and conducting the analyses were blinded, and rats were handled and euthanized in random order.

2.3. Preparation of Fish Meals

Two Norwegian factory trawlers, Havstrand (Havstrand AS) and Granit (Halstensen Granit AS), prepared presscake fish meals on board from residual materials from Atlantic cod (Gadus morhua) fished in the Barents Sea in July 2016. Havstrand headed and gutted the cod. The heads were ground before mixing with gut, heated in a continuous cooker and mechanical pressed. The press liquid were run over a three-phase decanter centrifuge to remove oil and suspended solids. The decanter solids were mixed with the presscake and dried to a presscake meal (PC-H). The decanter liquid (stickwater) was immediately frozen for further processing on land; i.e., heated to 90 °C, centrifuged to remove residual solids and oil, concentrated and freeze dried (SW-H). A blend of stickwater + presscake meal was prepared, containing 20% of the total dry matter from stickwater from Havstrand (SWPC-H). Granit produced skin free cod fillets. The residuals (head, gut, backbone, skin, and trimmings) were ground before heated in a continuous cooker and mechanical pressed. The presscake was dried to a press cake meal (PC-G). Skin free fillets from Granit were grinded, heated to 80 °C and freeze dried to produce a fillet meal (FM-G). All experimental fish meals were ground on a Retsch ZM-1 centrifugal mill (Retsch GmbH, Haan, Germany) with a ring sieve aperture of 1 mm before analysis and inclusion in diets.

The residual cod meal from Havstrand comprises only head and gut and contains approximately twice as much liver compared to the residual meal from Granit which contains head, gut, backbone, skin, and trimmings (calculated from the official conversion factors from the Norwegian Directorate of Fisheries, www.fiskeridir.no).

2.4. Diets

The rats were fed experimental diets based on the AIN-93G recommendation for growing rats [34] with addition of 1.6 g methionine/kg diet as recommended by Reeves [35] (Table 1). All diets contained 20 wt % proteins, and casein was the sole protein source in the Control diet. Cod meal from residual material or fillet were added to the other diets in amounts providing 25 wt % of total protein from cod, while casein constituted the remaining 75 wt % of protein. Five diets containing different cod meals were prepared, containing either stickwater from Havstrand (SW-H), presscake meal from Havstrand (PC-H), a blend of stickwater + presscake meal from Havstrand (SWPC-H), presscake meal from Granit (PC-G), or fillet meal from Granit (FM-G).

Table 1. Composition of the experimental diets.

g/kg Diet	Control Diet	SW-H Diet	PC-H Diet	SWPC-H Diet	PC-G Diet	FM-G Diet
Casein *	223.8	167.8	167.8	167.8	167.8	167.8
Stickwater from Havstrand †	-	82.2	-	-	-	-
Presscake meal from Havstrand ‡	-	-	81.9	-	-	-
Stickwater + Presscake mealfrom Havstrand §	-	-	-	84.6	-	-
Presscake meal from Granit ǀǀ	-	-	-	-	77.6	-
Fillet meal from Granit #	-	-	-	-	-	60.7
Soybean Oil	70.0	70.0	70.0	70.0	70.0	70.0
Cornstarch	504.1	477.8	478.2	475.5	482.5	499.3
Sucrose	90.0	90.0	90.0	90.0	90.0	90.0
Cellulose	50.0	50.0	50.0	50.0	50.0	50.0
Tert-butylhydroquinone	0.014	0.014	0.014	0.014	0.014	0.014
Mineral Mix (AIN-93MX)	35.0	35.0	35.0	35.0	35.0	35.0
Vitamin Mix (AIN-93VX)	10.0	10.0	10.0	10.0	10.0	10.0
L-Methionine	1.6	1.6	1.6	1.6	1.6	1.6
L-Cystine	3.0	3.0	3.0	3.0	3.0	3.0
Choline Bitartrate **	2.5	2.5	2.5	2.5	2.5	2.5
Growth and Maintenance Supplement ††	10.0	10.0	10.0	10.0	10.0	10.0

* contains 89.4% crude protein; † contains 60.8% crude protein; ‡ contains 61.1% crude protein; § contains 59.1% crude protein; ǀǀ contains 64.5% crude protein; # contains 82.3% crude protein; ** contains 41.1% choline; †† contains vitamin B12 (40 mg/kg) and vitamin K1 (25 mg/kg) mixed with sucrose (995 g/kg) and dextrose (5 g/kg); SW-H; Stickwater from Havstrand, PC-H; Presscake meal from Havstrand, SWPC-H; Stickwater + Presscake meal from Havstrand, PC-G; Presscake meal from Granit, FM-G; Fillet meal from Granit.

Casein was purchased from Sigma-Aldrich (Munich, Germany). All feed ingredients except cod meals and casein were purchased from Dyets Inc. (Bethlehem, PA, USA). Since the feeds were given as powder formulas, the rats always had access to wood chewing sticks. The rats were weighed every seventh day during the intervention period. Casein and cod meals were not hydrolyzed prior to use.

2.5. Analyses of Diets

Total energy in diets was measured using an IKA C6000 global standards calorimeter in isoperibol measurement mode (IKA®-Werke GmbH & Co, Staufen, Germany). Total amino acids, taurine, fatty acids, sodium, potassium and chloride in diets were analyzed by Nofima BioLab (Fyllingsdalen, Norway). Total amino acid composition and content of cysteine + cystine were measured according to the method of Cohen & Michaud [36], and tryptophan was determined by the method of Miller [37]. Taurine was quantified by HPLC using the Waters Pico-Tag method as described by Bidlingmeyer et al. [38]. Lipids were extracted according to the AOCS method Ce 1b-89, and fatty acids were quantified as described by Oterhals & Nygård [39]. Contents of sodium and potassium in the diets were determined by flame atomic absorption spectrometry in accordance with ISO6869:2000 [40] using Perkin Elmer Analyst 400 with an AS 90plus autosampler (PerkinElmer, Waltham, MA, USA). Chloride in diets was determined by volumetric method in accordance with AOAC Official Method 937.09, by boiling the sample in silver nitrate and nitric acid to precipitate silver chloride. The residual soluble silver ions were titrated with ammonium thiocyanate [41].

2.6. *In Vitro Inhibition of Angiotensin Converting Enzyme (ACE) and Renin*

Casein and cod protein meals were added Trizma buffer (50 mM, pH 8.0) and hydrolyzed using trypsin from bovine pancreas (T1426, from Sigma-Aldrich) at 45 °C for 4 h as recommended by Shalaby et al. [42]. ACE-inhibition was measured using the method by Shalaby et al. [42], as previously described [43]. Renin inhibition was measured using the Renin Assay Kit (MAK157, from Sigma-Aldrich) as described in the user manual. Protein in hydrolysates were quantified on the Cobas c111 system (Roche Diagnostics GmbH, Mannheim, Germany) using the TP2 kit from Roche.

2.7. *Analyses in Serum and Urine*

As a measure of nitric oxide we measured the stable metabolites of nitric oxide metabolism, i.e., nitrite and nitrate, in serum using the Nitrite/Nitrate Assay Kit (cat #23479, Sigma-Aldrich, Munich, Germany) based on the Griess assay. Serum was filtrated (Amicon Ultra-0.5 Centrifugal Filter Unit with Ultracel membrane 10K device, Merck KGaA, Darmstadt, Germany) to remove hemoglobin and proteins before analysis of nitrite and nitrate. Sodium in urine was analyzed on the Cobas c111 system (Roche Diagnostics GmbH, Mannheim, Germany) using the Ion-Selective Electrode module from Roche Diagnostics.

2.8. *Statistical Analyses*

Variables were evaluated for normality by the Shapiro-Wilk test, Q-Q plots and histograms. Most variables were within normal distribution, and variables that were not normally distributed were log-transformed before parametric statistical tests were performed. Variables were compared between groups using one-way analysis of variance (ANOVA) with Fisher's least significant difference (LSD) post-hoc test when appropriate. Changes in MAP from baseline to Day 14, and from baseline to endpoint within each group were tested using the paired sampled T-test, and the within-group changes were compared using ANOVA with LSD post-hoc test. Level of statistical significance were set at $p < 0.05$. Statistical analyses were performed using IBM SPSS Statistics 25 (SPSS, Inc., IBM Corporation, Armonk, NY, USA). Results from rat samples are presented as mean with standard deviations as a measure of variability. Results from in vitro inhibition of ACE and renin are presented as mean with standard error of mean as a measurement of the uncertainty of the mean measurements. Means with different letters are significantly different. One rat in the SW-H group had a lean phenotype and was excluded from all analyses, therefore results are presented for $n = 5$ rats in SW-H group, for $n = 6$ rats in the other cod meal diet groups, and for $n = 8$ rats in the control group.

3. Results

3.1. *Measurements of Blood Pressure*

Systolic and diastolic blood pressures were measured in conscious rats at baseline, on Day 14 and three days before endpoint (i.e., Day 25). MAP was similar in all groups at baseline; mean (SD) for all rats was 114 (9) mm Hg with p ANOVA = 0.41. One-way ANOVA analyses show differences between the groups for MAP at Day 14 (p ANOVA 6.8×10^{-4}) and at endpoint (p ANOVA 6.8×10^{-4}). The changes in MAP from baseline to Day 14, and from baseline to endpoint were significantly lower in PC-H group when compared to all other groups (Figure 1 and Table 2). A paired samples T-test for PC-H group reveal that there were no statistically significant changes in MAP throughout the study period ($p > 0.05$), meaning that the blood pressures were not changed from baseline to endpoint in this group. Changes in MAP in SW-H, SWPC-H, PC-G and FM-G groups from baseline to Day 14, and from baseline to endpoint were not changed, and were similar to those of control group. At Day 14 the change in MAP from baseline was significantly different between PC-G and FM-G groups, but no difference in MAP was seen between these groups at endpoint.

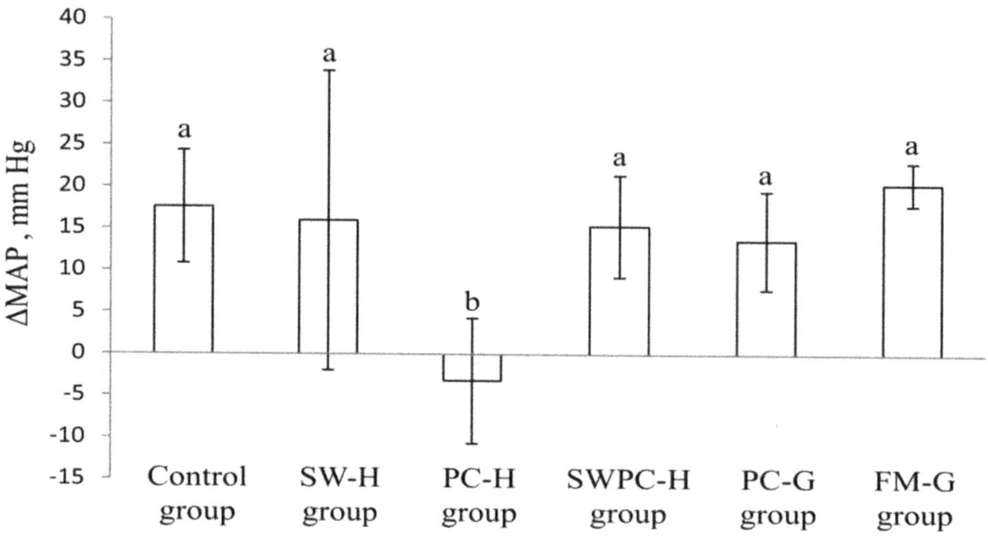

Figure 1. Changes in mean arterial pressure (MAP) from baseline to endpoint. Values are means, with standard error of mean represented as vertical bars. Values are shown for $n = 8$ in control group, $n = 5$ in SW-H, and $n = 6$ in all other groups. Groups are compared using one-way ANOVA with LSD post hoc test. Bars with different letters are significantly different ($p < 0.05$). BP; blood pressure, SW-H; stickwater from Havstrand, PC-H; presscake meal from Havstrand, SWPC-H; stickwater + presscake meal from Havstrand, PC-G; presscake meal from Granit, FM-G; fillet meal from Granit.

Table 2. Mean arterial pressure (MAP) measured at baseline, Day 14 and at endpoint.

	Control Group	SW-H Group	PC-H Group	SWPC Group	PC-G Group	FM-G Group
MAP baseline, mm Hg	111 ± 11	114 ± 5	120 ± 8	115 ± 10	110 ± 7	112 ± 8
MAP Day 14, mm Hg	126 ± 10	127 ± 7	115 ± 13	128 ± 8	127 ± 12	118 ± 8
MAP endpoint, mm Hg	128 ± 10	130 ± 18	117 ± 7	130 ± 13	124 ± 9	132 ± 10
p for change baseline to Day 14	4.5×10^{-4}	4.1×10^{-3}	0.22	0.051	0.011	6.4×10^{-3}
p for change baseline to endpoint	1.6×10^{-4}	0.12	0.35	0.0016	2.4×10^{-3}	6.5×10^{-6}
ΔMAP baseline to Day 14, mm Hg	15 ± 7 [ab]	12 ± 5 [ab]	−5 ± 9 [c]	13 ± 12 [ab]	17 ± 11 [a]	6 ± 3 [b]
ΔMAP baseline to endpoint, mm Hg	18 ± 7 [a]	16 ± 18 [a]	−3 ± 8 [b]	15 ± 6 [a]	14 ± 6 [a]	20 ± 3 [a]

Data are presented as mean ± standard deviation, $n = 8$ in Control group, $n = 5$ in SW-H, and $n = 6$ in all other groups. Changes in MAP from baseline to Day 14, and from baseline to endpoint within each group were tested using the paired sampled T-test, and the within-group changes were compared using ANOVA with LSD post-hoc test. Means in a row with different letters are significantly different ($p < 0.05$). SW-H; stickwater from Havstrand, PC-H; presscake meal from Havstrand, SWPC-H; stickwater + presscake meal from Havstrand, PC-G; presscake meal from Granit, FM-G; fillet meal from Granit.

3.2. Circulating Concentration of Nitrite + Nitrate

Serum concentration of nitrite + nitrate (p ANOVA = 0.022) was significantly higher in PC-H and SWPC-H when compared to Control group (p values 0.015 and 0.0049, respectively), and in addition serum nitrite+nitrate concentrations were significantly higher in PC-H and SWPC-H when compared to PC-G (p values 0.022 and 0.0081, respectively), with no differences between the other experimental groups (Figure 2).

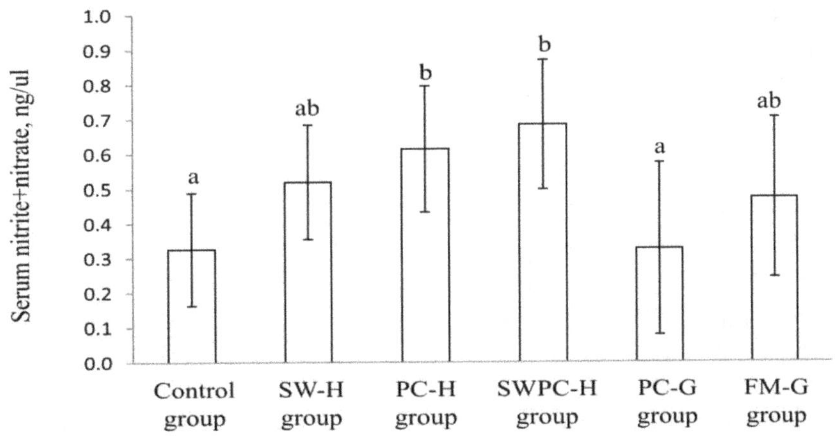

Figure 2. Serum concentration of nitrite + nitrate. Values are means, with standard error of mean represented as vertical bars. Values are shown for $n = 8$ in Control group, $n = 5$ in SW-H, and $n = 6$ in all other groups. Groups are compared using one-way ANOVA with LSD post hoc test when appropriate. Bars with different letters are significantly different ($p < 0.05$). SW-H; stickwater from Havstrand, PC-H; presscake meal from Havstrand, SWPC-H; stickwater + presscake meal from Havstrand, PC-G; presscake meal from Granit, FM-G; fillet meal from Granit.

3.3. *In Vitro Inhibition of ACE and Renin Activities*

The ACE and renin inhibiting capacities of the dietary proteins were measured after hydrolysis with trypsin by calculating IC50 concentrations. For ACE-inhibition (p ANOVA = 2.0×10^{-5}), the ACE-IC50 for SW-H protein was much higher (i.e., less potent) when compared to all other groups (Figure 3A), whereas ACE-IC50 concentrations for both PC-H and SWPC-H proteins were lower when compared to casein. In addition, ACE-IC50 for PC-H protein was lower when compared to SWPC-H protein, with no differences in ACE-IC50 between the other dietary proteins. For renin activity inhibition, no measurable inhibition was detected for casein, therefore casein was not included in the ANOVA analysis (Figure 3B). All cod meal proteins had different renin-IC50 from each other (p ANOVA = 1.5×10^{-7}), with the highest renin-IC50 observed for SW-H protein and the lowest renin-IC50 for PC-H protein.

3.4. *Growth and Dietary Intake*

All experimental groups had similar body weights at baseline, and no differences were seen in percent growth and body weight-to-square body length (without tail) ratio between the groups after four weeks' intervention (Table 3). Some differences were seen between the groups for mean daily energy intake (p ANOVA = 0.035), with higher intake in FM-G group when compared to control group, PC-H group and PC-G group, and higher intake in SWPC-H group when compared to PC-H group and PC-G group. Water intake and urine output per 24 h were similar between all groups (p ANOVA 0.19 and 0.41, respectively, data not presented).

Daily intakes of amino acids, taurine, fatty acids and electrolytes are presented relative to bodyweight in the Table S1. Intakes of most compounds are different between the groups, as demonstrated by low p-values after one-way ANOVA testing and subsequent post-hoc LSD tests. Intakes of alanine, arginine, aspartic acid + asparagine and glycine were higher in groups fed diets containing cod meal when compared to the control diet, which contained casein as the sole protein source. Of special interest in the present study are intakes of arginine which is a precursor of the vasodilator nitric oxide [8], taurine which is shown to have hypotensive effect [44], the long-chain n-3 PUFAs which may delay development of hypertension [45,46] and sodium which may act as a vasoconstrictor [9]. From calculations of dietary intake it is evident that arginine intake was not particularly high and the sodium intake was not particularly low in the PC-H group, which experienced a delay in the blood pressure increase compared to the other groups. Taurine and long-chain n-3

PUFAs were not detected in the control diet, but the comparisons between groups fed diets with cod meal/proteins show that taurine intake was not especially high in PC-H group, however the n-3 PUFA intake was similar to SW-PC group and higher compared to SW-H, PC-G and FM-G groups.

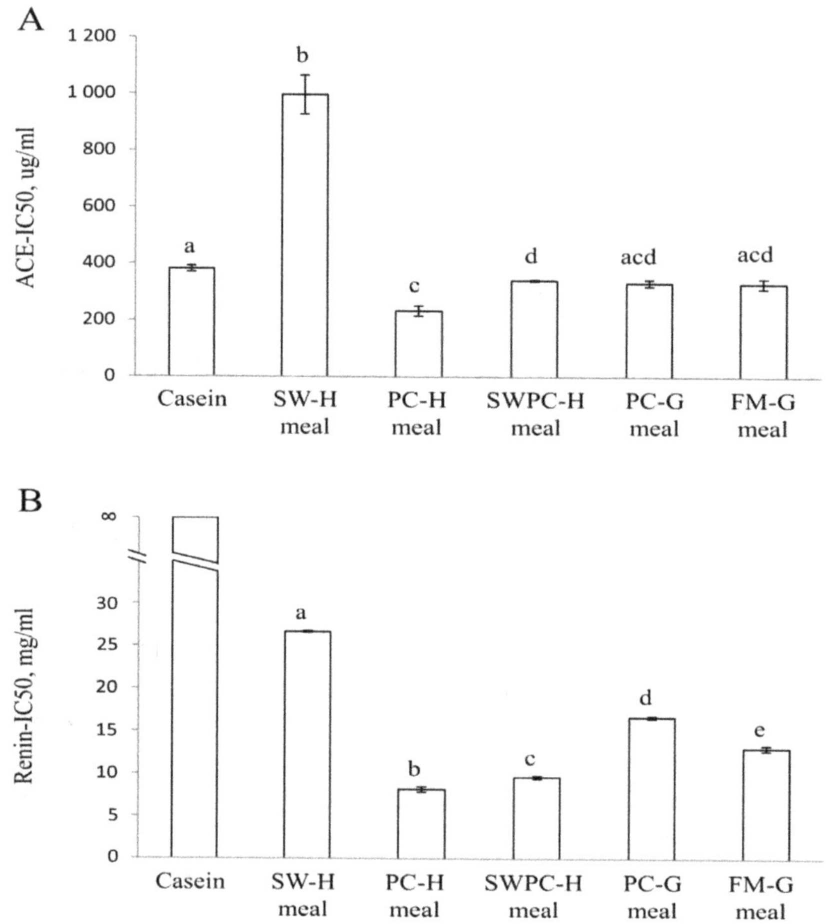

Figure 3. In vitro inhibition of activities of angiotensin-converting enzyme (**A**) and renin (**B**). Values are means, with standard error of mean represented as vertical bars. Values are shown for two or three measurements for casein and cod protein meals. Proteins are compared using one-way ANOVA with LSD post hoc test. Bars with different letters are significantly different ($p < 0.05$). SW-H; stickwater from Havstrand, PC-H; presscake meal from Havstrand, SWPC-H; stickwater + presscake meal from Havstrand, PC-G; presscake meal from Granit, FM-G; fillet meal from Granit.

Table 3. Bodyweight at baseline and growth at time of euthanasia, and energy intake at day 17.

	Control Group	SW-H Group	PC-H Group	SWPC-H Group	PC-G Group	FM-G Group	p Anova
Bodyweight at baseline, g	339 ± 16	345 ± 15	340 ± 11	334 ± 14	335 ± 13	342 ± 16	0.81
Body weight gain, %	31 ± 6	37 ± 5	35 ± 3	37 ± 5	30 ± 4	34 ± 6	0.053
Bodyweight-to-square body length without tail ratio, kg/m^2	8.4 ± 0.5	8.3 ± 0.4	8.3 ± 0.4	8.2 ± 0.4	8.3 ± 0.3	8.4 ± 0.3	0.94
Energy intake, kcal/kg bodyweight/24 h	219 ± 31 ^{ab}	238 ± 10 ^{abc}	209 ± 14 ^{a}	245 ± 20 ^{bd}	212 ± 36 ^{a}	248 ± 25 ^{cd}	0.035

Data are presented as mean ± standard deviation, $n = 8$ in Control group, $n = 5$ in SW-H, and $n = 6$ in all other groups; Groups are compared using one-way ANOVA with LSD post hoc test when appropriate; Means in a row with different letters are significantly different ($p < 0.05$); SW-H; stickwater from Havstrand, PC-H; presscake meal from Havstrand, SWPC-H; stickwater + presscake meal from Havstrand, PC-G; presscake meal from Granit, FM-G; fillet meal from Granit.

3.5. *Urine Sodium Excretion*

Urinary sodium excretion showed a large variation between the dietary groups (p ANOVA = 1.9×10^{-18}). The mean sodium excretion in urine (per 24 h) was higher in SW-H group compared to all other groups (Figure 4). Urinary sodium excretion was similar in PC-H and PC-G groups, whereas rats fed SWPC-H had a urine sodium excretion that was between SW-H and PC-H, as could be expected since SWPC-H meal is a mixture of these two meals. Sodium excretion was similar in rats fed FM-G diet and those fed the control diet.

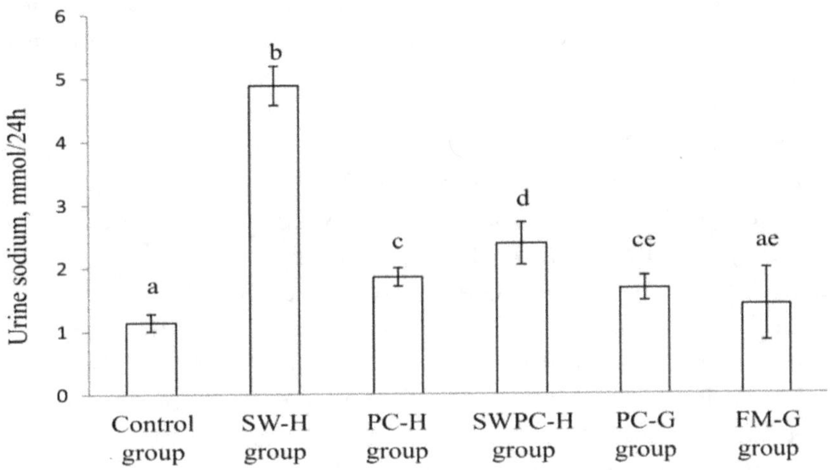

Figure 4. Urine 24 h sodium excretion. Values are means, with standard error of mean represented as vertical bars. Values are shown for $n = 8$ in Control group, $n = 5$ in SW-H, and $n = 6$ in all other groups. Groups are compared using one-way ANOVA with LSD post hoc test when appropriate. Bars with different letters are significantly different ($p < 0.05$). SW-H; stickwater from Havstrand, PC-H; presscake meal from Havstrand, SWPC-H; stickwater + presscake meal from Havstrand, PC-G; presscake meal from Granit, FM-G; fillet meal from Granit.

4. Discussion

In the present study we show for the first time that intake of cod presscake meal produced from residual materials with high content of gut prevented blood pressure increase in obese Zucker fa/fa rats. This effect was evident already after two weeks, and persisted until endpoint at four weeks. The other cod meal diets tested, containing either a residual stickwater, a mixture of residual presscake and stickwater, a residual presscake meal with low gut content, or fillet did not affect blood pressure development in this rat model. We chose to use obese Zucker fa/fa rats in this experiment, since this model resembles human obesity [29] and the rats spontaneously develop high blood pressure from a young age, that is, before the age of 10 weeks [31,32,47].

Renin and ACE are important enzymes for blood pressure control since they catalyze the conversion of angiotensinogen via angiotensin I to the vasoconstrictor angiotensin II, with renin as the rate determining enzyme [7]. Medications that inhibit either renin or ACE activity have been developed, although Skeggs et al. already in 1957 suggested that renin inhibition should be preferred to ACE inhibition [48]. Peptides with ACE inhibiting properties in vitro have been identified in fillet, skin, and backbone from various fish species [21–24] and in milk proteins such as casein [49]. Renin inhibitory effects of cod fillet has been demonstrated [50], however little is known about whether proteins from fish residual materials and milk may affect renin activity in vitro, and whether in vitro findings are transferable to live animals including humans.

In the present study we found that PC-H had significantly (although marginally) lower in vitro ACE-IC50 and renin-IC50 (i.e., the strongest ACE and renin inhibiting potencies) compared to casein and all other cod meals after trypsin digestion, and in line with this we found that the PC-H diet prevented the development of high blood pressure in the obese Zucker rats. This suggests that the postponed development of high blood pressure in PC-H fed rats could be regulated through the renin-angiotensin system; however, since ACE and renin activities are measured in vitro these may not be directly transferable to effects in the rats. We saw no associations between the in vitro ACE and renin inhibitory capacities and blood pressure development in the other experimental groups. The ACE-IC50 for FM-G meal, containing cod fillet meal, was not markedly different from the ACE-IC50 for casein, which was surprising since we recently demonstrated that proteins from cod fillet had a lower ACE-IC50 compared to a casein-whey (9:1) mixture [43].

ACE-IC50 and renin-IC50 were highest for SW-H, however the blood pressure development in rats fed SW-H diet was similar to the other experimental groups except for the PC-H group (where MAP was unchanged). Also, dietary sodium can act as a vasoconstrictor through its control of blood volume by increasing arterial constriction and peripheral vascular resistance [9]. Sodium intake was lowest in the control group, but still no difference was seen for blood pressure development between this group and SW-H, SWPC-H, PC-G, and FM-G groups. In the present study, the sodium intake was significantly higher in the SW-H diet compared to the other diets, and the high urinary output of sodium in rats fed this diet imply that the kidney coped well with this higher sodium load, and thus avoided development of hypervolemic high blood pressure.

Components other than sodium in the diets may also affect blood pressure development, such as arginine, taurine, and long-chain n-3 PUFAs. Arginine is a conditionally essential amino acid in rats [51], and is a precursor for the formation of the vasodilator nitric oxide [8]. It has been suggested by others that dietary fish proteins delays development of hypertension due to higher arginine content in fish proteins compared to casein [16]. We found no association between arginine intake, serum nitrite + nitrate concentration (as a measure of nitric oxide), and blood pressure development in the present study; however, we cannot exclude the possibility that the higher serum nitrite + nitrate in PC-H group compared to the control group may have beneficially contributed to the prevention of blood pressure increase in this group. Intake of taurine has been shown to have a hypotensive effect in prehypertensive humans [44] and to delay blood pressure increase in spontaneously hypertensive rats [52], but the mechanisms behind this is not fully elucidated. Since the taurine intake in the PC-H group was relatively low when compared to especially the SW-H diet, and only the former diet prevented an increase in blood pressure, the observed effects on blood pressure by the PC-H diet can probably not be ascribed to the taurine intake.

The gut residual includes liver in addition to intestines and other internal organs. Since the residual cod meal from Havstrand contains approximately twice as much liver compared to the residual meal from Granit, and since cod liver contains high amounts of long-chain n-3 PUFAs, the groups fed PC-H and SWPC-H diets had the highest intake of EPA, DPA, and DHA of the experimental diets. Studies in spontaneously hypertensive rats report a delay in the development of hypertension after intake of fish oil [45,46], and a negative association between fish fillet or fish oil intake and blood pressure has been observed in several studies [11–14,53,54]. A statement from the American Heart Association concludes that high doses of fish oil may reduce blood pressure in hypertensive individuals, but have no mention of fish oil or fish fillet intake for the prevention of development of high blood pressure [55]. In a recent paper [17] we show that feeding obese Zucker fa/fa rats a diet containing salmon fillet with low n-3 PUFA content prevented blood pressure increase, comparable to that observed in the PC-H group in the present experiment. Since only the PC-H diet prevented the blood pressure increase we cannot conclude if the dietary content of long-chain n-3 PUFA in PC-H diet played a role to prevent blood pressure increase in the present study.

There are some methodological limitations in the present study. This study was designed to investigate the effects of different cod meals on the development of high blood pressure using an experimental design that is relevant for human nutrition. We used a relevant rat model that develops high blood pressure and diets with 25% of protein from fish meal, and future studies should investigate if these findings are relevant for human hypertension. Blood pressure was measured using the non-invasive tail-cuff method (volume-pressure recording) at baseline and near endpoint of the intervention period instead of continuous intravascular blood pressure measured by telemetry, since comparison of these methods shows similar results in mice [56].

5. Conclusions

The present study demonstrates that presscake meal from cod residual materials with high gut content (PC-H) effectively prevented the increases in MAP that are normally observed in obese Zucker fa/fa rats, whereas the other cod meals tested did not influence the blood pressure development in these rats. In line with this, PC-H had the strongest effect on in vitro inhibition of ACE and renin activities of the cod meals tested.

Author Contributions: Conceptualization, I.V., A.D., Å.O., O.W., A.H., and O.A.G.; Methodology, validation, formal analysis, investigation, data curation and writing—original draft preparation, I.V., A.D., Å.O., A.H., and O.A.G.

Acknowledgments: We thank Jon Grimstad (Strand Havfiske AS), Ola Inge Grønnevet (Halstensen Management AS) and the crews that collected on-board samples on the trawlers Havstrand and Granit, Jørgen Borthen (Norwegian Seafood Center) for organizing and facilitating applications for funding and implementation of the study, and Margareth Kjerstad and Janne Kristin Stangeland (Møreforsking) for organizing practical aspects for obtaining the cod meals from the trawlers. We are also grateful for funding from the Norwegian Directorate of Fisheries.

References

1. Kearney, P.M.; Whelton, M.; Reynolds, K.; Muntner, P.; Whelton, P.K.; He, J. Global burden of hypertension: Analysis of worldwide data. *Lancet* **2005**, *365*, 217–223. [CrossRef]
2. Danaei, G.; Lu, Y.; Singh, G.; Stevens, G.; Cowan, M.; Farzadfar, F.; Lin, J.; Finucane, M.; Rao, M.; Khang, Y.; et al. Cardiovascular disease, chronic kidney disease, and diabetes mortality burden of cardiometabolic risk factors from 1980 to 2010: A comparative risk assessment. *Lancet* **2014**, 2, 634–647.
3. Olsen, M.H.; Angell, S.Y.; Asma, S.; Boutouyrie, P.; Burger, D.; Chirinos, J.A.; Damasceno, A.; Delles, C.; Gimenez-Roqueplo, A.P.; Hering, D.; et al. A call to action and a lifecourse strategy to address the global burden of raised blood pressure on current and future generations: The Lancet Commission on hypertension. *Lancet* **2016**, *388*, 2665–2712. [CrossRef]
4. Kannel, W.B. Blood pressure as a cardiovascular risk factor: Prevention and treatment. *JAMA* **1996**, *275*, 1571–1576. [CrossRef] [PubMed]
5. The World Health Organization. *A Global Brief on Hypertension: Silent Killer, Global Public Health Crisis*; WHO: Geneva, Switzerland, 2013.
6. Whelton, P.K.; Carey, R.M.; Aronow, W.S.; Casey, D.E., Jr.; Collins, K.J.; Dennison Himmelfarb, C.; DePalma, S.M.; Gidding, S.; Jamerson, K.A.; Jones, D.W.; et al. 2017 ACC/AHA/AAPA/ABC/ACPM/AGS/APhA/ASH/ASPC/NMA/PCNA Guideline for the Prevention, Detection, Evaluation, and Management of High Blood Pressure in Adults: A Report of the American College of Cardiology/American Heart Association Task Force on Clinical Practice Guidelines. *J. Am. Coll. Cardiol.* **2018**, *71*, e127–e248. [PubMed]
7. Zaman, M.A.; Oparil, S.; Calhoun, D.A. Drugs targeting the renin-angiotensin-aldosterone system. *Nat. Rev. Drug Discov.* **2002**, *1*, 621–636. [CrossRef] [PubMed]
8. Palmer, R.M.; Ashton, D.S.; Moncada, S. Vascular endothelial cells synthesize nitric oxide from L-arginine. *Nature* **1988**, *333*, 664–666. [CrossRef] [PubMed]
9. Blaustein, M.P.; Leenen, F.H.; Chen, L.; Golovina, V.A.; Hamlyn, J.M.; Pallone, T.L.; Van Huysse, J.W.; Zhang, J.; Wier, W.G. How NaCl raises blood pressure: A new paradigm for the pathogenesis of salt-dependent hypertension. *Am. J. Physiol. Heart Circ. Physiol.* **2012**, *302*, H1031–H1049. [CrossRef] [PubMed]
10. Davis, J.O.; Freeman, R.H. Mechanisms regulating renin release. *Physiol. Rev.* **1976**, *56*, 1–56. [CrossRef] [PubMed]

11. Panagiotakos, D.B.; Zeimbekis, A.; Boutziouka, V.; Economou, M.; Kourlaba, G.; Toutouzas, P.; Polychronopoulos, E. Long-term fish intake is associated with better lipid profile, arterial blood pressure, and blood glucose levels in elderly people from Mediterranean islands (MEDIS epidemiological study). *Med. Sci. Monit. Int. Med. J. Exp. Clin. Res.* **2007**, *13*, CR307–CR312.
12. Ramel, A.; Martinez, J.A.; Kiely, M.; Bandarra, N.M.; Thorsdottir, I. Moderate consumption of fatty fish reduces diastolic blood pressure in overweight and obese European young adults during energy restriction. *Nutrition* **2010**, *26*, 168–174. [CrossRef] [PubMed]
13. Zaribaf, F.; Falahi, E.; Barak, F.; Heidari, M.; Keshteli, A.H.; Yazdannik, A.; Esmaillzadeh, A. Fish consumption is inversely associated with the metabolic syndrome. *Eur. J. Clin. Nutr.* **2014**, *68*, 474–480. [CrossRef] [PubMed]
14. Ke, L.; Ho, J.; Feng, J.; Mpofu, E.; Dibley, M.J.; Feng, X.; Van, F.; Leong, S.; Lau, W.; Lueng, P.; et al. Modifiable risk factors including sunlight exposure and fish consumption are associated with risk of hypertension in a large representative population from Macau. *J. Steroid Biochem. Mol. Biol.* **2014**, *144*, 152–155. [CrossRef] [PubMed]
15. Torris, C.; Molin, M.; Cvancarova, M.S. Lean fish consumption is associated with lower risk of metabolic syndrome: A Norwegian cross sectional study. *BMC Public Health* **2016**, *16*, 347. [CrossRef] [PubMed]
16. Ait-Yahia, D.; Madani, S.; Savelli, J.L.; Prost, J.; Bouchenak, M.; Belleville, J. Dietary fish protein lowers blood pressure and alters tissue polyunsaturated fatty acid composition in spontaneously hypertensive rats. *Nutrition* **2003**, *19*, 342–346. [CrossRef]
17. Vikoren, L.A.; Drotningsvik, A.; Mwakimonga, A.; Leh, S.; Mellgren, G.; Gudbrandsen, O.A. Diets containing salmon fillet delay development of high blood pressure and hyperfusion damage in kidneys in obese Zucker fa/fa rats. *J. Am. Soc. Hypertens.* **2018**, *12*, 294–302. [CrossRef] [PubMed]
18. Ness, A.R.; Whitley, E.; Burr, M.L.; Elwood, P.C.; Smith, G.D.; Ebrahim, S. The long-term effect of advice to eat more fish on blood pressure in men with coronary disease: Results from the diet and reinfarction trial. *J. Hum. Hypertens.* **1999**, *13*, 729–733. [CrossRef] [PubMed]
19. Grieger, J.A.; Miller, M.D.; Cobiac, L. Investigation of the effects of a high fish diet on inflammatory cytokines, blood pressure, and lipids in healthy older Australians. *Food Nutr. Res.* **2014**, *58*, 20369. [CrossRef] [PubMed]
20. von Houwelingen, R.; Nordoy, A.; van der Beek, E.; Houtsmuller, U.; de Metz, M.; Hornstra, G. Effect of a moderate fish intake on blood pressure, bleeding time, hematology, and clinical chemistry in healthy males. *Am. J. Clin. Nutr.* **1987**, *46*, 424–436. [CrossRef] [PubMed]
21. Ngo, D.H.; Vo, T.S.; Ngo, D.N.; Wijesekara, I.; Kim, S.K. Biological activities and potential health benefits of bioactive peptides derived from marine organisms. *Int. J. Biol. Macromol.* **2012**, *51*, 378–383. [CrossRef] [PubMed]
22. Vercruysse, L.; Van Camp, J.; Smagghe, G. ACE inhibitory peptides derived from enzymatic hydrolysates of animal muscle protein: A review. *J. Agric. Food Chem.* **2005**, *53*, 8106–8115. [CrossRef] [PubMed]
23. Darewicz, M.; Borawska, J.; Vegarud, G.E.; Minkiewicz, P.; Iwaniak, A. Angiotensin I-converting enzyme (ACE) inhibitory activity and ACE inhibitory peptides of salmon (*Salmo salar*) protein hydrolysates obtained by human and porcine gastrointestinal enzymes. *Int. J. Mol. Sci.* **2014**, *15*, 14077–14101. [CrossRef] [PubMed]
24. Jensen, I.J.; Eysturskareth, J.; Madetoja, M.; Eilertsen, K.E. The potential of cod hydrolyzate to inhibit blood pressure in spontaneously hypertensive rats. *Nutr. Res.* **2014**, *34*, 168–173. [CrossRef] [PubMed]
25. Je, J.Y.; Park, P.J.; Byun, H.G.; Jung, W.K.; Kim, S.K. Angiotensin I converting enzyme (ACE) inhibitory peptide derived from the sauce of fermented blue mussel, Mytilus edulis. *Bioresour. Technol.* **2005**, *96*, 1624–1629. [CrossRef] [PubMed]
26. Qian, Z.J.; Je, J.Y.; Kim, S.K. Antihypertensive effect of angiotensin i converting enzyme-inhibitory peptide from hydrolysates of Bigeye tuna dark muscle, Thunnus obesus. *J. Agric. Food Chem.* **2007**, *55*, 8398–8403. [CrossRef] [PubMed]
27. Zhao, Y.; Li, B.; Dong, S.; Liu, Z.; Zhao, X.; Wang, J.; Zeng, M. A novel ACE inhibitory peptide isolated from Acaudina molpadioidea hydrolysate. *Peptides* **2009**, *30*, 1028–1033. [CrossRef] [PubMed]
28. Food and Agriculture Organization. *FAO Fisheries Department: The State of World Fisheries and Aquaculture*; Food and Agriculture Organization: Rome, Italy, 2014.
29. de Artinano, A.A.; Castro, M.M. Experimental rat models to study the metabolic syndrome. *Br. J. Nutr.* **2009**, *102*, 1246–1253. [CrossRef] [PubMed]

30. Franklin, S.S.; Gustin, W.t.; Wong, N.D.; Larson, M.G.; Weber, M.A.; Kannel, W.B.; Levy, D. Hemodynamic patterns of age-related changes in blood pressure. The Framingham Heart Study. *Circulation* **1997**, *96*, 308–315. [CrossRef] [PubMed]
31. Kurtz, T.W.; Morris, R.C.; Pershadsingh, H.A. The Zucker fatty rat as a genetic model of obesity and hypertension. *Hypertension* **1989**, *13*, 896–901. [CrossRef] [PubMed]
32. Luo, H.; Wang, X.; Chen, C.; Wang, J.; Zou, X.; Li, C.; Xu, Z.; Yang, X.; Shi, W.; Zeng, C. Oxidative stress causes imbalance of renal renin angiotensin system (RAS) components and hypertension in obese Zucker rats. *J. Am. Heart Assoc.* **2015**, *4*, e001559. [CrossRef] [PubMed]
33. Pinto, Y.M.; Paul, M.; Ganten, D. Lessons from rat models of hypertension: From Goldblatt to genetic engineering. *Cardiovasc. Res.* **1998**, *39*, 77–88. [CrossRef]
34. Reeves, P.G.; Nielsen, F.H.; Fahey, G.C., Jr. AIN-93 purified diets for laboratory rodents: Final report of the American Institute of Nutrition ad hoc writing committee on the reformulation of the AIN-76A rodent diet. *J. Nutr.* **1993**, *123*, 1939–1951. [CrossRef] [PubMed]
35. Reeves, P.G. AIN-93 purified diets for the study of trace element metabolism in rodents. In *Trace Elements in Laboratory Rodents*; Watson, R.R., Ed.; CRC Press Inc.: Boca Raton, FL, USA, 1996; pp. 3–37.
36. Cohen, S.A.; Michaud, D.P. Synthesis of a Fluorescent Derivatizing Reagent, 6-Aminoquinolyl-N-Hydroxysuccinimidyl Carbamate, and its Application for the Analysis of Hydrolysate Amino Acids via High-Performance Liquid Chromatography. *Anal. Biochem.* **1993**, *211*, 279–287. [CrossRef] [PubMed]
37. Miller, E.L. Determination of the tryptophan content of feedingstuffs with particular reference to cereals. *J. Sci. Food Agric.* **1967**, *18*, 381–386. [CrossRef] [PubMed]
38. Bidlingmeyer, B.A.; Cohen, S.A.; Tarvin, T.L.; Frost, B. A new, rapid, high-sensitivity analysis of amino acids in food type samples. *J. Assoc. Off. Anal. Chem.* **1987**, *70*, 241–247. [PubMed]
39. Oterhals, A.; Nygard, E. Reduction of persistent organic pollutants in fishmeal: A feasibility study. *J. Agric. Food Chem.* **2008**, *56*, 2012–2020. [CrossRef] [PubMed]
40. International Organization for Standardization. *Animal Feeding Stuffs—Determination of the Contents of Calcium, Copper, Iron, Magnesium, Manganese, Potassium, Sodium and Zinc—Method Using Atomic Absorption Spectrometry (ISO 6869:2000)*; International Organization for Standardization: Geneva, Switzerland, 2000.
41. Association of Official Agricultural Chemists. *AOAC Official Method 937.09 Salt (Chlorine as Sodium Chloride) in Seafood*; Association of Official Agricultural Chemists: Arlington, VA, USA, 2013.
42. Shalaby, S.M.; Zakora, M.; Otte, J. Performance of two commonly used angiotensin-converting enzyme inhibition assays using FA-PGG and HHL as substrates. *J. Dairy Res.* **2006**, *73*, 178–186. [CrossRef] [PubMed]
43. Drotningsvik, A.; Midttun, O.; McCann, A.; Ueland, P.M.; Hogoy, I.; Gudbrandsen, O.A. Dietary intake of cod protein beneficially affects concentrations of urinary markers of kidney function and results in lower urinary loss of amino acids in obese Zucker fa/fa rats. *Br. J. Nutr.* **2018**, *120*, 740–750. [CrossRef] [PubMed]
44. Sun, Q.; Wang, B.; Li, Y.; Sun, F.; Li, P.; Xia, W.; Zhou, X.; Li, Q.; Wang, X.; Chen, J.; et al. Taurine Supplementation Lowers Blood Pressure and Improves Vascular Function in Prehypertension: Randomized, Double-Blind, Placebo-Controlled Study. *Hypertension* **2016**, *67*, 541–549. [CrossRef] [PubMed]
45. van den Elsen, L.W.; Spijkers, L.J.; van den Akker, R.F.; van Winssen, A.M.; Balvers, M.; Wijesinghe, D.S.; Chalfant, C.E.; Garssen, J.; Willemsen, L.E.; Alewijnse, A.E.; et al. Dietary fish oil improves endothelial function and lowers blood pressure via suppression of sphingolipid-mediated contractions in spontaneously hypertensive rats. *J. Hypertens.* **2014**, *32*, 1050–1058. [CrossRef] [PubMed]
46. Frenoux, J.M.; Prost, E.D.; Belleville, J.L.; Prost, J.L. A polyunsaturated fatty acid diet lowers blood pressure and improves antioxidant status in spontaneously hypertensive rats. *J. Nutr.* **2001**, *131*, 39–45. [CrossRef] [PubMed]
47. Coimbra, T.M.; Janssen, U.; Grone, H.J.; Ostendorf, T.; Kunter, U.; Schmidt, H.; Brabant, G.; Floege, J. Early events leading to renal injury in obese Zucker (fatty) rats with type II diabetes. *Kidney Int.* **2000**, *57*, 167–182. [CrossRef] [PubMed]
48. Skeggs, L.T., Jr.; Kahn, J.R.; Lentz, K.; Shumway, N.P. The preparation, purification, and amino acid sequence of a polypeptide renin substrate. *J. Exp. Med.* **1957**, *106*, 439–453. [CrossRef] [PubMed]
49. FitzGerald, R.J.; Murray, B.A.; Walsh, D.J. Hypotensive peptides from milk proteins. *J. Nutr.* **2004**, *134*, 980S–988S. [CrossRef] [PubMed]

50. Girgih, A.T.; Nwachukwu, I.D.; Hasan, F.; Fagbemi, T.N.; Gill, T.; Aluko, R.E. Kinetics of the inhibition of renin and angiotensin I-converting enzyme by cod (*Gadus morhua*) protein hydrolysates and their antihypertensive effects in spontaneously hypertensive rats. *Food Nutr. Res.* **2015**, *59*, 29788. [CrossRef] [PubMed]
51. McCoy, R.H. Dietary requirements of the rat. In *The Rat in Laboratory Investigation*; Griffith, J.Q., Farris, E.J., Eds.; J. B. Lippincott Company: Philadelphia, PA, USA, 1949; pp. 67–101.
52. Trachtman, H.; Del Pizzo, R.; Rao, P.; Rujikarn, N.; Sturman, J.A. Taurine lowers blood pressure in the spontaneously hypertensive rat by a catecholamine independent mechanism. *Am. J. Hypertens.* **1989**, *2*, 909–912. [CrossRef] [PubMed]
53. Morris, M.C.; Sacks, F.; Rosner, B. Does fish oil lower blood pressure? A meta-analysis of controlled trials. *Circulation* **1993**, *88*, 523–533. [CrossRef] [PubMed]
54. Mori, T.A.; Woodman, R.J. The independent effects of eicosapentaenoic acid and docosahexaenoic acid on cardiovascular risk factors in humans. *Curr. Opin. Clin. Nutr. Metab. Care* **2006**, *9*, 95–104. [CrossRef] [PubMed]
55. Appel, L.J.; Brands, M.W.; Daniels, S.R.; Karanja, N.; Elmer, P.J.; Sacks, F.M.; American Heart, A. Dietary approaches to prevent and treat hypertension: A scientific statement from the American Heart Association. *Hypertension* **2006**, *47*, 296–308. [CrossRef] [PubMed]
56. Feng, M.; Whitesall, S.; Zhang, Y.; Beibel, M.; D'Alecy, L.; DiPetrillo, K. Validation of volume-pressure recording tail-cuff blood pressure measurements. *Am. J. Hypertens.* **2008**, *21*, 1288–1291. [CrossRef] [PubMed]

Permissions

All chapters in this book were first published by MDPI; hereby published with permission under the Creative Commons Attribution License or equivalent. Every chapter published in this book has been scrutinized by our experts. Their significance has been extensively debated. The topics covered herein carry significant findings which will fuel the growth of the discipline. They may even be implemented as practical applications or may be referred to as a beginning point for another development.

The contributors of this book come from diverse backgrounds, making this book a truly international effort. This book will bring forth new frontiers with its revolutionizing research information and detailed analysis of the nascent developments around the world.

We would like to thank all the contributing authors for lending their expertise to make the book truly unique. They have played a crucial role in the development of this book. Without their invaluable contributions this book wouldn't have been possible. They have made vital efforts to compile up to date information on the varied aspects of this subject to make this book a valuable addition to the collection of many professionals and students.

This book was conceptualized with the vision of imparting up-to-date information and advanced data in this field. To ensure the same, a matchless editorial board was set up. Every individual on the board went through rigorous rounds of assessment to prove their worth. After which they invested a large part of their time researching and compiling the most relevant data for our readers.

The editorial board has been involved in producing this book since its inception. They have spent rigorous hours researching and exploring the diverse topics which have resulted in the successful publishing of this book. They have passed on their knowledge of decades through this book. To expedite this challenging task, the publisher supported the team at every step. A small team of assistant editors was also appointed to further simplify the editing procedure and attain best results for the readers.

Apart from the editorial board, the designing team has also invested a significant amount of their time in understanding the subject and creating the most relevant covers. They scrutinized every image to scout for the most suitable representation of the subject and create an appropriate cover for the book.

The publishing team has been an ardent support to the editorial, designing and production team. Their endless efforts to recruit the best for this project, has resulted in the accomplishment of this book. They are a veteran in the field of academics and their pool of knowledge is as vast as their experience in printing. Their expertise and guidance has proved useful at every step. Their uncompromising quality standards have made this book an exceptional effort. Their encouragement from time to time has been an inspiration for everyone.

The publisher and the editorial board hope that this book will prove to be a valuable piece of knowledge for researchers, students, practitioners and scholars across the globe.

List of Contributors

Dohyun Yoo and Yongsoon Park
Department of Food and Nutrition, Hanyang University, 222 Wangsimni-ro, Seongdong-gu, Seoul 04763, Korea

Cecilia Guastadisegni, Chiara Donfrancesco, Luigi Palmieri, Serena Vannucchi, Graziano Onder and Simona Giampaoli
Department of Cardiovascular, Endocrine-metabolic Diseases and Aging, Istituto Superiore di Sanita, 00161 Rome, Italy

Sara Grioni and Vittorio Krogh
Epidemiology and Prevention Unit, Fondazione IRCCS Istituto Nazionale dei Tumori, 20133 Milan, Italy

Diego Vanuzzo
Associazione Nazionale Medici Cardiologi Ospedalieri (ANMCO), 50121 Florence, Italy

Pasquale Strazzullo
Department of Clinical Medicine and Surgery, ESH Excellence Centre of Hypertension, Federico II University of Naples Medical School, 80131 Naples, Italy

Ikuko Kashino, Takako Miki and Tetsuya Mizoue
Department of Epidemiology and Prevention, Center for Clinical Sciences, National Center for Global Health and Medicine, Tokyo 162-8655, Japan

Masafumi Eguchi, Takeshi Kochi and Isamu Kabe
Department of Health Administration, Furukawa Electric Corporation, Tokyo 100-8322, Japan

Akiko Nanri
Department of Epidemiology and Prevention, Center for Clinical Sciences, National Center for Global Health and Medicine, Tokyo 162-8655, Japan
Department of Food and Health Sciences, International College of Arts and Sciences, Fukuoka Women's University, Fukuoka 813-8529, Japan

Ana Luiza Amaral, Igor M. Mariano, Victor Hugo V. Carrijo, Tállita Cristina F. de Souza, Jaqueline P. Batista and Guilherme M. Puga
Laboratory of Cardiorespiratory and Metabolic Physiology, Federal University of Uberlândia, Uberlândia, MG 38400-678, Brazil

Anne M. Mendonça
Laboratory of Cardiorespiratory and Metabolic Physiology, Federal University of Uberlândia, Uberlândia, MG 38400-678, Brazil
School of Medicine, Federal University of Uberlândia, Uberlândia, MG 38400-902, Brazil
Department of Food and Human Nutritional Sciences, University of Manitoba, Winnipeg, MB R3T 2N2, Canada
Canadian Centre for Agri-Food Research in Health and Medicine, St. Boniface Hospital Research Centre, Winnipeg, MB R2H 2A6, Canada

Adriele V. de Souza, Douglas C. Caixeta, Renata R. Teixeira and Foued S. Espindola
Laboratory of Biochemistry and Molecular Biology, Institute of Biotechnology, Federal University of Uberlândia, Uberlândia, MG 38400-902, Brazil

Erick P. de Oliveira
School of Medicine, Federal University of Uberlândia, Uberlândia, MG 38400-902, Brazil

Cecilia Villa-Etchegoyen
Laboratory of Cardiovascular Surveillance of Drugs, Department of Toxicology and Pharmacology, School of Medicine, Universidad de Buenos Aires, Ciudad Autonoma de Buenos Aires, Buenos Aires 1121, Argentina

Mercedes Lombarte
Bone Biology Laboratory, School of Medicine, Rosario National University, Rosario, Santa Fe 3100, Argentina

Natalia Matamoros
Instituto de Desarrollo e Investigaciones Pediátricas "Prof. Dr. Fernando E. Viteri" Hospital de Niños "Sor María Ludovica de La Plata (IDIP), Ministerio de Salud/Comisión de Investigacines Científicas de la Provincia de Buenos Aires, La Plata, Buenos Aires 1900, Argentina

José M. Belizán
Department of Mother and Child Health Research, Institute for Clinical Effectiveness and Health Policy (IECS-CONICET), Ciudad Autonoma de Buenos Aires, Buenos Aires 1414, Argentina

Gabriela Cormick
Department of Mother and Child Health Research, Institute for Clinical Effectiveness and Health Policy (IECS-CONICET), Ciudad Autonoma de Buenos Aires, Buenos Aires 1414, Argentina
Departamento de Salud, Universidad Nacional de La Matanza, Florencio Varela, San Justo 1903, Argentina

Eleonora Poggiogalle, Anna Maria Giusti, Alessandro Pinto, Andrea Lenzi and Lorenzo Maria Donini
Department of Experimental Medicine-Medical Pathophysiology, Food Science and Endocrinology Section; Sapienza University of Rome, 00185 Rome, Italy

Mario Fontana
Department of Biochemical Sciences "A. Rossi-Fanelli"; Sapienza University of Rome, Piazzale Aldo Moro 5, 00185 Rome, Italy

Gino Iannucci
Department of Internal Medicine and Medical Specialties, Sapienza University of Rome, Viale del Policlinico 155, 00165 Rome, Italy

Alice Giontella, Sara Bonafini, Angela Tagetti, Pietro Minuz, Denise Marcon, Lorella Branz, Lara Nicolussi Principe and Cristiano Fava
Department of Medicine, University of Verona, 37129 Verona, Italy

Irene Bresadola, Rossella Gaudino, Paolo Cavarzere, Diego Alberto Ramaroli, Franco Antoniazzi and Claudio Maffeis
Department of Surgery, Dentistry, Paediatrics and Gynaecology, University of Verona, 37129 Verona, Italy

Dragana Komnenov
Department of Physiology, Wayne State University, 4160 John R Street #908, Detroit, MI 48201, USA
Department of Internal Medicine, Wayne State University, 4160 John R Street #908, Detroit, MI 48201, USA

Peter E. Levanovich
Department of Physiology, Wayne State University, 4160 John R Street #908, Detroit, MI 48201, USA

Noreen F. Rossi
Department of Physiology, Wayne State University, 4160 John R Street #908, Detroit, MI 48201, USA
Department of Internal Medicine, Wayne State University, 4160 John R Street #908, Detroit, MI 48201, USA
John D. Dingell VA Medical Center, 4646 John R Street, Detroit, MI 48201, USA

Kunanya Masodsai and Ai-Lun Yang
Institute of Sports Sciences, University of Taipei, Taipei 11153, Taiwan

Yi-Yuan Lin
Department of Occupational Therapy, Asia University, Taichung 41354, Taiwan
Graduate Institute of Clinical Medical Science, China Medical University, Taichung 40402, Taiwan

Rungchai Chaunchaiyakul
College of Sports Science and Technology, Mahidol University, Nakhonpathom 73170, Thailand

Chia-Ting Su
Department of Occupational Therapy, College of Medicine, Fu Jen Catholic University, New Taipei City 24205, Taiwan

Shin-Da Lee
Department of Occupational Therapy, Asia University, Taichung 41354, Taiwan
Department of Physical Therapy, Graduate Institute of Rehabilitation Science, China Medical University, Taichung 40402, Taiwan
School of Rehabilitation Science, Shanghai University of Traditional Chinese Medicine, Shanghai 201203, China

Francesco Fantin, Anna Giani, Elena Zoico, Andrea P. Rossi, Gloria Mazzali and Mauro Zamboni
Department of Medicine, Section of Geriatrics, University of Verona Healthy Aging Center, Verona, Piazzale Stefani 1, 37126 Verona, Italy

Daxiang Li, Ruru Wang, Jinbao Huang, Qingshuang Cai, Xiaochun Wan and Zhongwen Xie
State Key Laboratory of Tea Plant Biology and Utilization, School of Tea and Food Sciences and Technology, Anhui Agricultural University, Hefei 230036, China
International Joint Laboratory on Tea Chemistry and Health Effects of Ministry of Education, Anhui Agricultural University, Hefei 230036, China

Chung S. Yang
International Joint Laboratory on Tea Chemistry and Health Effects of Ministry of Education, Anhui Agricultural University, Hefei 230036, China
Department of Chemical Biology, Ernest Mario School of Pharmacy, Rutgers, The State University of New Jersey, Piscataway, NJ 08854-8020, USA

Paolo Coruzzi
Department of Medicine and Surgery, University of Parma, 43121 Parma, Italy

Byung Hyuk Han, Jung Joo Yoon, Hye Yoom Kim, You Mee Ahn, Mi Hyeon Hong, Ho Sub Lee, Yun Jung Lee and Dae Gill Kang
Hanbang Cardio-Renal Syndrome Research Center, Wonkwang University, 460, Iksan-daero, Iksan, Jeonbuk 54538, Korea
College of Oriental Medicine and Professional Graduate School of Oriental Medicine, Wonkwang University, 460, Iksan-daero, Iksan, Jeonbuk 54538, Korea

Lucia Salvi
IRCCS Policlinico San Matteo Foundation, University of Pavia, 27100 Pavia, Italy

So Young Eun
Hanbang Cardio-Renal Syndrome Research Center, Wonkwang University, 460, Iksan-daero, Iksan, Jeonbuk 54538, Korea
Department of Dental Pharmacology, School of Dentistry and Institute of Oral Bioscience, BK21 Plus, Chonbuk National University, 567 Baekje-daero, Jeonju, Jeonbuk 54896, Korea

Jae Geon Lee
Hanbang Cardio-Renal Syndrome Research Center, Wonkwang University, 460, Iksan-daero, Iksan, Jeonbuk 54538, Korea
Department of Physiology, Seoul National University College of Medicine, 103, Daehak-ro, Jongno-gu, Seoul 03080, Korea

Putcharawipa Maneesai, Upa Kukongviriyapan and Poungrat Pakdeechote
Department of Physiology, Faculty of Medicine, Khon Kaen University, Khon Kaen 40002, Thailand
Cardiovascular Research Group, Khon Kaen University, Khon Kaen 40002, Thailand

Sarawoot Bunbupha and Thewarid Berkban
Faculty of Medicine, Mahasarakham University, Maha Sarakham 44000, Thailand

Prapassorn Potue
Department of Physiology, Faculty of Medicine, Khon Kaen University, Khon Kaen 40002, Thailand

Veerapol Kukongviriyapan
Department of Pharmacology, Faculty of Medicine, Khon Kaen University, Khon Kaen 40002, Thailand

Parichat Prachaney
Cardiovascular Research Group, Khon Kaen University, Khon Kaen 40002, Thailand
Department of Anatomy, Faculty of Medicine, Khon Kaen University, Khon Kaen 40002, Thailand

Andrea Grillo and Paolo Salvi
IRCCS Istituto Auxologico Italiano, Cardiology Unit, 20100 Milan, Italy

Chang Seob Seo and Hyeun Kyoo Shin
K-herb Research Center, Korea Institute of Oriental Medicine, 1672 Yuseong-daero, Yuseong-gu, Daejeon 34054, Korea

Gianfranco Parati
IRCCS Istituto Auxologico Italiano, Cardiology Unit, 20100 Milan, Italy
Chair of Cardiovascular Medicine, Department of Medicine and Surgery, University of Milano-Bicocca, 20100 Milan, Italy

Sehar Iqbal, Norbert Klammer and Cem Ekmekcioglu
Department of Environmental Health, Center for Public Health, Medical University Vienna, Kinderspitalgasse 15, 1090 Vienna, Austria

Iselin Vildmyren
Dietary Protein Research Group, Department of Clinical Medicine, University of Bergen, 5021 Bergen, Norway
K. Halstensen AS, P.O. Box 103, 5399 Bekkjarvik, Norway

Aslaug Drotningsvik
Dietary Protein Research Group, Department of Clinical Medicine, University of Bergen, 5021 Bergen, Norway
TripleNine Vedde AS, 6030 Langevåg, Norway

Åge Oterhals
Nofima AS, P.B. 1425 Oasen, 5844 Bergen, Norway

Ola Ween
Møreforsking Ålesund AS, Ålesund, Norway

Alfred Halstensen
K. Halstensen AS, Bekkjarvik, Norway
Department of Clinical Science, University of Bergen, 5021 Bergen, Norway

Oddrun Anita Gudbrandsen
Dietary Protein Research Group, Department of Clinical Medicine, University of Bergen, 5021 Bergen, Norway

Index

www.ingramcontent.com/pod-product-compliance
Lightning Source LLC
LaVergne TN
LVHW081028210926
848485LV00004B/973